616.85882 AUT
Autism frontiers   OCT   2008

D1365635

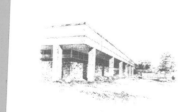

Presented By:

KILGORE MEMORIAL LIBRARY FOUNDATION
MILDRED McCLOUD BEQUEST

KILGORE MEMORIAL LIBRARY YORK, NE 68467

Autism Frontiers

Autism Frontiers
Clinical Issues and Innovations

edited by

Bruce K. Shapiro, M.D.
The Johns Hopkins University School of Medicine
Kennedy Krieger Institute
Baltimore

and

Pasquale J. Accardo, M.D.
Virginia Commonwealth University
Richmond

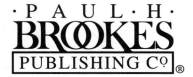
·P A U L·H·
BROOKES
PUBLISHING C? ®

Baltimore • London • Sydney

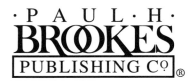

Paul H. Brookes Publishing Co.
Post Office Box 10624
Baltimore, Maryland 21285-0624
USA

www.brookespublishing.com

Copyright © 2008 by Paul H. Brookes Publishing Co.
All rights reserved.

"Paul H. Brookes Publishing Co." is a registered trademark
of Paul H. Brookes Publishing Co., Inc.

Typeset by Spearhead Global, Inc., Bear, Delaware.
Manufactured in the United States of America by
Sheridan Books, Inc., Chelsea, Michigan.

The information provided in this book is in no way meant to substitute for a medical or
mental health practitioner's advice or expert opinion. Readers should consult a health or
mental health professional if they are interested in more information. This book is sold
without warranties of any kind, express or implied, and the publisher and authors disclaim
any liability, loss, or damage caused by the contents of this book.

Purchasers of *Autism Frontiers: Clinical Issues and Innovations* are granted permission to pho-
tocopy the blank forms in the appendices found at the end of Chapter 7 and Chapter 13.
None of the forms may be reproduced to generate revenue for any program or individual.
Photocopies may only be made from an original book. *Unauthorized use beyond this privilege is
prosecutable under federal law.* You will see the copyright protection notice at the bottom of
each photocopiable page.

Library of Congress Cataloging-in-Publication Data
Autism frontiers : clinical issues and innovations / edited by Bruce K. Shapiro and
Pasquale J. Accardo.
     p. ; cm.
   Includes bibliographical references and index.
   ISBN-13: 978-1-55766-957-5 (hardcover)
   ISBN-10: 1-55766-957-0 (hardcover)
   1. Autism.   I. Shapiro, Bruce K.   II. Accardo, Pasquale J.   III. Title. [DNLM: 1. Autistic
Disorder—Congresses.   2. Asperger Syndrome—Congresses.   WM 203.5 A93725 2008]
RC553.A88.A848 2008
616.85′882—dc22   2008000616

British Library Cataloguing in Publication data are available from the British Library.

2012   2011   2010   2009   2008
10   9   8   7   6   5   4   3   2   1

Contents

Editors and Contributors

Editors

Bruce K. Shapiro, M.D.
Professor of Pediatrics
The Johns Hopkins University School of
  Medicine
The Arnold J. Capute, M.D., M.P.H. Chair
  in Neurodevelopmental Disabilities
Vice President, Training
Kennedy Krieger Institute
707 North Broadway
Baltimore, MD 21205

Pasquale J. Accardo, M.D.
Professor of Pediatrics
Virginia Commonwealth University
9000 Stony Point Parkway
Richmond, VA 23235

Contributors

Thomas D. Challman, M.D.
Assistant Professor of Pediatrics
Jefferson Medical College
Neurodevelopmental Pediatrician
Geisinger Health System
100 North Academy Avenue
Danville, PA 17822

Martha J. Coutinho, Ph.D.
Professor
Special Education Program
Department of Human Development and
  Learning
East Tennessee State University
Box 70548
Johnson City, TN 37614

Andrew L. Egel, Ph.D.
Professor
Department of Special Education
University of Maryland–College Park
1308 Benjamin Building
College Park, MD 20742

Deborah Fein, Ph.D.
Board of Trustees Distinguished
  Professor
Department of Psychology
University of Connecticut
406 Babbidge Road
Storrs, CT 06268

Jesse "Woody" Johnson, Ed.D.
Associate Professor
Department of Teaching and Learning
Northern Illinois University
DeKalb, IL 60115

Rebecca Landa, Ph.D.
Associate Professor of Psychiatry
The Johns Hopkins University School of
  Medicine
Director, Center for Autism and Related
  Disorders
Kennedy Krieger Institute
3901 Greenspring Avenue
Baltimore, MD 21211

Jennifer H. Larson, M.Ed.
Research Analyst, Project ASSESS
Department of Human Development and
   Learning
East Tennessee State University
Box 70548
Johnson City, TN 37614

Thomas M. Lock, M.D.
Associate Professor of Pediatrics
The University of Oklahoma School of
   Medicine
Child Study Center
1100 NE 13th Street
Oklahoma City, OK 73117

John F. Mantovani, M.D.
Medical Director and Division Chief Child
   Neurology
St. John's Mercy Children's Hospital
Associate Professor Child Neurology and
   Pediatrics
Washington University School of Medicine
621 South New Ballas #5009
St. Louis, MO 63141

Carla A. Mazefsky, Ph.D.
Assistant Professor of Pediatrics and
   Psychiatry
University of Pittsburgh School of Medicine
Child Development Unit
Children's Hospital of Pittsburgh
3705 Fifth Avenue
Pittsburgh, PA 15213

Deepa U. Menon, M.D., M.B.B.S.
Instructor in Neurology
The Johns Hopkins University School of
   Medicine
Assistant Medical Director
Center for Autism and Related Disorders
Kennedy Krieger Institute
3901 Greenspring Avenue
Baltimore, MD 21211

Scott M. Myers, M.D.
Assistant Professor of Pediatrics
Jefferson Medical College
Philadelphia, PA 19107
Neurodevelopmental Pediatrician
Janet Weis Children's Hospital

Geisinger Health System
100 North Academy Avenue
Danville, PA 17822

Donald P. Oswald, Ph.D.
Professor
Department of Psychiatry
Virginia Commonwealth University
Box 980489
Richmond, VA 23298

Juhi Pandey, M.A.
Clinical Psychology Intern
Department of Psychology
University of Connecticut
406 Babbidge Road, Unit 1020
Storrs, CT 06269

Isabelle Rapin, M.D.
Professor Neurology and Pediatrics
   (Neurology)
Albert Einstein College of Medicine and
   Affiliated Hospitals
K 807 Albert Einstein College of Medicine
1300 Morris Park Avenue
Bronx, NY 10461

Janet E. Turner, Ph.D.
Assistant Professor of Physical Medicine
   and Rehabilitation
The Johns Hopkins University School of
   Medicine
Director of Speech-Language and Assistive
   Technology
Kennedy Krieger Institute
707 North Broadway
Baltimore, MD 21205

Alyssa Verbalis, B.A.
Graduate Student
Department of Psychology
University of Connecticut
406 Babbidge Road, Unit 1020
Storrs, CT 06269

Leandra Wilson, M.A.
Doctoral Candidate
Department of Psychology
University of Connecticut
406 Babbidge Road, Unit 1020
Storrs, CT 06269

Foreword

Over the past two decades there has been an increase in public awareness of autism and its associated disorders. This has resulted in changing concepts of autism—from a categorical to a spectral disorder. Bringing autism to the forefront has expanded the boundaries, led to earlier diagnosis, and resulted in the proliferation of treatment programs.

The need to progress beyond the behavioral descriptions of autism spectrum disorders (ASDs) and to define the mechanism responsible for the clinical symptoms has resulted in the application of neuroscience approaches to the problems of children with ASDs. Neuroimaging and other neurometric techniques, genetics, epidemiology, and immunology are but some of the methods employed to enhance our understanding. Debates have evolved over the etiology of ASDs—whether they are genetic or acquired, whether secondary autism and idiopathic autism are the same disorders, why some children seem to "outgrow" their autism, and whether autism can be prevented.

We are at a crossroads in our understanding of the autism syndromes. The progress in understanding the mechanism will depend on the ability to define distinctive clinical syndromes. Defining the mechanism will lessen the dependence on behavioral characteristics. It is time to develop a consensus that delineates and quantifies the characteristics that are used to study the mechanisms of ASDs.

This book approaches the issue from the clinical perspective. It selectively focuses on topics presented at recent Spectrum of Developmental Disabilities conferences. The editors have compiled a series of papers that review ASDs and focus on diagnosis, developmental aspects, overlapping syndromes, and management. They have sought to place the ASDs within the broader spectrum of neurodevelopmental disorders.

Mark L. Batshaw, M.D.
Chief Academic Officer
Children's National Medical Center
Professor and Chair, Department of Pediatrics
Associate Dean for Academic Affairs
The George Washington University School of Medicine and Health Sciences

Preface

In 1943, Leo Kanner described 11 children with a unique behavioral disorder that came to be known as autism. In addition to describing the cardinal characteristics of the syndrome—"impairment of social interaction manifesting an inability to relate themselves in the ordinary way to people and situations . . ." (p. 242) and behavior dominated by profound aloneness, impaired language development, and restricted, stereotypic behavior—Kanner noted that these children showed many other dysfunctions. He distinguished this disorder from intellectual disability (ID) and schizophrenia, disorders with which he was familiar.

In the 1970s, the diagnosis of autism had to be proved beyond a reasonable doubt. Children with the diagnosis of autism had to meet the criteria of Kanner and be significantly impaired. Occasionally, a child would receive the diagnosis of mental retardation and "autistic features." The operational diagnosis, however, was mental retardation. It was the best forecaster of outcome and the behavioral dysfunction could be managed in segregated special education settings.

Dr. Arnold Capute was among those who questioned the specificity of the autism diagnosis (Capute, Derivan, Chauvel, & Rodriguez, 1975). He felt that autism was not a unique condition and that the diagnosis did not add to the management of the patient, to our understanding of the mechanism of dysfunction, or to the prognosis. From his work with developmental assessment, he recognized the developmental aspects of symptoms of autism and the need to distinguish them from more typical development. For example, pronomial reversal and echolalia was associated with language development in children younger than 30 months. His extensive clinical experiences caused him to question the validity of an autism diagnosis. He knew that restricted, stereotypic behavior was not uncommon in children with severe ID and that perseveration was seen often in children with cerebral palsy and other brain injury. Finally, the close linkage between language and social interaction caused him to question whether deficient socialization could exist as an independent factor. Subsequent studies have validated this viewpoint.

In the 1980s, the focus on early identification and early intervention extended to autism. As the diagnostic criteria were applied increasingly to younger children, the diagnostic margins blurred. Autism moved from a categorical to a dimensional disorder. During this epoch, there was an increased appreciation of the role of pragmatics in developmental language disorders. Frequent debates centered on whether the child had a developmental language disorder or autism.

The authors of the *Diagnostic and Statistical Manual of Mental Disorders, Fourth Edition* (*DSM-IV*; American Psychiatric Association, 1994) recognized the dimensional nature of autism and changed the diagnostic criteria from "significant impairment" to "qualitative abnormalities." Unfortunately, they failed to appreciate that all neurodevelopmental disorders are on a spectrum. Every child with a neurodevelopmental disorder has elements of every dysfunction. Children with attention-deficit/hyperactivity disorder (ADHD) have motor coordination deficits. Those with speech-language impairments have academic difficulties. Children with motor coordination disorders have language deficits. All neurodevelopmental dysfunction is associated with impairments in social interactions.

Since the early 1990s, there has been an explosion of interest in the area of autism. This is in part fueled by the increased number of children who have been diagnosed with autism, the desperation of these children's parents and grandparents to find effective treatment, and the parallel explosion in genetics and neuroscience that generates the hope that understanding the mechanism of autism will make it possible to learn how to treat or prevent it.

The current state of affairs is confused. Absolute proof is no longer required to establish the diagnosis. The boundaries of autism extend into ID, ADHD, and receptive-expressive language disorders (Howlin, Mahwood, & Rutter, 2000). Indeed, the term *autism spectrum disorders (ASDs)* has become the default diagnosis for a variety of reasons. The parental stigma is less, the outcome is more hopeful, and resolution of symptoms has been documented.

ABOUT THE BOOK

Autism Frontiers: Clinical Issues and Innovations is based on the Spectrum of Developmental Disabilities conference. This conference, marking its 30th year in 2008, focuses on an aspect of neurodevelopmental disabilities. It brings together experts to provide an interdisciplinary focus on neurodevelopmental and related disorders. Presentations address the public health aspects, diagnostic issues, neuroscience advances, developmental aspects, and current management strategies. Speakers blend current research with clinical expertise to delineate the boundaries of our knowledge in diagnosis, research, and management.

The 2006 conference focused on autism from a number of perspectives and helped clarify the state of knowledge. It addressed the epidemiology and concomitant implications for service provision, diagnostic criteria and overlaps, and clinical management and treatment. *Autism Frontiers: Clinical Issues and Innovations* explores

three clinical aspects of autism: diagnosis, management, and associated dysfunctions. It is not a textbook about autism but a compendium of chapters that examines aspects of this disorder, reflects current thinking on the topic, and identifies the limits of clinical knowledge.

Shapiro, Menon, and Accardo synthesize a large body of material to derive a clinical approach to ASDs that can be employed in a primary care setting. Lock uses his experiences in delivering early intervention services to children with ASDs to demonstrate the overlaps in diagnosis and service delivery needs. Rapin expands upon these findings and addresses the milder end of the autism spectrum. In her discussion of Asperger syndrome, the syndrome of nonverbal learning disability, and "Einstein children," she illustrates the rigor of thought and method needed to establish disorders as distinctive entities. She provides a neurologist's insights to gene–behavior interactions.

Language issues are addressed in separate chapters by Mantovani, Shapiro, and Turner. Mantovani addresses the dual clinical entities of regression and seizures and distinguishes isolated language regression from more generalized regression. He reviews the relationship between ASDs and epilepsy and concludes that epileptic encephalopathy is rare. He provides clinical suggestions to guide the ordering of electroencephalograms in children with ASDs. Shapiro focuses broadly on language dysfunction in preschool children. He notes that these disorders have effects on function in cognitive, academic, social/behavioral, and motor function. In this chapter, he raises the question of the specificity of the diagnosis of receptive-expressive language disorder. Turner takes a novel approach to the language of children with ASDs and addresses the impact of nonliteral language on pragmatics. She reviews humor, irony, inferencing, and figurative language. She also addresses the interactive aspects of conversation and notes how children with ASDs have difficulty with being conversational partners. The implications of these findings for function, assessment, and treatment are discussed.

Landa and Accardo each address the possibility of earlier diagnosis of ASDs. Early identification is a prelude to early intervention. Landa reviews the possibility of identifying children between 12 and 36 months. She posits that ASDs can be detected by 14 months of age. Her chapter also provides an approach to intervention that can be used for toddlers who have been identified as having ASDs. Accardo speaks to the issues of early identification and diagnosis, notes the early overlaps between ASDs and other developmental disorders, and uses this knowledge to propose a two-level screen that would be easily adapted to well-child care of 18- to 24-month-olds.

Egel focuses on treating the primary behavioral dyfunctions of autism in the classroom. His discussion recognizes the important role that school plays in the lives of children with ASDs. His chapter operationalizes some of the precepts discussed by Turner. Oswald, Coutinho, Johnson, Larson, and Mazefsky address the special issues that children with Asperger syndrome encounter in the classroom. They present qualitative data derived from a project that investigated the implementation of a team-based approach to supporting students with Asperger syndrome in the classroom. They illustrate the barriers and challenges that confront students and provide suggestions for clinicians who interact with school personnel, students with Asperger syndrome, and students' families in school settings.

Myers, in a comprehensive review of psychopharmacology of ASDs, makes the important point that there is no drug therapy that addresses the core symptoms of ASDs. His chapter outlines the spectrum of challenging behaviors that may be encoun-tered by clinicians who care for children and adults with ASDs. He underlines the need for individualization of pharmacologic approaches and reinforces the primacy of educational and behavioral approaches for the management of ASDs.

Challman addresses attempts to treat ASDs with complementary and alternative medicine (CAM). He reviews the rationale for the popularity of various CAM approaches and provides a reasoned approach that professionals can share with parents who ask about CAM. Challman also notes that the placebo effect plays a prominent role in determining therapeutic effectiveness in both CAM and traditional intervention. Finally, he notes that interventions must be proven both safe and effective.

Pandey, Wilson, Verbalis, and Fein raise the provocative question, "Can autism resolve?" They review the literature and amplify it with their own experience based on longitudinal studies. They conclude that some children may eventually lose their diagnosis, but residual difficulties in attention, language, and socialization may persist in children who have achieved an "optimal" outcome.

REFERENCES

American Psychiatric Association. (1994). *Diagnostic and statistical manual of mental disorders* (4th ed.). Washington, DC: Author.

Capute, A.J., Derivan, A.T., Chauvel, P.J., & Rodriguez, A. (1975). Infantile autism. I: A prospective study of the diagnosis. *Developmental Medicine and Child Neurology, 17*(1), 58–62.

Howlin, P., Mawhood, L., & Rutter, M. (2000). Autism and developmental receptive language disorder—a follow-up comparison in early adult life. II: Social, behavioural, and psychiatric outcomes. *Journal of Child Psychology and Psychiatry, 41*(5), 561–578.

Kanner, L. (1943). Autistic disturbances of affective contact. *The Nervous Child*, 2, 217–250.

To Arnold Capute, who taught us neurodevelopmental disabilities,
to our patients, from whom we continue to learn,
and to our spouses, who support us in the process

Clinical Overview
of the Autism Spectrum

Bruce K. Shapiro, Deepa U. Menon, and Pasquale J. Accardo

In 1943, Leo Kanner described 11 children who exhibited a disorder of development that resulted in a failure to establish typical social interactions, unusual language features, and a markedly restricted repertoire of behaviors. Kanner proposed that the children's inability to relate to people and situations was the fundamental disorder. The children failed to anticipate being picked up. Profound aloneness dominated their behavior. Although they were aware of others, the children did not interact with anyone, isolated themselves, and did not discriminate family members from strangers.

Eight of the children developed speech, but three did not; those who did speak did not use language for communication, and their language usage tended to be literal or concrete. Personal pronouns were repeated as heard. For instance, a child would refer to him- or herself as "you" and the person addressed as "I" (i.e., pronominal reversal). Word meanings were inflexible and thus words could not be used in different connotations. A concept such as *yes* was difficult, so the children would use repetition (i.e., echolalia) for affirmation. The children did not generalize concepts and meanings associated with particular situations.

The children evidenced "monotonously repetitious" performances (i.e., echopraxia) that reflected a severely diminished behavioral repertoire. Their behavior was governed by an "anxiously obsessive desire for the maintenance of sameness" (Kanner, 1943, p. 245). Indeed, the children were noted to relate better to objects than to people.

Although the syndrome was defined by extreme aloneness, obsessiveness, stereotypy, and echolalia, Kanner (1943) reported additional developmental dysfunctions. He also distinguished this group of children from those with mental retardation, now termed *intellectual disability* (ID), noting that they "are all unquestionably endowed with good *cognitive potentialities*" (p. 247). Subsequent to Kanner's description, there has been much debate about exactly what constitutes autism.

Once thought to be rare, autism spectrum disorders (ASDs) now affect approximately 1 in 150 children (Autism and Developmental Disabilities Monitoring Network Surveillance, Year 2002 Principal Investigators, 2007). Some have interpreted this increase as an "autism epidemic." Others have related the increasing prevalence to 1) changing diagnostic criteria, 2) different data collection, and 3) diagnostic substitution (Gernsbacher, Dawson, & Goldsmith, 2005).

There have been significant changes in diagnostic criteria between the *Diagnostic and Statistical Manual of Mental Disorders, Third Edition, Revised* (*DSM-III-R;* American Psychiatric Association [APA], 1987) and the *Diagnostic and Statistical Manual of Mental Disorders, Fourth Edition (DSM-IV;* APA, 1994). Asperger syndrome (AS; i.e., high-functioning abilities with features of autism but intact language skills at the age of 3 years) was not included in the earlier *DSM* versions, and pervasive developmental disorder-not otherwise specified (PDD-NOS; i.e., milder autism in which the severity of symptoms does not reach the diagnostic level in one or more areas) was not incorporated into the *DSM* until 1987. These last two disorders account for nearly 75% of current ASD diagnoses.

Another source of the apparent increase in autism prevalence is the Individuals with Disabilities Education Act (IDEA) reports from the U.S. Department of Education (2002). Children receiving special education services under IDEA are counted and reported each year. The number of children classed as having autism increased substantially after the 1991–1992 report was released. However, there was no category for autism before that report. Similar increases have occurred when other new conditions causing educational impairment (traumatic brain injury and developmental delay) were included in IDEA.

Diagnostic substitution has also contributed to the increase in the number of individuals diagnosed with ASDs. Between autism and specific learning disabilities, mild ID has almost disappeared. There is reason to prefer an ASD diagnosis over one of ID, especially when both coexist. Parents are more accepting of the term *autism* than they are of terms such as *mental retardation* and *intellectual disability*. The prognosis for children with ASDs may also be better than that of children with ID. Children with ASDs receive more intensive developmental and educational services than children who are diagnosed with ID or developmental delays.

Because of an eight-fold increase in the prevalence of ASDs from 1983 to 1997 (Barbaresi, Katusic, Colligan, Weaver, & Jacobsen, 2005), ASDs diagnoses are straining public service systems. Children diagnosed with ASDs are receiving an increasing amount of developmental and educational services. Current manpower resources are insufficient for meeting the needs of all children with ASDs. Many providers have little experience diagnosing and treating children with such diagnoses.

Increasingly, primary care providers are being asked to assume responsibility for children with ASDs. They are asked to identify disorders, make early diagnoses, delineate associated dysfunctions, arrange for developmental consultations, participate in the prioritization of a comprehensive management plan, provide continuing care through each child's lifespan, and serve as advocates for children with ASDs and their families. The purpose of this chapter is to provide primary care providers with an overview for addressing the issues regarding children with ASDs.

DIAGNOSTIC CONSIDERATIONS

ASDs are neurobehavioral syndromes defined by their behavioral phenotypes. The most commonly used classification system is the text revision of the *Diagnostic and Statistical Manual of Mental Disorders, Fourth Edition, Text Revision* (*DSM-IV-TR*; APA, 2000). Autistic Disorder, Asperger's Disorder, Rett's Disorder, Childhood Disintegrative Disorder, and Pervasive Developmental Disorder Not Otherwise Specified (PDD-NOS) are classed in the overall category of Pervasive Developmental Disorders (PDDs) (Figure 1.1).

Deciding where to draw the line that defines ASDs has become difficult. This is due to 1) a lack of reliable behavioral definitions, 2) poor quantification of the target behaviors, and 3) failure to allow for the effects of maturation and intervention on the clinical presentation. Comorbid diagnoses, such as ID and deafness, also complicate the diagnostic process.

Diagnostic schemas rely on unclear behavioral definitions. Similar behaviors may be called by different names. When does "persistence" become "perseveration"?

Diagnostic criteria for 299.00 Autistic Disorder

A. A total of six (or more) items from (1), (2), and (3), with at least two from (1) and one each from (2) and (3):
  (1) Qualitative impairment in social interaction, as manifested by at least two of the following:
    (a) marked impairment in the use of multiple nonverbal behaviors such as eye-to-eye gaze, facial expression, body postures, and gestures to regulate social interaction
    (b) failure to develop peer relationships appropriate to developmental level
    (c) a lack of spontaneous seeking to share enjoyment, interests, or achievements with other people (e.g., a lack of showing, bringing, or pointing out objects of interest)
    (d) lack of social or emotional reciprocity
  (2) qualitative impairments in communication as manifested by at least one of the following:
    (a) delay in, or total lack of, the development of spoken language (not accompanied by an attempt to compensate through alternative modes of communication such as gesture or mime)
    (b) in individuals with adequate speech, marked impairment in the ability to initiate or sustain a conversation with others
    (c) stereotyped and repetitive use of language or idiosyncratic language
    (d) lack of varied, spontaneous make-believe play or social imitative play appropriate to developmental level
  (3) restricted repetitive and stereotyped patterns of behavior, interests, and activities, as manifested by at least one of the following:
    (a) encompassing preoccupation with one or more stereotyped and restricted patterns of interest that is abnormal either in intensity or focus.
    (b) apparently inflexible adherence to specific, nonfunctional routines or rituals
    (c) stereotyped and repetitive motor mannerisms (e.g., hand or finger flapping or twisting, or complex whole-body movements)
    (d) persistent preoccupation with parts of objects

B. Delays or abnormal functioning in at least one of the following areas, with onset prior to age 3 years: (1) social interaction, (2) language as used in social communication, and/or (3) symbolic or imaginative play.

C. The disturbance is not better accounted for by Rett's Disorder or Childhood Disintegrative Disorder.

Diagnostic criteria for 299.80 Asperger's Disorder

A. Qualitative impairment in social interaction, as manifested by at least two of the following:
  (1) marked impairment in the use of multiple nonverbal behaviors such as eye-to-eye gaze, facial expression, body postures, and gestures to regulate social interaction
  (2) failure to develop peer relationships appropriate to developmental level
  (3) a lack of spontaneous seeking to share enjoyment, interests, or achievements with other people (e.g., by a lack of showing, bringing, or pointing out objects of interest)
  (4) lack of social or emotional reciprocity

B. Restricted repetitive and stereotyped patterns of behavior, interests, and activities, as manifested by at least one of the following:
  (1) encompassing preoccupation with one or more stereotyped and restricted patterns of interest that is abnormal either in intensity or focus
  (2) apparently inflexible adherence to specific, nonfunctional routines or rituals
  (3) stereotyped and repetitive motor mannerisms (e.g., hand or finger flapping or twisting, or complex whole-body movements)
  (4) persistent preoccupation with parts of objects

(continued)

Figure 1.1. *Diagnostic and Statistical Manual of Mental Disorders, Fourth Edition, Text Revision (DSM-IV-TR)*, criteria for Autistic Disorder, Asperger's Disorder, and Pervasive Developmental Disorder Not Otherwise Specified. (*Note:* The *DSM-IV-TR* category of Pervasive Developmental Disorders [PDDs] also includes Rett's Disorder and Childhood Disintegrative Disorder. Because of its specific genetic etiology, Rett's Disorder will be deleted from subsequent editions of the *DSM.* Most child neurologists and many child psychiatrists consider Childhood Disintegrative Disorder [i.e., Heller syndrome] to be more appropriately placed in the category of neurodegenerative disorders rather than PDDs.) (From American Psychiatric Association. [2000]. *Diagnostic and statistical manual of mental disorders* [4th ed., tex rev., pp. 75, 84]. Washington, DC: Author. Reprinted with permission from the *Diagnostic and Statistical Manual of Mental Disorders, Fourth Edition, Text Revision* [Copyright © 2000]. American Psychiatric Association.)

Figure 1.1.   *(continued)*

C.   The disturbance causes clinically significant impairment in social, occupational, or other important areas of functioning.

D.   There is no clinically significant general delay in language (e.g., single words used by age 2 years, communicative phrases used by age 3 years).

E.   There is no clinically significant delay in cognitive development or in the development of age-appropriate self-help skills, adaptive behavior (other than in social interaction), and curiosity about the environment in childhood.

F.   Criteria are not met for another specific Pervasive Developmental Disorder or Schizophrenia.

299.80 Pervasive Developmental Disorder Not Otherwise Specified (Including Atypical Autism)

This category should be used when there is a severe and pervasive impairment in the development of reciprocal social interaction or verbal and nonverbal communication skills or with the presence of stereotyped behavior, interests, and activities, but the criteria are not met for a specific Pervasive Developmental Disorder, Schizophrenia, Schizotypal Personality Disorder, or Avoidant Personality Disorder. For example, this category includes "atypical autism"—presentations that do not meet the criteria for Autistic Disorder because of late age at onset, atypical symptomatology, or subthreshold symptomatology, or all of these.

Do children who flap their hands when they get excited exhibit stereotypy, synkinesia, or overflow? In addition, different behaviors may have the same name. Are the stereotypies seen in Tourette syndrome the same as the stereotypies seen in ASDs? Kanner (1943) defined the term *autism* by the constellation of symptoms but did not claim that the individual symptoms were specific to autism. Most symptoms that characterize ASDs have been noted in other disorders. Children with ID, deafness, blindness, and severe receptive-expressive language disorders evidence symptoms that overlap those of ASDs (Capute, Derivan, Chauvel, & Rodriguez, 1975).

The symptoms described in the *DSM-IV-TR* are not well quantified. The children described by Kanner (1943) represented the extreme end of a spectrum, but in the absence of quantification, it will become difficult to distinguish typical variations from pathology at the mild end of the autism spectrum. For example, how much social impairment is required to cause consideration of the diagnosis of an ASD? Many children exhibit symptoms of ASDs but do not meet the full diagnostic criteria. A dimensional approach to diagnosis risks classifying almost all children with developmental dysfunction (and many children with typical development as well) as having ASDs.

The *DSM-IV-TR* criteria for the diagnosis of the PDDs do not allow for changes in symptoms that result from maturation or intervention. The early symptoms of the children described by Kanner (1943) diminished with age. Between 5 and 6 years of age, the echolalia ended, pronouns were used appropriately, language became more spontaneous, panic tantrums subsided, repetition became more like obsessive preoccupation, and contact with people began to emerge.

ASDs have been associated with many different etiologies (e.g., fragile X syndrome [FXS], tuberous sclerosis, Down syndrome, congenital rubella, untreated phenylketonuria) (Rapin, 1997), but the criteria for ASDs do not distinguish autism that is associated with a known etiology from idiopathic forms. The impact of such etiologies on the diagnosis, presentation, management, and outcome remains unclear. Certain etiologies may increase the expression of ASD symptoms whereas others may mask them.

PRESENTATIONS

The most common reason for referral is the failure to meet age-appropriate expectations. Consequently, most children with ASDs are not diagnosed until they are at least preschool age. Research is being conducted to develop techniques for earlier identification (see Chapters 7, 12, and 13). One technique recommended for early identification is the use of autism-specific screening questionnaires for children who have failed routine developmental screening procedures (e.g., the Modified Checklist for Autism in Toddlers [M-CHAT; Robins, Fein, Barton, & Green, 2001] in 18-month-old infants; the Autism Screening Questionnaire [Berument, Rutter, Lord, Pickles, & Bailey, 1999] for children 4 years of age and older) (Filipek et al., 2000).

Language and Behavior Disorders

The most common presentation of an ASD is a child's failure to achieve language milestones on time coupled with behavioral disturbance. The language delay may assume four forms.

1. A decreased number of words
2. Regression
3. Nonverbal language
4. Aberrant language

The decreased number of words may be due to the slow rate of language achievement, with the child steadily increasing his or her vocabulary size. Language delay associated with ASDs usually involves receptive as well as expressive language. Consequently, the child may not follow commands or point to objects or pictures. Absence of pointing has been highlighted as a possible early marker for ASDs.

Alternatively, a decrease in words may be the result of a plateau or regression in language abilities, both of which may be seen in ASDs. Regression occurs in as many as one third of children with ASDs in the second year of life. It may be restricted to language or it may affect other developmental areas, especially social interaction and interest. If regression is noted in both language and nonlanguage areas, a full neurogenetic evaluation is warranted. The assessment of isolated language regression is less intense.

Children who are nonverbal do not consistently use words or sound approximations (e.g., "ba" for *ball*). They merit further evaluation because the mutism is rare in isolated ASDs. Children who are nonverbal will often have significant ID, but the possibility of communicatively disabling hearing loss should be excluded via a formal audiologic evaluation.

Aberrant language may manifest as developmental deviance. Some children with several hundred words may not use two-word combinations. Others may use sentences but never vary the words. Still others may use programmed speech, reciting language taken from television, radio, or the playground, but not utilizing it in a fashion that implies understanding. A rare few may use their language in an idiosyncratic fashion (e.g., invented words or phrases). The use of rote stems (e.g., "I want. . . .") as the child's first sentences may occur spontaneously or may be programmed.

Behavioral disturbance often accompanies language delays. Meltdowns composed of resistance, noncompliance, temper tantrums, aggression (e.g., hitting, hair pulling, biting), and self-injurious behavior may be seen if routines are violated. Often, challenging behavioral outbursts occur as a result of communication failure. Children with ASDs typically become frustrated less over communication difficulties when compared with children with severe expressive language disorders; instead, children with

ASDs are more likely to become frustrated by the failure to obtain what they want. Hyperactivity is common and may be extreme; sleep disturbances are the rule.

Children with ASDs may have difficulty modulating their responses to sensory stimuli. Loud noises from lawn mowers, vacuum cleaners, thunder, or the barber's shears may send the child scurrying for safety. The discomfort caused by clothing tags, woolens, or socks may be to the level that the tags must be removed, cotton clothes must be exclusively used, or shoes and socks must not be worn even in the winter. Food temperature, texture, aroma, taste, color, or even position on the plate (e.g., different foods may not be allowed to mix with each other) may also evoke an excessive response. Extremely restrictive diets with the child eating only a half dozen solid foods are not unusual, as children with ASDs seem to prefer foods on the white-tan-yellow-brown color spectrum (e.g., chicken nuggets, French fries, macaroni and cheese); rarely does this lead to growth failure, weakness, or nutritional deficiency. Some have proposed that these symptoms represent sensory integrative disorders and should be included as a fourth—if optional—category of deficits in ASDs.

"Little Professors"

Some early school-age children with ASDs are perceived as "little professors" who offer a tremendous amount of information about a single limited topic. Cars, dinosaurs, and weather phenomena are common topics upon which little professors often focus. (Oddly, a subject that is frequently obsessed upon by people without ASDs—sports statistics—is almost never encountered.) Sometimes children with ASDs will focus on idiosyncratic topics such as the physical structure of their school buildings. Little professors shift conversations to their topic of interest and speak at great length in excruciating detail. Their pragmatic language becomes more a lecture "at" rather

than a conversation "with" the listener. They will be socially ostracized because of their single focus, which prevents others from participating in their conversations. Two mechanisms may be responsible for this phenomenon: 1) the topic area is the only thing that the child knows and, in order to communicate, he or she has to speak on this particular topic, or 2) the child uses a large amount of information to control the situation, limit the participation of others, and thereby decrease anxiety.

Attention-Deficit/Hyperactivity Disorder and Lack of Friendships

There is substantial overlap between ASDs and attention-deficit/hyperactivity disorder (ADHD). Many children with ADHD show increased ASD traits (Reiersen, Constantino, Volk, & Todd, 2007). Some children are initially diagnosed as having ADHD, but when social demands become less structured and predictable, they encounter difficulty with the subtleties of language (e.g., tone of voice, irony, subtle humor, puns), fail to sustain conversations, and demonstrate poor turn-taking skills, the latter of which typically occurs around the age of 10. Their poorly graded responses may adversely affect social interactions so that they perform adequately in the classroom but poorly in the gymnasium or cafeteria. They are often excluded from birthday parties, sleepovers, and similar group activities.

Decoding and Comprehension Dissociations

Some children with ASDs present with a precocious onset of reading (Grigorenko, Klin, & Volkmar, 2003). Parents report these children to be decoding fluently at the age of 3–4 years and deny that they spend time drilling their children on reading skills. The children seem to have a voracious appetite for "reading." The exact mechanism is not clear, but some have noted that children with hyperlexia have an intact phonological system and excellent rote memory. Consequently, they are able to decode text to a level that exceeds their chronological, cognitive, and language abilities. Early on, until the comprehension deficit is appreciated, these children may be misperceived as being academically talented.

Reading progresses from decoding through literal comprehension to inferential comprehension. Children with high-functioning autism (HFA), AS, and PDD-NOS usually do not present with reading problems in early elementary school. They often have sufficient decoding and literal comprehension skills, but they eventually experience difficulty when confronting inferential material. For example, children with ASDs will have little trouble reading (i.e., decoding) a paragraph that reads, "Six boys set up a tent by the river. They went into the tent to sleep. During the night, a cow came by the tent. The boys were afraid it was a bear." They would be able to tell (i.e., literally comprehend) the number of boys involved, the location where the tent was set up, the place where the boys slept, and the creature that came by the tent at night. They would have difficulty, however, concluding (i.e., inferring) what made the boys afraid.

ASSOCIATED DISABILITIES

Brain dysfunction in childhood has diffuse manifestations that are often reflected in multiple diagnoses. Associated dysfunctions are also common in ASDs. It is important to identify such disorders because they have implications for treatment and prognosis.

Intellectual Disability

ID is the most common dysfunction associated with ASDs. ID may be seen in approximately 70% of children with ASDs—approximately 30% in the mild range and 40% in the severe to profound range (Frombonne, 2003). ID is rare in AS (Gillberg & Coleman, 2000), however.

The best predictor of outcome in ASDs is the child's intelligence quotient (IQ). A diagnosis of an ASD contributes minimally to the predictive value of the individual's IQ score. This ID is nevertheless often overlooked when a management program is crafted and therapeutic goals are set. Treating the ASD symptoms without recognizing the impact of the ID will result in treatment failure.

IQ tests must be interpreted with caution. A child's IQ correlates with the severity of the ASD symptoms, but it has limited predictive value. Young children may have IQ scores that fall in the typical range, but their performance often declines into the range of ID with maturation. This is not because they are losing function, but because they are not acquiring the abstract skills at the same rate as their age peers. Occasionally, children with ASDs will show acceleration of their intellectual growth (Rapin, 1997).

Anxiety

Anxiety is common in children with ASDs. Hyperactivity, perseveration, inattention, and compliance may all be adversely affected by anxiety. Excessive fears, transition-related stress, altered reactivity, obsessions and compulsions, and even self-injury may be manifestations of anxiety. If severe, anxiety may affect all phases of function. The etiology and mechanism of such anxiety are unknown.

Attention-Deficit/ Hyperactivity Disorder

As noted previously, some symptoms of ASDs and ADHD overlap. Children with ASDs often demonstrate developmentally inappropriate levels of hyperactivity and impulsivity. Although ASDs focus on perseveration, children with ASDs also show difficulty sustaining attention (e.g., distractibility, inattention). Even though the

DSM-IV-TR precludes the diagnosis of ADHD in children who have PDDs, almost all children with ASDs meet the diagnostic criteria for ADHD (Yoshida & Uchiyama, 2004).

Seizures

Seizures occur more frequently in children who have ASDs than in the general population. Between one quarter and one third of children with ASDs will have at least two unprovoked seizures by adulthood (Rapin, 1997). Seizures are about half as frequent in children with AS. Seizure onset is most common in early childhood, with a second peak occurring during adolescence (Gillberg & Coleman, 2000). Partial complex seizures are common in children with prepubertal onset. There may be substantial underreporting of more subtle seizure patterns.

The relationship of seizures to ASDs is complex in part because ASDs form a heterogeneous group of disorders. Some of the disorders that are associated with ASDs are also associated with seizures (e.g., tuberous sclerosis, anomalous brain development, infantile spasms). Abnormal electroencephalograms are common in ASDs even without seizures, so the EEG should not represent the deciding factor in determining whether seizures exist. Epilepsy is not thought to cause ASDs, but some epilepsy syndromes (e.g., Landau Kleffner syndrome, see Chapter 4) may be misdiagnosed as ASDs because of the language regression.

Differential Diagnosis

As the preceding sections show, ASDs overlap with other disorders; thus, many areas require differential diagnosis. Table 1.1 lists the major manifestations of ASDs and the alternative diagnoses that may show those symptoms.

Table 1.1. Differential diagnosis regarding features of autism spectrum disorders

Diminished social interaction
  Receptive-expressive language disorders
  Intellectual disability
  Anxiety
  Affective disorders
  Adjustment disorders
  Deafness
  Neurodegenerative disorders

Delayed language development
  Receptive-expressive language disorders
  Intellectual disability
  Hearing loss
  Elective mutism

Stereotypies
  Tourette syndrome
  Blindness
  Deafness
  Severe deprivation

Hyperactivity
  Attention-deficit/hyperactivity disorder (primary)
  Anxiety
  Situational factors
  Tourette syndrome
  Neurodegenerative disorders

EVALUATION

The American Academy of Neurology and the Child Neurology Society Subcommittee on Quality Standards developed a practice parameter that addressed the screening and diagnosis of ASDs (Table 1.2) (Filipek et al., 2000). They also endorsed a number of instruments with which to diagnose ASDs. The first group of assessment instruments, based on parental reports, included the Gilliam Autism Rating Scale (GARS; Gilliam, 1995), the Parent Interview for Autism (Stone & Hogan, 1993), the Pervasive Developmental Disorders Screening Test–Stage 3 (Siegel, 1998, 2004a, 2004b), and the Autism Diagnostic Interview–Revised (ADI-R; Le Couteur, Rutter, & Lord, 1989; Lord, Rutter, & Le Couteur, 1994). The second group of assessment instruments, using data from direct observation of the child, included the Childhood Autism

Table 1.2.　Diagnosis and evaluation of autism spectrum disorders (ASDs)

Recommendation	Level of endorsement	Comment
Diagnostic process should include the use of an instrument with at least moderate sensitivity and good specificity for ASDs	Consensus	*Diagnostic parent interview* 　Gilliam Autism Rating Scale (GARS; Gilliam, 1995) 　Parent Interview for Autism (Stone & Hogan, 1993) 　Pervasive Developmental Disorders Screening Test–Stage 3 (Siegel, 1998, 2004a, 2004b) 　Autism Diagnostic Interview–Revised (ADI-R; Le Couteur, Rutter, & Lord, 1989; Lord, Rutter, and Le Couteur, 1994) *Diagnostic observation instruments* 　Childhood Autism Rating Scale (CARS; Schopler, Reicheler, & Rochen-Renner, 1988) 　Screening Tool for Autism in Two-Year-Olds (STAT; Stone, 1988a, 1988b) 　Autism Diagnostic Observation Schedule–Generic (ADOS-G; DiLavore, Lord, & Rutter, 1995; Lord, 1998; Lord et al., 1989)
Complete medical and neurological examination should be performed	Consensus	*History* 　Perinatal and developmental history 　Evidence of regression 　Encephalopathic events 　Attentional deficits 　Seizure disorder 　Depression or mania 　Behaviors such as irritability, self-injury, sleep and eating disturbances, and pica *Physical examination* 　Longitudinal measurements of head circumference 　Examination for unusual features suggesting the need for genetic evaluation 　Particular attention to skin for neurocutaneous disorders 　Neurologic evaluation to include assessment of gait, tone, reflexes, and cranial nerves 　Determination of cognitive status, including verbal and nonverbal language and play
Audiologic evaluation	Guideline	Behavioral audiometric measures, assessment of middle ear function, and electrophysiologic measures, as needed, conducted by an experienced pediatric audiologist using current testing methods and technology
Speech language and communication evaluation	Consensus	Recommended for all new diagnoses
Cognitive and adaptive behavior evaluation	Consensus	Recommended for all new diagnoses
Sensorimotor and occupational therapy evaluation	Consensus	Should be considered Indicated when deficits exist in functional skills

(continued)

Table 1.2. *(continued)*

Recommendation	Level of endorsement	Comment
Neuropsychological assessment	Consensus	To supplement cognitive and speech-language evaluations and to focus on specific domains such as Learning style, motivation, and reinforcement Sensory functioning and self-regulation Social skills and relationships Problematic behaviors Educational function Assessment of family resources
Electroencephalogram	Guideline	Inadequate evidence to recommend electroencephalogram (EEG) study for all individuals with ASDs; indications for EEG include seizures, concern about subclinical seizures, and regression
Neuroimaging	Guideline	No clinical evidence to support the role of routine clinical neuroimaging, even in the presence of megalencephaly
Event-related potentials	Guideline	Research tool; no evidence of clinical utility
Magnetoencephalography	Guideline	Research tool; no evidence of clinical utility
Genetic testing	Standard	High-resolution chromosome analysis and DNA analysis for fragile X syndrome should be performed if intellectual disability present
Metabolic testing	Standard	Selective metabolic testing should be initiated by the presence of suggestive clinical and physical findings
Lead testing	Guideline	Recommended for children with developmental delays and pica
Hair analysis	Guideline	Inadequate supporting evidence for routine use in the absence of specific clinical indications
Celiac antibodies	Guideline	Inadequate supporting evidence for routine use in the absence of specific clinical indications
Allergy testing	Guideline	Inadequate supporting evidence for routine use in the absence of specific clinical indications
Evaluation of immunologic or neurochemical abnormalities	Guideline	Inadequate supporting evidence for routine use in the absence of specific clinical indications
Micronutrients levels	Guideline	Inadequate supporting evidence for routine use in the absence of specific clinical indications
Intestinal permeability	Guideline	Inadequate supporting evidence for routine use in the absence of specific clinical indications
Stool analysis	Guideline	Inadequate supporting evidence for routine use in the absence of specific clinical indications
Urinary peptides	Guideline	Inadequate supporting evidence for routine use in the absence of specific clinical indications
Mitochondrial disorders (including lactate and pyruvate)	Guideline	Inadequate supporting evidence for routine use in the absence of specific clinical indications
Thyroid function tests	Guideline	Inadequate supporting evidence for routine use in the absence of specific clinical indications
Erythrocyte glutathione peroxidase studies	Guideline	Inadequate supporting evidence for routine use in the absence of specific clinical indications
Evaluation and monitoring	Consensus	Reevaluation within 1 year that addresses current issues Continued monitoring

Source: Filipek, Accardo, Ashwal, Baranek, Cook, Jr., Dawson, G., et al. (2000).

Rating Scale (CARS; Schopler, Reicheler, & Rochen-Renner, 1988), the Screening Tool for Autism in Two-Year-Olds (STAT; Stone, 1988a, 1988b), and the Autism Diagnostic Observation Schedule–Generic (ADOS-G; DiLavore, Lord, & Rutter, 1995; Lord, 1998; Lord et al., 1989). Table 1.3 lists the instruments commonly used in the evaluation of ASDs. The endorsed instruments had at least moderate sensitivity and good specificity.

Table 1.3. Instruments used in the evaluation of autism spectrum disorders (ASDs)

Instrument	Age of administration	Description
Checklist for Autism in Toddlers (CHAT; Baron-Cohen, Allen, & Gillberg, 1992; Baron-Cohen et al., 1996)	18 months	14 questions: 9 parent report and 5 observations; 3 key questions: eye gaze, pretend play, and protodeclarative pointing Sens 0.20–0.38; Spec 0.83
Modified Checklist for Autism in Toddlers (M-CHAT; Robins, Fein, Barton, & Green, 2001)	16–30 months	23-item parent report with yes/no answers; 6 critical items: interest in children, protodeclarative pointing, bringing object to parent, imitating; engaging in reciprocal communication and following point Sens 0.87; Spec 0.99
Checklist for Autism in Toddlers (CHAT-23) for Chinese children (Wong et al., 2004)	18–24 months	Normed on Chinese children; Combines 23 Questions of the M-CHAT and the observational section of the CHAT. 23 questions scored on 4-point Leikert Scale (i.e., Never 0%; Seldom <25%; Usual 25%–50%; Often >50%) Sens 0.93; Spec 0.77
Autism Diagnostic Observation Schedule–Generic (ADOS-G; DiLavore, Lord, & Rutter, 1995; Lord, 1998; Lord et al., 1989)	18 months and older	Semistructured, including observations and structured activities; four modules: preverbal/single words; phrase speech; fluent speech as a child); fluent speech as an adolescent or adult
Autism Diagnostic Interview–Revised (ADI-R; Le Couteur, Rutter, & Lord, 1989; Lord, Rutter, & Le Couteur, 1994)		93-item parent questionnaire; takes 1.5–3 hours to administer; historical and current functioning of language and communication; social play and development; interests and behaviors; general behaviors
Pervasive Developmental Disorders Screening Test–II (PDDST-II; Siegel, 1998, 2004a, 2004b)	12–48 months	Three-stage questionnaire; Stage I: 22 items; if positive in > 5, further screening for ASDs is recommended; Sens 0.92; Stage II: 14 questions; Sens 0.73 and Spec 0.49; Stage III: 12 items; Sens 0.58 and Spec 0.60
Gilliam Autism Rating Scale (GARS; Gilliam, 1995)	3–22 years	56-item questionnaire divided into 4–14 questions (i.e., stereotyped behavior, communication, social interaction, and other developmental milestones) 4-point Leikert scale derives ASD quotient (AQ); Sens 0.48; Spec 0.90
Childhood Autism Rating Scale (CARS; Schopler, Reicheler, & Rochen-Renner, 1988)		Based on *DSM-III* criteria; 15 items on 4-point Leikert scale (i.e., typical–severely atypical); total scores > 30 high likelihood of ASD; 30–36 mild ASD; 37 moderate–severe ASD; Sens 0.44; Spec 0.92

Key: Sens = sensitivity, Spec = specificity; *DSM-III = Diagnostic and Statistical Manual of Mental Disorders, Third Edition* (American Psychiatric Association, 1980).

Assessment based on both parental report and observation of the child can structure the diagnosis and provide important information that assists the clinical formulation. Scales, however, cannot replace clinical judgment in diagnosis.

The medical evaluation of ASDs consists of a history that addresses the key diagnostic points, identifies other significant disorders, delineates areas of strength and weakness, and evaluates etiologic factors. The history should include birth and neonatal history, developmental history—particularly language milestones and regression, functional abilities (e.g., feeding, dressing, and toileting in young children; cooking, cleaning, and chores in older children), encephalopathic events, seizures, play and socialization, affective symptoms (e.g., depression, irritability), attentional symptoms, anxiety, dysmodulation (e.g., mania, tantrums, aggression, sensory overload), stereotypies, and unusual behaviors relating to sleep, food, pica, and self-injury. Family history should be reviewed for ASDs, language disorders, ID, psychiatric disorders (e.g., bipolar disorder, depression), and genetic disorders. Special attention should be focused on the function of siblings.

The physical examination should include longitudinal plotting of head circumference measurements and a "clothes off" examination for dysmorphic features and neurocutaneous markers. The neurodevelopmental assessment should be appropriate for the child's functional age. Generally, the child should be given sufficient time to warm up before trying to engage him or her. Success is more likely to be achieved if items requiring cooperation are completed before the physical examination.

Mild axial hypotonia, oral postures (e.g., open mouth, drooling), fine motor clumsiness (e.g., reach, pencil grasp, and peg board performance in younger children), and equinus gait may all reflect various degrees of hypotonia. Occasionally, there may be some tightness of the heel cords, but this may be difficult to distinguish from volitional resistance.

Gait abnormalities are common. Toe walking due to hypotonia should be distinguished from that due to mild spasticity. Functionally insignificant asymmetries of gait may also be noted.

Deep tendon reflexes are difficult to quantify in children with ASDs because of the inability of the examiner to acquire consistent cooperation. Absent reflexes and sustained clonus are not typical. Several beats of ankle clonus in an anxious child should not be cause for concern.

Cranial nerve abnormalities are not criteria for ASDs. When seen, they reflect the associated or underlying pathology and merit further evaluation. Additional consultation from ophthalmology, a feeding team, or speech-language professionals may be needed to incorporate specific data into a comprehensive management plan.

Verbal, nonverbal, and play behavior may be observed in the waiting area. Free play, spontaneous speech, and interaction with parents and other children provide useful diagnostic information. Such direct observation may be supplemented by video recordings of the child's behavior at home and at school.

All children with ASDs should have 1) a formal audiologic evaluation, 2) a comprehensive speech-language assessment, and 3) a cognitive and adaptive behavior assessment by a psychologist. Occupational therapy, neuropsychological testing, educational evaluations, and other behavioral assessments are recommended on an "as dictated by the clinical situation" basis.

Many children with ASDs show substantial discrepancies between their measured cognitive, language/communication, and adaptive behavior abilities, which is an uncoupling of the usual association between these streams of development. Given this variability, attempts at formal measures of cognition, communication, and adaptive behavior are indicated. Measuring adaptive behavior using instruments such as the Vineland Adaptive Behavior Scales (Sparrow, Balla, & Cicchetti, 1984), the Scales of Independent Behavior–Revised (SIB-R; Bruininks, Woodcock, Weatherman, & Hill, 1996), the Adaptive Behavior Assessment System–Second Edition (ABAS-Second Edition; Harrison & Oakland, 2003), or the AAMR Adaptive Behavior Scales–School Edition: Second Edition (ABS-S:2; Lambert, Leland, & Nihira, 1993; Nihira, Leland, & Lambert, 1993) can help determine how the "whole package" functions in the real world and identify treatment goals.

Electroencephalograms, neuroimaging (even in the presence of macrocephaly or megaloencephaly), and selective metabolic testing were not endorsed and are not routinely indicated, but they may address specific clinical findings or indications. Magnetoencephalography and evoked potentials are research tools without clinical application at this time.

Karyotyping and FXS testing should be done in the presence of ID. Routine lead testing is indicated for all children with developmental delay and pica. There is inadequate evidence to support hair analysis, allergy testing (particularly food allergies for gluten, casein, candida, and other molds), celiac antibodies, immunologic or neurochemical abnormalities, micronutrients (including vitamins), intestinal permeability studies, stool analysis, urinary peptides, mitochondrial disorders, thyroid function, or erythrocyte glutathione peroxidase studies.

MANAGEMENT

The management of children with ASDs has been reviewed recently (Myers, Johnson, & Council on Children with Disabilities, 2007). Dawson and Osterling (1997) identified the characteristics of successful programs for children with ASDs.

1. A curriculum with a scope and sequence relevant to the child's capacities; a structured curriculum that teaches methods for paying attention to environmental stimuli and other people, motor and verbal imitation, the child's ability to comprehend and use language, his or her ability to play with toys in an appropriate manner, and his or her ability to socially interact with others

2. A supportive teaching environment with strategies and opportunities for generalization of skills; skills taught in a highly structured environment with a low staff-to-child ratio

3. Presentation of material in a predictable manner; children with ASDs become more open to learning and more attentive when material is presented in a structured, predictable routine

4. A functional approach to behavioral problems; inappropriate and disruptive behaviors should be evaluated by a functional assessment of the problem behavior and by teaching alternative appropriate behaviors that serve the same function for the child

5. Transition planning as the child progresses through school

6. Involving family members as part of the therapeutic team

Behavior therapy can be used to foster desired behaviors and decrease challenging behaviors. Applied behavioral analysis (ABA) is the best-studied intervention for children with ASDs (Anderson & Romanczyk, 2000). ABA involves setting goals for the child and mastering skills by breaking them down into small steps. It may be implemented through discrete trials, individualized instruction, group interventions, or incidental learning. Developmental therapies focus on fundamental developmental processes (e.g., social referencing, self-regulation) that underlie particular symptoms and serve as the foundations for future cognitive, social, and emotional growth. The TEACCH (Treatment and

Education of Autistic and related Communi-
cation-handicapped Children) program
uses a structured teaching curriculum and
extensive environmental modifications and
supports. It attends to skill deficits, but
emphasizes capitalizing on the individual's
strengths. "Floor Time" is a child-directed
therapy in which parents are asked to set
aside short, regularly scheduled periods to
play with their children and encourage purposeful and positive reciprocal exchanges.
Research provides the strongest support for
the use of ABA for children younger than
5 years of age. If, however, one closely examines the details of TEACCH and Floor Time,
it becomes obvious that a large part of these
latter programs qualify as ABA.

Enhancing communication is a major
therapeutic goal. Direct speech training
using discrete trials, natural language, or
incidental learning may be used when a
child evidences some language. Augmentative communication techniques (e.g., picture exchange systems) do not delay
language development. It is interesting to
note that in contrast to its successes in children with hearing impairments and other
severe communication disorders, sign language rarely makes much progress.

Impaired self-help skills increase the
burden of care for families and limit the
participation of individuals with ASDs in
society. Occupational therapists can facilitate the development of self-help skills
through sensory and instructional activities
that address related symptoms and deficits
in children with sensorimotor problems.

A successful comprehensive management plan carefully addresses associated
dysfunctions because these dysfunctions
may prove even more limiting to a child's
life than the actual ASD. Anxiety, hyperactivity, or seizures can preclude achievement of therapeutic goals. There is no
specific remedy for ID, but management
plans must accommodate limitations in
learning, judgment, and socialization that
are part of ID.

The management of young children
with ASDs should focus on the achievement
of competence in communication, behavior,
and self-help domains. Specifically, the goals
are to reduce problem behaviors that interfere with learning and foster growth in communication, cognition, and self-help skills.
Speech pathologists, occupational therapists, educators, and psychologists may all be
involved. There is such substantial overlap
that no single discipline can claim priority.
Interdisciplinary approaches prioritize and
coordinate the therapies included in the
management program.

Despite governmental endorsement of
early intervention programs, wide access to
therapeutic interventions through schools,
and the proliferation of varied treatment
approaches, there are no cures for ASDs.
Anecdotal testimonials aside, the vast majority of children with ASDs will not achieve the
functional levels of typical adults. The goal
of a management program is not to achieve
typical function, but to limit the disability
resulting from the language and socialization impairments and to enhance social participation.

Appropriate treatment goals are critical
to a successful outcome for the child with an
ASD. Goals must reflect current function
and project long-term achievement. They
must be revised as the child matures, capa-
bilities improve, situational demands alter,
or the family or social situation changes.
Unattainable goals will result in failed programs, an unhappy child, disillusioned therapists, and parental sorrow and anger.

Pharmacotherapy is often used for children with ASDs as part of a comprehensive
management program. Table 1.4 provides
an overview of this topic; see Chapter 10 for
more information.

Complementary approaches flourish
when there is no single therapy. Their use by
parents is well motivated. Chapter 11 provides detailed information on complementary approaches. In brief, however, it can be
noted that children with ASDs who are

Table 1.4. Considerations in the pharmacotherapy of children with autism spectrum disorders (ASDs)

1. Pharmacotherapy does not address the core symptoms of ASDs. Core symptoms are best addressed through psychoeducational approaches.
2. Associated dysfunctions such as anxiety, hyperactivity, and seizures are appropriately addressed with pharmacologic agents.
3. Children with ASDs seem to respond to pharmacologic agents in the same ways as other children. Stimulants aid hyperactivity, selective serotonin reuptake inhibitors (SSRIs) aid anxiety and obsessive-compulsive features, and antiepileptic drugs may be used to treat seizures.
4. Monitoring of drug effects is more complex because of the child's limited communicative skills, intellectual disability, and atypical behaviors.
5. Environmental manipulation may be more effective in addressing problem behaviors than pharmacotherapy.
6. Monotherapy is preferred.
7. Side effect profiles, including the frequency and magnitude of side effects, should be considered when choosing a pharmacologic agent.
8. Children with ASDs seem to have an increase in potential behavioral side effects with the use of psychopharmacologic medications.
9. Stimulants have the best effect to side effect ratio, followed by SSRIs and then atypical neuroleptics.
10. Therapeutic objectives that can be clearly measured should be developed before a pharmacotherapy program is undertaken.
11. If the pharmacotherapy program is not successful, the possibility of a previously unrecognized significant associated dysfunction or incomplete information should be considered.

treated with one or several components of complementary therapy all get better—some dramatically, and a few actually lose their ASD diagnoses. At the same time, children with ASDs who do not undergo complementary therapies also get better—some dramatically, and a few actually lose their ASD diagnoses.

ADVOCACY

Parents may choose to obtain services for their children in many different ways. Care for children with ASDs is often fragmentary if not incoherent. For example, some health insurance carriers only cover limited developmental services to children with ASDs. Some insurance policies contractually exclude services for ASDs, classifying them as contractually uncovered mental health services due to the *DSM* coding of ASDs as psychiatric disorders. Regardless, therapy services can be very costly in dollars as well as in time.

Most therapeutic services are received through the school systems. IDEA states that all children are entitled to a free and appropriate education in the least restrictive environment. The education of children older than the age of 3 years is governed by Part B, whereas the education of children younger than the age of 3 years is governed by Part C. The requirements and approaches in these two parts are different. Younger children must evidence a 25% delay in a developmental domain, exhibit atypical behavior, or have a condition that is determined to place the child at high risk for developmental dysfunction. Older children must have a condition that adversely affects educational performance in order to receive services.

The most contentious interactions with schools center on two points—defining the least restrictive environment and discriminating between *appropriate* and *optimal*. Schools are mandated to provide services in the least restrictive environment. For most children, these services can be provided in general education classrooms. Children with ASDs may do poorly in such classrooms, but schools may be unwilling to place them in a "more restrictive" environment. Although schools are required to provide only "appropriate" services, what is "appropriate" is determined by the school.

Parents confront this challenge in different ways. Some are able to successfully negotiate with the school interdisciplinary team to achieve their objectives; some supplement the school program with private therapy; some choose home schooling; some opt to appeal and pursue due process. This last approach is becoming more difficult with each reauthorization of IDEA.

To deal successfully with schools, insurance companies, and governmental agencies, parents must learn to advocate for their children (Accardo & Shapiro, 2006). Providers need to be knowledgeable in order to advocate and, occasionally, turn down parental requests. See Table 1.5 for guidelines regarding successful advocacy.

OUTCOMES

The follow-up studies of Kanner's original cohort (1973) showed that almost all the patients with ASDs lived with their parents. Eleven percent had secured outside employment. More recent studies have shown that 75%–85% (Seltzer, Shattuck, Abbeduto, & Greenberg, 2004) of individuals with ASD diagnoses in childhood maintain those diagnoses in adolescence and adult life. Children diagnosed with PDD-NOS and AS may outgrow their diagnoses. Although some children with HFA and AS may succeed in their studies during higher education, they still have difficulty functioning in the workplace. Very few individuals with ASDs marry or have sexual relationships.

Social impairments continue to be ongoing deficits in patients on the spectrum. Howlin, Mawhood, and Rutter (2000) showed that only 16.7% of adult patients scored in the average range on the social domain of the Vineland Adaptive Behavior Scales. More than half had very few or no social contacts, and one third were described as awkward. Approximately 15% had close friendships, and 10% had typical social interactions. Wing (1997) described four social phenotypes of individuals with ASDs—aloof, passive, active but odd, and loner. She observed that passive people tended not to interact spontaneously in social settings, but would accept approaches by others; loners preferred to be alone but had subtle social deficits; active but odd people attempted to interact socially, but they were socially awkward and sometimes inappropriate; aloof individuals would interact with familiar people, but they were usually indifferent to others, especially their peers. This has raised the possibility that unlike the other groups, the active but odd group may experience loneliness and depression.

Table 1.5.   Successful advocacy

1. Parents must be knowledgeable about their children's disorders.
2. Parents must understand the rules of the game. They need to know the requirements of the various laws and regulations.
3. Parents need to know the course of action for proceeding if the initial answer is no.
4. Parents cannot advocate alone. They must forge alliances with supportive professionals (e.g., educators, therapists, parent groups, lawyers).
5. Parent groups may provide core information, inform the parents of their rights under law, and identify providers who are knowledgeable and helpful.
6. The parent and health provider should periodically review the child's longitudinal course.
7. Health providers must be up to date in their knowledge of the child's disorders and the acceptable strategies for managing the disorder.
8. Health providers may arrange for consultations that will support the parents' objectives or provide alternative methods of meeting the therapeutic goal.
9. Health providers may share their insights about the child and participate in interdisciplinary team meetings that make decisions about the child's treatment. Alternatively, they may discuss these issues with education officials in the child's school or district.
10. Health providers should strive to keep emotions out of the decision-making process.

Age of language acquisition is a potent predictor of long-term outcome. Kanner (1943); Rutter, Greenfeld, and Lockyer (1967); and Gillberg and Steffenburg (1987) showed that poor nonsocial language at the age of 5–6 years is associated with poor adult outcomes. As a group, those with better verbal and communication skills had more favorable functional outcomes. Approximately one third of children with ASDs improve their communication skills, but they still have persistent idiosyncratic use of language (Howlin, Goode, Hutton, & Rutter, 2004; Mawhood, Howlin, & Rutter, 2000; see also Chapter 6). In multiple studies, there is a persistence of communication difficulties in about 78% of the patients, and one fifth have repetitive language (Anagnostou & Shevell, 2006).

IQ score is the best predictor of long-term outcome. Rutter et al. (1967) reported the relationship between IQ and outcome. They noted that children with ASDs and IQ scores of > 50 had better adaptive skills, whereas those with IQs > 70 had more friends and had secured gainful employment. Szatmari, Bartolucci, Bremner, Bond, and Rich (1989) followed a sample of individuals with IQs of > 90, which demonstrated that one third maintained regular employment and half were completely independent. IQ may not be a stable construct in children with ASDs. Recent studies (Howlin et al., 2004; Mawhood et al., 2000) have noted that while full-scale IQ scores remain stable in people with ASDs, verbal IQ scores tend to rise and performance IQ scores decline.

Sensory overload symptoms tend to improve with age, but most severe behavior problems will not resolve without intervention. Behavioral, educational, pharmacologic, and communicative strategies may be employed. Persistence of repetitive behaviors into adulthood is common (Howlin et al., 2004; Seltzer et al., 2003). The course of problematic behaviors suffers from a lack of study, but it seems that those behaviors remain a serious problem into adulthood (Ballaban-Gil, Rapin, Tuchman, & Shinnar, 1996).

Improved outcomes depend in part on appropriate treatment. Table 1.6 outlines some general principles of care that must be individualized in accordance with each child's characteristics, the family's capacities, and the community's resources.

CONCLUSION

More than half a century after Kanner's first description, the understanding of ASDs con-

Table 1.6.   The role of the primary care physician in autism spectrum disorders (ASDs)

1. Maintain a high index of suspicion for the possibility of ASDs throughout the child's infancy and early childhood.
2. In the presence of any developmental delay, consider the possibility of an ASD.
3. Closely monitor language development between 18–30 months of age as a major indicator of a possible ASD.
4. Rapid head growth late in the first year, persistent toe walking, extremely restricted diet, echolalia, and a family history of ASDs or bipolar disorder should increase one's index of suspicion for an ASD.
5. Utilize an autism-specific screening test (e.g., M-CHAT) at 18–24 months of age.
6. When an ASD is suspected, refer the child to an agency, program, or professional that has the tools to finalize or rule out that diagnosis.
7. Support the family of a child with an ASD by familiarizing oneself with local resources (e.g., schools, therapists, sitters, reading materials, parent support groups).
8. Learn about the medications used to treat challenging behaviors in children, as well as their effects and possible side effects, even if they are not actually being prescribed, to assess their impact on the child's general health.
9. Help the family maintain a positive attitude over what will be a long course of treatment.

Key: M-CHAT = Modified Checklist for Autism in Toddlers (Robins, Fein, Barton, & Green, 2001).

tinues to evolve. The diagnostic issues are still hotly debated. It is doubtful that society is experiencing an epidemic of ASDs. The neural mechanisms await elucidation. Current studies do not support a major role for immunization as an etiology for ASDs. Unfortunately, there are no cures for ASDs. Therapies focus on diminishing functional limitations, increasing participation in society, and addressing associated dysfunctions. Outcomes are related to language function, IQ, and the severity of behavior dysfunction.

REFERENCES

Accardo, J.A., & Shapiro, B.K. (2006). Beyond the diagnosis: Management of neurodevelopmental disabilities. *Seminars in Child Neurology, 12,* 242–249.

American Psychiatric Association. (1980). *Diagnostic and statistical manual of mental disorders* (3rd ed.). Washington, DC: Author.

American Psychiatric Association. (1987). *Diagnostic and statistical manual of mental disorders* (3rd ed., rev.). Washington, DC: Author.

American Psychiatric Association. (1994). *Diagnostic and statistical manual of mental disorders* (4th ed.). Washington, DC: Author.

American Psychiatric Association. (2000). *Diagnostic and statistical manual of mental disorders* (4th ed., text rev.). Washington, DC: Author.

Anagnostou, E., & Shevell, M. (2006). Outcomes of children with autism. In R. Tuchman & I. Rapin (Eds.), *Autism: A neurological disorder of early brain development* (pp. 308–322). Mac Keith Press.

Anderson, S., & Romanczyk, R.G. (2000). Early intervention for young children with autism. *Journal of the Association of Persons with Severe Handicaps, 24,* 162–173.

Autism and Developmental Disabilities Monitoring Network Surveillance, Year 2002 Principal Investigators, Centers for Disease Control and Prevention. (2007). Prevalence of autism spectrum disorders: Autism and developmental disabilities monitoring network, 14 sites, United States. *Morbidity and Mortality Weekly Report Surveillance Summaries 56*(1), 12–28.

Ballaban-Gil, K., Rapin, I., Tuchman, R., & Shinnar, S. (1996). Longitudinal examination of the behavioral, language, and social changes in a population of adolescents and young adults with autistic disorder. *Pediatric Neurology, 15,* 217–223.

Barbaresi, W.J., Katusic, S.K., Colligan, R.C., Weaver, A.L., & Jacobsen, S.J. (2005). The incidence of autism in Olmsted County, Minnesota, 1976–1997: Results from a population-based study. *Archives of Pediatric and Adolescent Medicine, 159*(1), 37–44.

Baron-Cohen, S., Allen, J., & Gillberg, C. (1992). Can autism be detected at 18 months? The needle, the haystack, and the CHAT. *British Journal of Psychiatry, 161,* 839–843.

Baron-Cohen, S., Cox, A., Baird, G., Swettenham, J., Nightingale, N., Morgan, K., et al. (1996). Psychological markers in the detection of autism in infancy in a large population. *British Journal of Psychiatry, 168,* 158–163.

Berument, S.K., Rutter, M., Lord, C., Pickles, A., & Bailey, A. (1999). Autism Screening Questionnaire: Diagnostic validity. *British Journal of Psychiatry, 175,* 444–451.

Bruininks, R.H., Woodcock, R.W., Weatherman, R.F., & Hill, B.K. (1996). *Scales of Independent Behavior–Revised (SIB-R).* Itasca, IL: Riverside Publishing.

Capute, A.J., Derivan, A.T., Chauvel, P.J., & Rodriguez, A. (1975). Infantile autism. I. A prospective study of the diagnosis. *Developmental Medicine and Child Neurology, 17,* 58–62.

Dawson, G., & Osterling, J. (1997). Early intervention in autism. In M.J. Guralnick (Ed.), *The effectiveness of early intervention* (pp. 302–326). Baltimore: Paul H. Brookes Publishing Co.

DiLavore, P.C., Lord, C., & Rutter, M. (1995). The pre-linguistic Autism Diagnostic Observation Schedule. *Journal of Autism and Developmental Disorders, 25,* 355–379.

Filipek, P.A., Accardo, P.J., Ashwal, S., Baranek, G.T., Cook, Jr., E.H., Dawson, G., et al. (2000). Practice parameter: Screening and diagnosis of autism—Report of the Quality Standards Subcommittee of the American Academy of Neurology and the Child Neurology Society. *Neurology, 55,* 468–479.

Frombonne, E. (2003). Epidemiological surveys of autism and other pervasive development disorders: An update. *Journal of Autism and Developmental Disorders, 33,* 365–382.

Gernsbacher, M.A., Dawson, M., & Goldsmith, H.H. (2005). Three reasons not to believe in an autism epidemic. *Current Directions in Psychological Science, 14,* 55–58.

Gillberg, C., & Coleman, M. (2000). *The biology of the autistic syndromes* (3rd ed.). London: Mac Keith Press.

Gillberg, C.C., & Steffenburg, S. (1987). Outcomes and prognostic factors in infantile autism and similar conditions: A population based study of 46 cases followed through puberty. *Journal of Autism and Developmental Disorders, 17*, 273–287.

Gilliam, J.E. (1995). *Gilliam Autism Rating Scale (GARS)*. Austin, TX: PRO-ED.

Grigorenko, G., Klin, A., & Volkmar, F. (2003). Annotation: Hyperlexia: Disability or superability? *Journal of Child Psychology and Psychiatry, 44*, 1079–1091.

Harrison, P., & Oakland, T. (2003). *Adaptive Behavior Assessment System–Second Edition (ABAS-Second Edition)*. San Antonio, TX: Harcourt Assessment.

Howlin, P., Goode, S., Hutton, J., & Rutter, M. (2004). Adult outcomes in children with autism. *Journal of Child Psychology and Psychiatry, 45*, 212–229.

Howlin, P., Mawhood, L., & Rutter, M. (2000). Autism and developmental receptive language disorder: A follow-up comparison in early adult life. II: Social, behavioral, and psychiatric outcomes. *Journal of Child Psychology and Psychiatry, 41*, 561–578.

Kanner, L. (1943). Autistic disturbances of affective contact. *Nervous Child, 2*, 217–250.

Kanner, L. (1973). *Childhood psychosis: Initial studies and new insights*. New York: Kluwer Academic/Plenum.

Lambert, N., Leland, H., & Nihira, K. (1993). *AAMR Adaptive Behavior Scales–School Edition: Second Edition (ABS-S:2)*. Los Angeles: Western Psychological Services.

Le Couteur, A., Rutter, M., & Lord, C. (1989). Autism Diagnostic Interview: A standardized investigator-based instrument. *Journal of Autism and Developmental Disorders, 19*(3), 363–387.

Lord, C. (1998, June 15–17). *The Autism Diagnostic Observation Schedule–Generic (ADOS-G)*. Paper presented at the NIH State of the Science in Autism: Screening and Diagnosis Working Conference, Bethesda, MD.

Lord, C., Rutter, M., Goode, S., Heemsbergen, J., Jordan, J., Mawhood, L., et al. (1989). Autism Diagnostic Observation Schedule: A standardized observation of communicative and social behavior. *Journal of Autism and Developmental Disorders, 24*, 659–685.

Lord, C., Rutter, M., & Le Couteur, A. (1994). *Autism Diagnostic Interview–Revised (ADI-R)*. Los Angeles: Western Psychological Services.

Mawhood, L., Howlin, P., & Rutter, M. (2000). Autism and developmental receptive language disorder: A comparative follow up in early adult life. I. Cognitive and language outcomes. *Journal of Child Psychology and Psychiatry, 41*, 547–559.

Myers, S.M., Johnson, C.P., & Council on Children with Disabilities. (2007). Management of children with autism spectrum disorders. *Pediatrics, 120*(5), 1162–1182.

Nihira, K., Leland, H., & Lambert, N. (1993). *AAMR Adaptive Behavior Scales–Residential and Community Edition: Second Edition (ABS-RC:2)*. Los Angeles: Western Psychological Services.

Rapin, I. (1997). Autism. *The New England Journal of Medicine, 377*, 97–104.

Reiersen, A.M., Constantino, J.N., Volk, H.E., & Todd, R.D. (2007). Autistic traits in a population-based ADHD twin sample. *Journal of Child Psychology and Psychiatry, 48*(5), 464–472.

Robins, D., Fein, D., Barton, M., & Green, J. (2001). The Modified Checklist for Autism in Toddlers: An initial study investigating the early detection of autism and pervasive developmental disorders. *Journal of Autism and Developmental Disorders, 31*(2), 131–144.

Rutter, M., Greenfeld, D., & Lockyer, L. (1967). A five to fifteen-year follow-up study of infantile psychosis. II. Social and behavioral outcome. *British Journal of Psychiatry, 113*, 1183–1199.

Schopler, E., Reicheler, R., & Rochen-Renner, B. (1988). *The Childhood Autism Rating Scale (CARS)*. Los Angeles: Western Psychological Services.

Seltzer, M.M., Krauss, M.W., Shattuck, P.T., Orsmond, G., Swe, A., & Lord, C. (2003). The symptoms of autism spectrum disorder in adolescence and adulthood. *Journal of Autism and Developmental Disorders, 33*, 565–581.

Seltzer, M.M., Shattuck, P., Abbeduto, L., & Greenberg, J.S. (2004). Trajectory of development in adolescents and adults with autism. *Mental Retardation and Developmental Disabilities Research Reviews, 10*, 234–247.

Siegel, B. (1998, June 15–17). *Early screening and diagnosis in autism spectrum disorders: The Pervasive Developmental Disorders Screening Test (PDDST)*. Paper presented at the NIH State of the Science in Autism: Screening and Diagnosis Working Conference, Bethesda, MD.

Siegel, B. (2004a). *Early screening for autism using the PDDST-II. Developmental and behavioural news.* Elk Grove Village, IL: American Academy of Pediatrics.

Siegel, B. (2004b). *Pervasive Developmental Disorders Screening Test–II (PDDST-II).* San Antonio, TX: Harcourt Assessment.

Sparrow, S., Balla, D., & Cicchetti, D. (1984). *Vineland Adaptive Behavior Scales.* Circle Pines, MN: AGS Publishing.

Stone, W.L. (1998a, June 15–17). *Descriptive information about the Screening Tool for Autism in Two-Year-Olds (STAT).* Paper presented at the NIH State of the Science in Autism: Screening and Diagnosis Working Conference, Bethesda, MD.

Stone, W.L. (1998b, June 15–17). *STAT Manual: Screening Tool for Autism in Two-Year-Olds.* Paper presented at the NIH State of the Science in Autism: Screening and Diagnosis Working Conference, Bethesda, MD.

Stone, W.L., & Hogan, K.L. (1993). A structured parent interview for identifying young children with autism. *Journal of Autism and Developmental Disorders, 23,* 639–652.

Szatmari, P., Bartolucci, G., Bremner, R., Bond, S., & Rich, S. (1989). A follow-up study of high-functioning autistic children. *Journal of Autism and Developmental Disorders, 19*(2), 213–225.

U.S. Department of Education. (2002). *Twenty-fourth annual report to Congress on the implementation of the Individual with Disabilities Education Act.* Washington DC: Author.

Wing, L. (1997). The autism spectrum. *Lancet, 350,* 1761–1766.

Wong, V., Hui, L.H., Lee, W.C., Leung, L.S., Ho, P.K., Lau, W.L., et al. (2004). A modified screening tool for autism (Checklist for Autism in Toddlers [CHAT-23]) for Chinese children. *Pediatrics, 114*(2), e166–e176.

Yoshida, Y., & Uchiyama, T. (2004). The clinical necessity for assessing attention-deficit/hyperactivity disorder (ADHD) symptoms in children with high-functioning pervasive developmental disorder (PDD). *European Child and Adolescent Psychiatry, 13*(5), 307–214.

2

Autism in the Spectrum of Developmental Disabilities

Thomas M. Lock

We could consider autism in a number of ways related to other developmental disabilities, "within the spectrum." We could consider the functional relationship to other disorders. What sets autism apart from other disorders? How is it similar? In a related vein, we could consider its differential diagnosis. We could ask what are its associated disabilities or comorbidities? On a health systems level, we could consider the relative burden of care compared with other disabilities. Do people with autism require different or similar services than people with other disabilities? Since the mid-1980s, our assessments of all of these aspects of autism have evolved. Once considered a rare disorder, autism has become a central concern.

The terminology used to refer to autism and related disorders has changed as part of this evolution (Levy, Hyman, & Pinto-Martin, 2008). Kanner presented a narrowly defined group of children with severe symptoms. The multiple revisions and various editions of the American Psychiatric Association (APA)'s *Diagnostic and Statistical Manual of Mental Disorders* created a broader group of "Pervasive Developmental Disorders." The World Health Organization's *International Classification of Diseases* has another categorization system that has also gone through multiple revisions. The Individuals with Disabilities Education Act (IDEA) of 2004 (PL 108-446) has a third definition that stresses educational needs over medical specificity. In the literature review section of this chapter, the reader is referred to the individual studies cited for the definitions used by the authors. For the Oklahoma case study section of the chapter, *Diagnostic and Statistical Manual of Mental Disorders, Fourth Edition* (*DSM-IV*; APA, 1994) criteria are used, except that the umbrella term *autism spectrum disorders (ASDs)* is used instead of *pervasive developmental disorders*.

HOW IS AUTISM RELATED TO OTHER DEVELOPMENTAL DISABILITIES?

Before the 1980s, autism was thought to be rare. Although many considered autism to be a developmental disorder, others considered it a mental health disorder with an environmental origin (Lewis, 1971). Autism's place within the spectrum of developmental disabilities at that time could have been viewed as illustrated in Figure 2.1. In this scheme, autism was conceptualized as a disorder of social interaction, and its relationship to other disorders was not clear or specific. This was reflected in the common clinical practices of the time, such as appending the phrase "with autistic features" to a diagnosis of mental retardation, now often termed *intellectual disability* (ID), or ascribing a diagnosis of "atypical psychosis." Beginning in the 1980s, the features

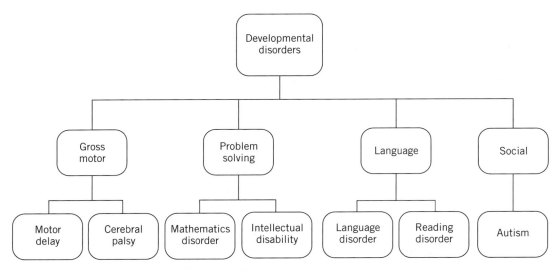

Figure 2.1.   Place of autism in developmental disabilities, 1970s–1980s. (*Note:* Autism appears in the lower right-hand corner, related to the social interaction stream of development. Its connection to other disorders is not clear.)

of autism were better delineated, and the disorder was eventually considered a condition that affects primarily language and social development, as well as motor and cognitive components. Thus, its place within the spectrum is more accurately illustrated in Figure 2.2.

HOW COMMON IS AUTISM?

Before 1985, population-based samples estimated the prevalence of ASDs at 4–5/10,000. More narrowly defined classic autism (i.e., Kanner's autism) was estimated at 2/10,000. Over the past 25 years, esti-

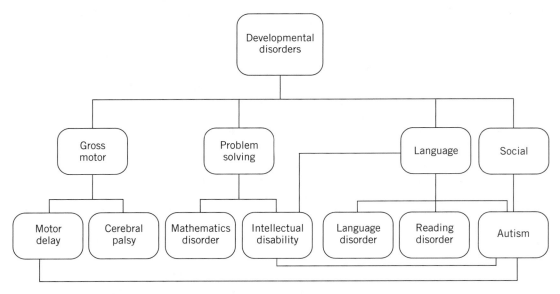

Figure 2.2.   Place of autism in developmental disabilities, 2006. (*Note:* All disorders are more interrelated. Autism is considered primarily related to both language and social streams of development with lesser connections to cognitive and motor disorders. Similar connections could also be drawn for cerebral palsy.)

mates have increased and are currently in the area of 34–67/10,000 (Bertrand et al., 2001; Chakrabarti & Fombonne, 2001; Yeargin-Allsopp et al., 2003). The most recent estimate from the Centers for Disease Control and Prevention in a multisite monitoring was 67/1,000 (Autism and Developmental Disabilities Monitoring Network Surveillance Year 2000 Principal Investigators, 2007). The cause of this increase has been controversial and has raised many important questions. Has there been an actual increase in the prevalence related to changes in maternal and child health? Has the expansion of the concept of autism resulted in the consideration of children who would have been otherwise classified or gone undetected resulted in the identification of more children with developmental disorders? Has the movement to include more children in typical community settings required different supports for children who would receive them under a different rationale in special segregated settings? Has the creation of an IDEA category for autism resulted in more children claiming this status? Is there a change in the way we, as a society, deal with disability that results in more people being identified, regardless of neurological dysfunction? Whatever the cause, there has clearly been an increase in the number of children who qualify for services under the category of autism.

SOCIETAL IMPACT

Recent studies have calculated the costs of autism (Ganz, 2007; Leslie & Martin 2007). Health care expenditures are increasing per affected person, as well as the treated prevalence. Average health care expenditures for individuals with ASDs have increased 20.4% from the year 2000 to $5,979 per patient in 2004 even after adjustment for inflation. When combined with rising ASD prevalence rates, total expenditures per 10,000 covered lives associated with ASDs increased 142.1%

over the 5-year period to approximately $114,710 per year in the U.S. (Leslie & Martin, 2007). Ganz (2007) calculated the lifetime per capita incremental societal cost of autism at $3,200,000 per case. Clearly autism has a major societal impact.

FITTING AUTISM INTO DEVELOPMENTAL SERVICES: A CASE STUDY IN OKLAHOMA

In response to the increase in the recognized impact of autism within the population of Oklahoma, the Section of Developmental and Behavioral Pediatrics has begun a number of initiatives at the University of Oklahoma Child Study Center aimed at improving access to diagnosis and treatment in young children with ASDs. Although the Child Study Center had been long established, it had undergone a great contraction of services after the oil crash of the 1980s. It also faced a number of challenges that are particular to providing services in a large, predominantly rural state.

Great geographical distance exists between patients in most of the state. Oklahoma has a land area of 68,667 square miles, and in the year 2000, it had a population of 3,511,532, a population density of 51 people per square mile. With the prevalence of autism estimated at 67/1,000, there would likely be a density of three people of any age with autism per square mile. In contrast, during the same time frame, Maryland, with a geographic area of 9,774 square miles, had a population of 5,508,909, making for a population density of 564 people per square mile. Many counties in western Oklahoma had population densities of 1–4 people per square mile, whereas the most rural counties in Maryland had densities of 25–50 people per square mile. Thus, in Oklahoma, there may be only one child with autism in a school grade or even in an entire school district, making it unreasonable to expect that many communities would develop special-

24   Lock

ized programs with staff dedicated solely to services for children with autism.

As of 2005, there were 1,268 children ages 8–21 receiving school services for autism in the state of Oklahoma. Data for younger children are not available, and many children receive services under the noncategorical designation of "child with a disability." There has been a steady increase in the number of children served since the establishment of the special designation in 1998 (see Figure 2.3). Although this accounts for 16.8% of children in Oklahoma receiving special education, it is still less than one identified student per 5 square miles.

Based on these considerations, we adopted a two-pronged approach. First, we would develop evaluation teams to assist with the early identification of children with disabilities, autism in particular. Second, we would develop a "school support services" team with the ability to provide training in evidence-based interventions for autism and other disorders recommended by the teams or requested by the schools.

Properties of a Practical Evaluation Service in Oklahoma

Based on the previously stated considerations, we concluded that there was a need for a centralized team. The very low density of children in most of the state made even regional clinics seem impractical. Given that the children and their families would have to travel long distances—often more than 4 hours—it was important that a child's evaluation be designed to take no more than a day and be completed in one visit, if possible. The visit had to provide both diagnosis and treatment recommendations. It also had to be affordable, covered in large part by insurance, either private or state.

Pilot Programs: Jumpstart and Autism Disorder Clinics

We simultaneously started two preschool diagnostic clinics, one designed to serve children with suspected developmental delays and another designed specifically for children believed to have ASDs. Each inter-

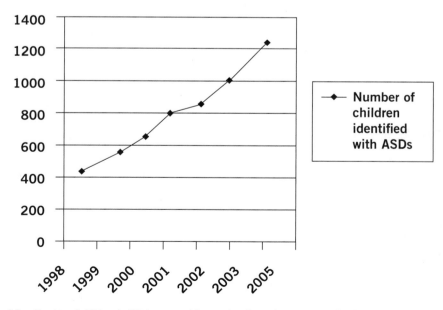

Figure 2.3. Number of children in Oklahoma receiving services for autism spectrum disorders (ASDs) by year.

disciplinary team met independently to organize services.

The team for children with delays, named the Jumpstart team, consisted of a psychologist, a speech-language pathologist, a physical therapist, a developmental pediatrician, and a family partner. The family partner was the mother of a child with a disability who was active in the Oklahoma Family Network, a statewide organization of families of children with disabilities. The team agreed on a format in which members would obtain a child's history as a group to minimize repetition and would then cooperate to plan and perform developmental testing. The team would meet, formulate a summary of findings and recommendations, and present the results to the family. It was assumed that intakes would be screened and that children with ASDs would be uncommon in this clinic.

The Autism team consisted of a psychologist, a speech-language pathologist, an occupational therapist, a social worker, a developmental pediatrician, and a family partner. This family partner was the mother of a young woman with autism. Team members determined that they would need to screen for children likely to have autism, and then the social worker would obtain an Autism Diagnostic Interview–Revised (ADI-R; Rutter, Le Couteur, & Lord, 2003) before each patient came in. The visit would otherwise be similar to the Jumpstart visit except that preparations would be made for an Autism Diagnostic Observation Schedule

(ADOS; Lord, Rutter, DiLavore, & Risi, 1999) to be performed.

Individuals Seen in the Programs

The children seen in the Autism clinic were older than those seen in the Jumpstart clinic (i.e., mean age 53.7 months versus 25.7 months). The diagnoses of the children evaluated are summarized in Table 2.1. Children with ASD diagnoses composed 30% of those evaluated. Despite great efforts to prescreen patients, 55% of those children evaluated in the clinic did not have ASD diagnoses, and 12% of those seen in Jumpstart did. If the clinics were not prepared to make diagnoses of both autism spectrum and other disorders, a significant proportion of children were required to return for second visits for further evaluation. In addition, prescreening, especially in the Autism clinic, resulted in significant delays while further data were collected.

Cognitive morbidity was significant in both groups, underscoring the need for developmental assessment of all children identified with developmental delays. Seventy-six percent of children with ASDs and 23% of children with other diagnoses had scores in the delayed range on nonverbal cognitive assessments (see Table 2.2).

Despite extensive efforts to separate children with autism spectrum symptoms from those without, a significant number of children ended up with the wrong evaluation. This added to extended waiting

Table 2.1.   Diagnoses of patients evaluated in the University of Oklahoma Child Study Center Clinics for Preschoolers

	Autism clinic	Jumpstart clinic	Combined clinics	Total
Autism	20 (37%)	7 (12%)	8 (13%)	35 (20%)
Pervasive developmental disorder	4 (7%)	0	6 (10%)	10 (6%)
Intellectual disability/developmental delay	7 (13%)	8 (13%)	16 (26%)	31 (18%)
Communication disorder	14 (26%)	20 (33%)	9 (15%)	43 (24%)
Attention-deficit/hyperactivity disorder	4 (7%)	0	7 (11%)	11 (6%)
Motor impairment	0	9 (15%)	5 (8%)	14 (8%)
Other	5 (9%)	17 (28%)	11 (18%)	33 (19%)

Table 2.2.   Cognitive morbidity in children evaluated in the University of Oklahoma Child Study Center Clinics for Preschoolers

	Autism clinic	Jumpstart clinic	Combined clinics	Total
Autism/pervasive developmental disorder	18 (75%)	6 (86%)	10 (71%)	34 (76%)
Other	7 (23%)	8 (15%)	16 (33%)	31 (23%)
Total	25 (46%)	14 (27%)	16 (33%)	65 (37%)

times while staff obtained interviews, application forms, and information from prior evaluations. Both teams had to be prepared to perform both cognitive and standardized autism evaluations on any given evaluation. In response to this, the two teams were combined, and one team was established to handle all evaluations for preschoolers. In addition to shortening waiting times and adding to scheduling flexibility, this provided a larger pool of team members to cover for those who were on vacation or were taking time off to treat an illness, thus resulting in more total available appointments.

The extensive data obtained from an Autism Diagnostic Interview in the absence of the child was not particularly helpful. We felt this was particularly true when children exhibited positive symptoms (e.g., tantrums, mood dysregulation, motor stereotypy) that overlapped other early childhood behavioral disorders (e.g., language disorders not related to autism, oppositional behavior disorders, anxiety disorders). In contrast, negative symptoms (e.g., the lack of joint attention, an absence of initiation of interaction, the lack of variability in interests) often went unreported by family members. The team screened children using the Modified Checklist of Autism in Toddlers (M-CHAT; Robins, Fein, Barton, & Green, 2001) and the Social Communication Questionnaire (Rutter, Bailey, & Lord, 2003). However, the team members found that the opportunities for joint attention and nonverbal communication in speech-language and cognitive testing could raise suspicion in children who would otherwise screen

negative. Similarly, it was often difficult to convince clinic staff to perform an ADOS on a child who shows these skills in abundance during cognitive or language evaluation, even if the child was referred specifically for an autism evaluation.

Differences in Treatment Recommendations for Children with Autism Spectrum Disorders and Those Without

Once a diagnosis was made, augmentive communication techniques were recommended for children with a number of communication problems, irrespective of the clinics in which they were seen or the disorders with which they were diagnosed. Similarly, visual supports such as visual schedules were recommended in both situations. Behavior therapy, usually in the form of Parent–Child Interaction Therapy, was rarely recommended for children with ASDs (see Table 2.3).

CONCLUSION

Autism is increasingly recognized in schools, communities, and clinics as a developmental disability in children, and the demand for services for these children continues to rise. In a clinically important number of cases, clinicians at the University of Oklahoma's Autism, Jumpstart, and combined clinics were unable to clinically separate children with autism from those without unless we performed a clinical eval-

Table 2.3.   Treatment recommendations for children with and without autism for the Autism, Jumpstart, and combined clinics

	Augmentative communication	Visual supports	Behavioral therapy	Total
Autism clinic recommendations				
Autism or pervasive developmental disorder	15 (63%)	5 (21%)	3 (13%)	24
Other	9 (30%)	16 (53%)	19 (63%)	30
Jumpstart clinic recommendations				
Autism or pervasive developmental disorder	7 (100%)	3 (43%)	0	7
Other	13 (24%)	18 (33%)	19 (35%)	54
Combined clinic recommendations				
Autism or pervasive developmental disorder	7 (50%)	5 (36%)	3 (21%)	14
Other	14 (29%)	19 (40%)	13 (27%)	48

uation. The special services recommended for both groups of children overlapped. Teams of clinicians who evaluate preschool children for developmental and behavioral problems need to be prepared for children with and without autism spectrum symptoms. As observed in our clinics, autism is a "primary color" in the spectrum of developmental disabilities.

REFERENCES

American Psychiatric Association. (1994). *Diagnostic and statistical manual of mental disorders* (4th ed.). Washington, DC: Author.

Autism and Developmental Disabilities Monitoring Network Surveillance Year 2000 Principal Investigators. (2007). Prevalence of autism spectrum disorders: Autism and Developmental Disabilities Monitoring Network, six sites, United States, 2000. *Morbidity and Mortality Weekly Report, 56*(SS1), 1–11.

Bertrand, J., Mars, A., Boyle, C., Bove, F., Yeargin-Allsopp, M., & Decoufle, P. (2001). Prevalence of autism in a United States population: The Brick Township, New Jersey investigation. *Pediatrics, 108*, 1155–1161.

Chakrabarti, S., & Fombonne, E. (2001). Pervasive developmental disorders in preschool children. *Journal of the American Medical Association, 285*, 3093–3099.

Ganz, M.L. (2007). The lifetime distribution of the incremental societal costs of autism. *Archives of Pediatrics and Adolescent Medicine, 161*(4), 343–349.

Individuals with Disabilities Education Improvement Act (IDEA) of 2004, PL 108-446, 20 U.S.C. §§ 1400 *et seq.*

Leslie, D.L., & Martin, A. (2007). Health care expenditures associated with autism spectrum disorders. *Archives of Pediatrics and Adolescent Medicine, 161*(4), 350–355.

Levy, S.E., Hyman, S.L., & Pinto-Martin, J.A. (2008). Autism spectrum disorders: Overview and diagnosis. In P.J. Accardo (Ed.), *Capute and Accardo's neurodevelopmental disabilities in infancy and childhood: Vol. II. The spectrum of neurodevelopmental disabilities* (3rd, pp. 495–511). Baltimore: Paul H. Brookes Publishing Co.

Lewis, M. (1971). *Clinical aspects of child development: An introductory synthesis of psychological concepts and clinical problems.* Philadelphia: Lea and Febiger.

Lord, C., Rutter, M., DiLavore, P., & Risi, S. (1999). *Autism Diagnostic Observation Schedule (ADOS): Manual.* Los Angeles: Western Psychological Services.

Robins, D.L., Fein, D., Barton, M.L., & Green, J.A. (2001) The Modified Checklist for Autism in Toddlers: An initial study investigating the early detection of autism and pervasive developmental disorders. *Journal of Autism and Developmental Disorders, 31*(2), 131–144.

Rutter, M., Bailey, A., & Lord, C. (2003). *Social Communication Questionnaire.* Los Angeles: Western Psychological Services.

Rutter, M., Le Couteur, A., & Lord, C. (2003). *Autism Diagnostic Interview, Revised.* Los Angeles: Western Psychological Services.

Yeargin-Allsopp, M., Rice, C., Karapurkan, T., Doernberg, N., Boyle, C., & Murphy, C. (2003). Prevalence of autism in a US metropolitan area. *Journal of the American Medical Association, 289,* 49–55.

3

Classification Issues in the Milder Developmental Disorders

Asperger Syndrome, the Syndrome of Nonverbal Learning Disability, and "Einstein Children"

Isabelle Rapin

Classification of behaviorally defined syndromes, including the developing disorders of the immature brain, is dimensional, not categorical. This means that their margins are inherently fuzzy and that overlaps between related syndromes are frequent, especially for individuals in the tails of their continuum of severity. There is no one-to-one relationship between etiology (i.e., biologic causation), be it acquired or genetic, and phenotype. Most developmental disorders are influenced by both multigenic and environmental factors. Demonstrating this point are three developmental disorders that overlap with the mild end of the pervasive developmental disorders (i.e., autism spectrum) and, in some cases, typical development: 1) Asperger syndrome (AS) and high-functioning autism (HFA), 2) Rourke's syndrome of nonverbal learning disability (NVLD), and 3) the precociously nonverbally bright "Einstein children" with delayed speech described by Thomas Sowell (1997, 2001). The appropriate application of each of these labels can be confusing for both parents and professionals. This chapter compares their similarities and differences, concluding that, in some individuals, variability and overlaps are such that expediency plays a decisive role in choosing the appropriate label.

Parents and professionals alike are often confused by the complexities of the conflicting labels clinicians are likely to apply when their children's development does not follow expected norms. Parents are particularly at a loss when the labels change with age or when different professionals with different knowledge bases assign several labels as they focus on different aspects of one child's profile of abilities and disabilities. School systems and insurance companies require that practitioners give one unequivocal diagnosis to children because their services are predicated on one categorical diagnosis. The purpose of this chapter is to consider why it is so often difficult to provide crisp diagnoses or even to decide whether a particular child should be considered impaired. These issues are epitomized by the comparison of the three diagnostic labels—AS, the syndrome of NVLD, and Einstein children.

DEVELOPMENTAL DISORDERS ARE DIMENSIONAL DIAGNOSES

All developmental disorders, be they dyslexia, intellectual disability (ID), attention-deficit/hyperactivity disorder (ADHD), autism, or any other, are diagnosed on the basis of their behavioral features, not on the basis of any blood, imaging, or electro-physiologic test result. Behavioral diagnoses stand in stark contrast to dichotomous medical diagnoses such as a broken leg or a strep infection that can be validated or dismissed definitively by an objective bio-logic test (Kraemer, 1992a, 1992b). Behav-ioral diagnoses are driven by quantitative criteria. They are based on the nature and size of deviations of criterion behaviors from agreed upon norms. Behavioral diag-noses thus have somewhat fuzzy margins. Diagnosis based on dimensional criteria is not unique to the developmental disor-ders, as solidly "medical" conditions like arterial hypertension, obesity, type II dia-betes, and Alzheimer disease are also dimen-sional despite their unequivocally biologic correlates.

Who does or does not meet a behav-iorally defined diagnosis depends on whether the individual's impairment is above or below an agreed upon—thus arbi-trary—threshold in a continuous range of symptom severity. Often, there is nearly unanimous agreement as to whether an individual is or is not affected when severity is well above or below this threshold. The problem is that agreement deteriorates when severity is close to the threshold. Indi-viduals affected by dimensionally defined conditions fit under a bell-shaped curve of severity in which there are few individuals at the very severe end and few at the mild end of the distribution. The majority are found to be in the middle, where disorders are pro-totypical. These individuals fit diagnostic cri-teria and are easily diagnosable, and thus interobserver agreement is good. Diagnostic agreement for individuals in the tails of the distribution deteriorates because the least severely affected blend with the typical pop-ulation, whereas those in both tails share symptoms with other disorders.

Behavioral diagnoses are born from the repeated observation of individuals who present with a reasonably uniform cluster of abnormalities or deviations from expecta-tion. Clinicians catalog these deficits and agree upon their required number and severity to justify a syndromic diagnosis, and then upon exclusionary criteria that pre-clude it, they give it a name. Ideally, investi-gators submit the identified syndrome to field trials to determine how well the diag-nostic criteria apply to a new set of individu-als. Once a consensus has been reached and the criteria refined and validated statistically, the syndrome becomes accepted as a "real" diagnosis. This is the procedure to which the autism spectrum disorders (ASDs) were iter-atively submitted between the revised third edition of the *Diagnostic and Statistical Man-ual of Mental Disorders* (*DSM-III-R*; American Psychiatric Association [APA], 1987) and the text revision of the fourth edition (*DSM-IV-TR*; APA, 2000). The problem is that a siz-able proportion of individuals do not fit neatly into these diagnostic boxes, owing to the fuzzy margins and comorbidities inher-ent in quantitatively defined diagnoses, not to mention the fact that behavioral diag-noses rarely arise from a single cause.

COMPLEXITIES OF RELATIONSHIPS OF GENE TO BRAIN TO BEHAVIOR IN DEVELOPMENTAL DISORDERS

Human behavior is extraordinarily complex, and this complexity is made possible by the phenomenal complexity of the brain. It is the result of an enormously large number of interconnected and interacting cortico-cortical and cortico-subcortical circuits with billions of interneuronal synapses. Simplistic ideas about discrete circuits and specific cor-tical areas dedicated to particular complex behaviors such as language are no longer tenable. They are not even tenable for sim-ple voluntary movements or sensory percep-tions, as even the spinal cord relays for final motor outputs and first order sensory inputs are already richly interconnected to a num-ber of local, ascending, and descending brain circuits. Modern functional imaging shows that any task activates a number of distinct, widely distributed cortical and subcortical nodes. In addition, different tasks may activate some of the same nodes (and others), and activations for a given task vary during the acquisition of a skill or depend on the focus of attention during performance. Although this does away with simplistic localizationist views of how the brain is organized, it does not resurrect unsustainable equipotentiality theories or deny that at a sufficiently gross level of magnification like functional imaging, particular tasks such as reading or evoking unpleasant thoughts are correlated with predictable and partially selective cortical and subcortical activations. Functional imaging can help differentiate some deviant behaviors from typical behaviors, identify differences among diagnostic groups, and provide clues about underlying neural pathophysiology, but it does not explain behavior.

Functional brain imaging and electrophysiology that identify activated brain circuitry are more likely to illuminate behavioral phenotypes than the identification of the mutated gene or genes responsible for maldevelopment or malfunction of the circuitry. The reason is that *genes do not control behavior, the brain does*. Genes control the synthesis and degradation of proteins that contribute either to the structure of cells or to their functional chemical economy. During intrauterine development, precisely timed schedules of activation and silencing of the genes that synthesize a particular protein are orchestrated by many other genes and are also influenced by nongenetic factors such as the provision of nutrients. Extremely complex interactions of many genes turned on and off in precisely timed sequences controlled by noncoding RNAs sensitive to environmental influences are thus required to build the brain and its circuitry (Mehler & Mattick, 2007). Postnatal brain maturation continues to be influenced by both the individual's genes and the unique influences of unpredictable environmental experiences.

It is said that maybe 50% of human genes are concerned with brain development and function. With the one exception of monozygotic twins, no two individuals—even those closely related genetically—inherit more than 50% of the same genes because of gene exchanges at meiosis. Most genes have accumulated many mutations over the eons of evolution. Some of these mutations, referred to as *polymorphisms*, have no effect or neutral effects on gene function. Other mutations exert positive or negative effects on RNA transcription and translation and thus the synthesis and degradation of proteins, some of which are enzymes and receptors for neurotransmitters that have subtle or blatant effects on brain structure and function. The unique genetic background of each individual therefore modulates favorable or deleterious consequences of mutated genes. Consequently, the phenotypic expression of any given expressed mutation can vary significantly from individual to individual.

No human behavior is under the control of a single gene, as each behavior is influenced by the integrated activity of many brain circuits. This statement does not imply that the mutation or silencing of a single gene may not result in a complex yet easily recognizable phenotype that deserves to be called a diagnosis or syndrome, given that affected individuals who are carriers of the mutation share a large enough number of phenotypic commonalities, despite the lack of complete clinical uniformity. For example, mutation of the *FOXP2* gene is linked to a severe developmental language disorder in an extended British family (Fisher, Vargha-Khadem, Watkins, Monaco, & Pembrey, 1998; Liegeois et al., 2003; Vargha-Khadem et al., 1998) but, as all members of the family are not equally affected, it is clear that both different background genes and unique environmental experiences have influenced the phenotypic expression of the mutated gene among the affected family members (Lai, Gerrelli, Monaco, Fisher, & Copp, 2003; Macdermot et al., 2005).

Although the underlying cause of genetic developmental disorders is static and likely to have started its influence on brain development prenatally, its effects on the trajectory of behavioral development are not static. One of the reasons for change in phenotypic expression of a static genetic condition is the profound influence of the environment on maturation of both the brain and behavior. Perhaps the best clinical example of diagnostic change over time is that thanks to continuous exposure to language, a preschooler's language disorder may improve so much that by kindergarten it is liable to have been dismissed as a transient delay rather than a disorder, only to be reincarnated as dyslexia at school age (Bishop & Adams, 1990; Shaywitz, 2003). The consequence of this change in phenotype of an underlying static genetic disorder is that the child will receive two distinct diagnostic labels at different ages.

Single gene defects whose effects are strong enough to be expressed as a uniquely recognizable phenotype (e.g., "disease" or syndrome) are likely to affect the economy of cells in multiple organs. Therefore, in addition to their effects on the brain and behavior, some are responsible for widespread somatic effects, some of which may not be apparent in early life. This is the case in fragile X syndrome (FXS), whose characteristic facial features and enlarged testicular size do not develop until adolescence (Hagerman & Hagerman, 2004b). In tuberous sclerosis, cardiac rhabdomyomas may be present at birth and then regress, facial "adenoma sebaceum" that were absent at birth may appear in mid-childhood, and interstitial lung lesions may develop in adults (Curatolo, 2003).

Most mutations and their phenotypes are stable from generation to generation, but a few are not, resulting in drastically different lifespan phenotypes across genera-

tions. A good illustration is the mutation resulting in variable amplification of trinucleotide (CGG) repeats in FXS. Depending on the number of repeats in the individual, FRX mutation impairs more or less severely the development not only of cognition, language, attention, and sociability in boys; it may also cause slowly progressive degeneration of cerebellar and basal ganglia pathways, with the appearance of an incapacitating movement disorder late in the life in some of their until-then asymptomatic maternal grandfathers (Hagerman & Hagerman, 2004a).

Why certain nodes or pathways in the brain circuitry (or somatic organs) may be exquisitely susceptible to particular genetic or nongenetic deficits is not well understood; moreover, a consequence of the brain's massive interconnectedness is that the consequences of deficient function in any one biochemical pathway or functional circuit will almost invariably cascade onto other circuits. The result is that the dysfunction is likely to affect what are considered dissociable aspects of human behavior because they are not invariably linked. For example, some—but by no means all—symptoms of Tourette syndrome (e.g., obsessive-compulsive tendencies) overlap those of AS (Nass & Gutman, 1997). Because these symptoms do not always coexist with either disorder, and because there are sufficient differences between syndromes to consider them distinct, such overlaps are referred to as comorbidities when an individual has symptoms of both disorders.

In short, although developmental disorders may arise from single-gene defects, their phenotypic expression is under polygenic influence. They are the behavioral consequences of mutations affecting the timing of activation or silencing of one or several genes. The effects of the mutation are modulated by both the individual's unique genetic background (i.e., by polymorphisms or mutations in the many other genes that influence brain development and function), as well as by the equally unique environmental circumstances of that individual's life. The phenotypic consequences of static gene mutations are likely to change drastically over the span of the individual's life. Therefore, it is easy to understand why the relationship between genotype and behavioral phenotype is so far from uniform.

COMORBIDITY: DEVELOPMENTAL DISORDERS ARE CLASSIFIED BY THEIR MOST SALIENT SYMPTOM BUT ARE RARELY PURE

Developmental disorders are labeled according to their most salient deficit—for example, language → developmental language disorder (DLD), dysphasia, specific language impairment (SLI); reading → dyslexia; motor skills → clumsiness or dyspraxia; attention → ADD with or without hyperactivity; and so forth. Developmental disorders are rarely pure in the sense that deficits other than the most salient one are frequent. These are labeled *comorbidities* when behavioral impairments involve what are considered distinct aspects of behavior presumed to involve discrete brain circuitry. One example is the frequent cooccurrence of disorders of reading and attention (Shaywitz, Fletcher, & Shaywitz, 1995), each of which is considered a specific diagnosis. Another is overlap of the severe end of the language disorder spectrum with mild ID (Stevenson & Richman, 1976), and still another of autism with severe to profound ID. Overlap with typical development creates ambiguity at the mild end of the autism spectrum, ADHD, and other developmental disorders. Behavioral overlaps (i.e., comorbidities) are not limited to the extremes of the severity distribution but instead exist throughout its range.

There are two types of comorbidity. *Coincidental comorbidity* involves two independent disorders that occur fortuitously at the same time in one individual, such as the proverbial measles and broken leg. More common in the developmental disorders is *related comorbidity*—that is, the cooccurrence of two disorders considered to be distinct because each can occur in isolation but which overlap so often as to suggest that this is no mere coincidence. Examples are obsessive-compulsive behavior with both AS and Tourette syndrome, clumsiness with mixed receptive-expressive dysphasia and AS, and ADHD with dyscalculia and dyslexia.

There are many reasons for related comorbidity. A potentially detectable one is a chromosomal duplication or microdeletion that implicates a number of adjacent genes; the result is generally somatic effects, as well as involvement of a number of brain circuits resulting in a quite distinct behavioral syndrome. Examples are Down, Angelman (Cassidy, Dykens, & Williams, 2000), Shprintzen velo-cardio-facial (Shprintzen et al., 2005), and Williams (Bellugi, Lichtenberger, Mills, Galaburda, & Korenberg, 1999) syndromes, among many others. Second, related comorbidity may arise because the mutated gene affects the development of several distinct brain circuits. An example of single-gene mutation with widespread effects is the *MECP2* gene, which is responsible for Rett syndrome in girls and controls the methylation (i.e., turning off) of many genes at different times during development; as a consequence, it has early and delayed clinical effects such as early autistic regression (AR) and later epilepsy (Zoghbi, 2003). A third cause of related comorbidity is the relative nonselectivity of certain malformations like hydrocephalus and especially of exogeneous insults to the brain like anoxia, infection, or trauma. A fourth is the secondary behavioral consequences of a developmental deficiency; for example, the inability to fully understand what others are saying will interfere with the acquisition of a variety of academic and social skills, very likely resulting in secondary behavioral problems.

OVERLAPS IN AUTISM SPECTRUM DISORDERS OR PERVASIVE DEVELOPMENTAL DISORDERS

In this chapter, the term *autism* refers to the entire severity range of the autism spectrum, which encompasses the *DSM–IV-TR* diagnoses Autistic Disorder, Asperger's Disorder, and Pervasive Developmental Disorder Not Otherwise Specified (PDD-NOS). Omitted here are the *DSM-IV-TR* diagnoses Childhood Disintegrative Disorder, a delayed catastrophic AR that may or may not be distinct from the much more prevalent early AR, and Rett's Disorder, a specific genetic cause of AR.

As alluded to earlier, the severe end of the autism spectrum overlaps with severe ID. The *DSM–IV-TR* (APA, 2000) specifies that autism symptomatology must be out of proportion to the severity of the ID for a diagnosis of Autistic Disorder to apply, yet the autism literature contains innumerable descriptions of people with intelligence quotients (IQs) of 20–30 who clearly have both severe ID and an ASD. A visit to any program for people with severe intellectual disabilities illustrates that most of the patients are socially withdrawn, nonverbal, and rigid and that they engage in many stereotypic and often self-injurious behaviors, all of which are defining characteristics of autism. Yet not every child with severe ID has an ASD. A counterexample in point is Cockayne syndrome, in which the brain may weigh as little as a third of its expected weight and an individual's IQ is almost always well below 50, yet affected children are very sociable and communicative and clearly do not have autism (Cockayne, 1936; Nance & Berry, 1992). Many children with Down syndrome whose IQ falls in the same 50–70 range that characterizes classic Autistic Disorder are generally friendly and clearly do not have autism (Chapman & Hesketh, 2000), although occasionally a child with Down syndrome also has autism.

PDD-NOS is the box for those individuals who do not fit into the defined subtypes of the autism spectrum; it differs from AS by delayed development of expressive language, in some cases with less verbal fluency and syntactic complexity, by more overt social deficits, and perhaps more blatant stereotypies. High-functioning children on the spectrum do not have ID by definition but, like children with AS, they are likely to have uneven cognitive abilities. When they have reached midchildhood, they may be indistinguishable from children with AS were it not for the history of delayed emergence of speech (Wing, 1991). Comparing these descriptions indicates that any differences between these three subgroups of the autism spectrum are dimensional and not categorical.

It is the upper end of the distribution that is particularly relevant here. Does a gauche individual who interacts better with his computer than with people, who prefers solitude, who has little insight into what others may think of him (whose "theory of mind" [Baron-Cohen, Leslie, & Frith, 1985] is weak), who is intolerant of suggestions for a switch of activities, and who speaks endlessly of his or her preferred topic have HFA or AS, or is this person simply a harmless but lovable "nerd" who needs advice on how to dress?

THREE OVERLAPPING SYNDROMES: ASPERGER SYNDROME, THE SYNDROME OF NONVERBAL LEARNING DISABILITY, AND EINSTEIN CHILDREN

Children with Asperger syndrome, children with the syndrome of NVLD, and Einstein children share certain characteristics but not others. This has led to much controversy regarding the specificity and even the nosologic reality of these clinical syndromes.

Asperger Syndrome

AS refers to individuals on the autism spectrum—up to 6 boys to 1 girl (Gillberg, 2002)—whose IQ is by definition above 70; whose verbal IQ is typically equal to or superior to his or her performance IQ; whose expressive language, again by definition, developed at the expected age; and who may be clumsy. As with more severely affected children on the autism spectrum, the level of social inadequacy required for this diagnostic label must be sufficiently severe to be impairing. As children, they are at a loss on how to interact with peers but tend to do better with less demanding younger children or infants and with the more tolerant and accommodating adolescent and adult who resonates with their strengths and overlooks or excuses their peculiarities. The fact that young children with AS spoke at the expected age does not mean that their language is entirely unaffected, as the large size of their vocabularies tends to be out of proportion to their comprehension of discourse, their prosody is likely to be atypical, and their conversational skills are grossly deficient (Tager-Flusberg, 2003). Some—although not all—have the semantic-pragmatic language disorder syndrome (Allen, 1988; Rapin & Allen, 1998). Like other children on the autism spectrum, the play of children with AS tends to be impoverished, their interests narrow, and they are likely to have stereotypies. They are rigid and set in their ways. Clearly, this is a subgroup carved out of the autism spectrum. Whether AS does or does not have a specific biologic—presumably genetic—substrate is not known at this point.

Rourke's Syndrome of Nonverbal Learning Disability

Rourke is a neuropsychologist educated in the classic tradition of quantitative analysis of behaviors, the goal of which is detecting patterns of cognitive deficit that point to diffuse or focal brain pathology in adults. Rourke applied this quantitative approach to the developmental disorders of school-age children (and adults). His influential book *Nonverbal Learning Disabilities: The Syndrome and the Model* (Rourke, 1989) described in detail the neuropsychologic and behavioral profiles of children whose academic deficits are not in reading but in calculation. The children had salient impairments of their visual/spatial/constructional and organizational skills; markedly deficient reasoning and problem-solving abilities in the face of an often outstanding rote memory; fluent, even verbose perseverative speech; and inadequate social skills.

This syndrome shares features with developmental deficits attributed to right hemisphere pathology because of its similarities to acquired right hemispheric lesions in adults (Weintraub & Mesulam, 1983). More recent papers detailing the consequences of lateralized or focal congenital or very early static brain lesions of the right hemisphere confirm that they share some features with the syndrome of NVLD (Nass & Trauner, 2004). In a second book, *Syndrome of Nonverbal Learning Disabilities: Neurodevelopmental Manifestations* (Rourke, 1995), Rourke and others reported that they identified this syndrome in agenesis of the corpus callosum, hydrocephalus, Williams syndrome, and a variety of other genetic and acquired disorders, most of which predominantly affect the white matter. The book has a chapter that juxtaposes the neuropyschologically defined syndrome of NVLD with the behaviorally defined Asperger syndrome. A paper appeared that same year acknowledging the overlaps between the two (Klin, Volkmar, Sparrow, Cichetti, & Rourke, 1995).

Sowell's Einstein Children

Sowell's book *Late-Talking Children* (1997) is dedicated to his son John, "who was late in talking but early in thinking." Together with his second book, *The Einstein Syndrome:*

Bright Children Who Talk Late (2001), it illus-trates the diagnostic dilemmas developmen-tal disorders raise at the edges of typical development (Rapin, 2002).

The first book grew out of an article that Sowell had written in 1993 for a syndicated newspaper column describing his family's frustration during John's early years, his subsequent improvement, and his success as a computer programmer. This article elicited spontaneous communications and telephone calls from several dozen parents of children who had encountered similarly frustrating experiences of multiple evalua-tions for lack of speech by many profession-als who often provided conflicting diagnoses, one of the most common being an ASD. Sowell and the parents organized a support group to share experiences and resources. The book starts with variably detailed case vignettes of 19 children, then provides a compilation of answers to two questionnaires completed by 44 families about 46 children, 39 (i.e., 85%) of them boys. Sowell acknowl-edges that the group was heterogeneous and skewed toward highly educated parents as 77% of mothers and 69% of fathers were col-lege graduates, more than half of them also having a postgraduate education. All the listed occupations of close relatives were in quantitative fields—accountants, computer experts, engineers, scientists, and so forth—or in music. Indeed, all but 9% of these 80 close relatives were said to be musical, and 12 (i.e., 15%) were professional musicians. Sow-ell also provided a vignette of an acknowl-edged Australian musician with autism, Trevor Tao, about whom his educator, Jean Bryant (1993), had written a book titled *The Opening Door.*

As to the 46 children, their language was indeed very delayed, as only 1 of the 37 who were verbal had said a sentence before the age of 3 years. Twenty-four percent were not able to converse until age 3–4 years, 38% until 4–5 years, and 38% until after 5 years. In some children, when language appeared, it started suddenly and unexpect-edly in clear sentences with large vocabular-

ies, but that was not the case of all the chil-dren. Some were still nonverbal at the time of the report, and others utilized speech that was unclear and impoverished. Sowell stated that although some children had comprehension deficits, others did not. One third of the children had been given a diag-nosis of autism, 70% had below-average social skills, and 36% were reported to have had inadequate gestures and facial expres-sions when speaking. Two thirds of the group was fascinated with water, spinning wheels, and other objects; the same propor-tion was described as being extremely good at puzzles, and a few individuals were chess players. All the parents reported above-aver-age memories—outstanding in 59% of the children—and it was clear that some of the children were extremely bright, usually with nonverbal skills and reasoning greatly advanced compared with their verbal abili-ties. Some had learned to recognize letters and numbers at a very young age and some read early. One third of the children were judged to be clumsy, but 44% were judged to have better than average motor skills. Toi-let training was one area of virtually univer-sal deficit, with 39% trained for bladder and 48% for bowel after the age of 4 years.

Sowell is aware that this was a heteroge-neous group of children and that the out-come was not uniformly favorable. He gave the group the nickname "3 M" (i.e., memory, mathematics, and music). This syndrome overlaps in some of its features with Gillberg's DAMP syndrome (i.e., deficits in attention, motor control, and per-ception) (Landgren, Pettersson, Kjellman, & Gillberg, 1996), which is encountered in children with a variety of developmental dis-orders, including AS.

Sowell's second book (2001) added to the same sample descriptive informa-tion about 239 late speakers compiled by Dr. Camarata, a professor of speech and language pathology at Vanderbilt University in Nashville, Tennessee. The second book also contained some vignettes, including those of the two Nobelists—Einstein and

Feynman—both of whom were evidently late speakers and, needless to say, uniquely brilliant. The book provides tables that compare characteristics of the first and second cohorts. The Camarata cohort was similar to the Sowell cohort in many ways except that it seemed more representative of the general population of late talkers, as it was less skewed toward gifted children. Camarata stated that he intends to systematically follow-up his sample, but probably not enough time has elapsed for papers to be published as of the date this chapter was written (i.e., May 2006). Sowell discussed how difficult it was to determine how many of the social problems of the clearly gifted children were a reaction to their being misfits among ordinary people rather than to their having innate deficits, although he clearly favored the former. He was not a proponent of remedial programs or of most interventions, including early schooling, for this type of child because he predicted a favorable outcome and doubted the need or effectiveness of available interventions. This favorable view of outcome contrasts with an article about AS in *The New York Times* (Harmon, 2004), in which even high-achieving adults described major adaptive difficulties in the job and social arenas.

COMPARISONS AMONG THE THREE DIAGNOSES

Einstein children and children with the diagnosis of Asperger syndrome or the syndrome of NVLD can be compared across many different areas. Table 3.1 gives an overview of the characteristics of each one, and the following sections provide more in-depth discussion.

Subjects

One of the difficulties with the comparison is that the emphasis and interest of the authors who defined the syndromes differed, with the result that the information available on each is incomplete in some way.

AS has been the subject of intense research by mainstream investigators who have also recruited high-functioning volunteers with classic autism; they have carried out morphometric brain measurements, functional MRI studies of facial recognition, studies of eye movements, scanning of faces, and many others. They have also obtained language, cognitive, and social profiles, mostly on adolescent or adult subjects selected to fulfill research diagnostic criteria, compared to typical controls. Some of the studies do not make a clear distinction between individuals with AS and those with HFA (i.e., those who are verbal and of average or above-average intelligence). Because individuals who fit either of these diagnoses have so much in common by mid-childhood and adulthood—with the exception of delayed language and worse social deficits in classic autism—no attempt is made to separate AS from HFA in this discussion.

Most studies of the syndrome of NVLD were performed on school-age children referred for formal neuropsychologic testing because of difficulties in school; neurologic tests like brain imaging were available on some of them. Others were selected from neurologic clinics and underwent neuropsychologic testing because of a known genetic disease or acquired brain pathology to validate the existence and postulated neurologic basis of the syndrome of NVLD.

In stark contrast, information on the children with Einstein syndrome rests on the reports by their self-selected parents, many of whom had advanced educations. The emphasis of the reports was on delayed expressive language without systematic information on comprehension, on the troublesome problem of very delayed toilet training, and on unusual talents in memory, nonverbal problem solving, mathematics, and music. No neuropsychologic or neurologic information or formal information on social skills was available. Many of the children were considerably younger than most of those in the other two groups, most of whom were school-age children or adoles-

Table 3.1. Comparisons of Asperger syndrome, syndrome of nonverbal learning disabilities, and "Einstein children"

	Asperger syndrome (including HFA)	Syndrome of NVLD	Einstein children
Predominant age at description	Adolescents/adults	School age	Preschool age
Gender	Largely males	Equally distributed?	Largely males
Cause	Developmental, nonlesional disorder; presumed genetic	Developmental, nonlesional disorder (generally); known genetic/nongenetic conditions	Developmental, non-lesional condition; presumed genetic
Anatomy	Enlarged white matter	White matter (connectionist) hypothesis, right hemisphere worse than left	No information
Gross motor	May be clumsy	Possibly more impaired on the left	26% clumsy
Fine motor	Apraxia (e.g., handwriting, dressing, tying); deficits in oculomotor control and scanning faces	Impaired	May be excellent
Perception			
Visuospatial	Variable, including interpersonal space issues	Poor visuospatial sense, including interpersonal space, drawing, and constructional skill	Excellent
Faces	Impaired processing of facial expression, gaze avoidance	Possibly impaired	No information
Somatosensory	No information	Impaired tactile and body image, especially on the left	No information
Auditory	Some individuals have perfect pitch and a very good memory for music; many lack sensitivity to and have difficulty interpreting prosody	Excellent, some (e.g., individuals with Williams syndrome) have hyperacute auditory perception and perfect pitch	Interest in and, in some, talent for music
Memory	Good to excellent rote, auditory, and visual; "calendar calculators"	Good to excellent rote (verbatim) auditory; poor visual and tactile, especially on the left	Excellent visual ($\pm$ auditory)
Attention	Hyperfocused on self-generated activities; impaired joint attention	Impaired visual, tactile	Hyperfocused on self-generated activities
Flexibility	Inflexibility, resistance to change	Impaired adaptation to novel situations	No information
Language			
Onset and character	No delay in development; large vocabulary; often semantic-pragmatic language disorder; perseveration	May be delayed, then fluent; often semantic-pragmatic language disorder; perseveration	Very delayed; when/if it starts, it may progress very rapidly to fluency
Phonology and syntax	Okay	Okay	Impaired in some
Prosody	Impaired, singsong, poorly modulated voice	Impaired	No information
Comprehension	Comprehension of discourse and questions impaired early on	Good to excellent	Comprehension of discourse typical in some, impaired in others
Humor and incongruities	Appreciation often impaired	Appreciation impaired	No information

	Asperger syndrome (including HFA)	Syndrome of NVLD	Einstein children
Pragmatics	Pragmatics and conversational skills impaired; insistence on own topic	Pragmatics and conversational skills impaired; verbose	May use pointing/gestures to make up for lack of speech
Cognition	Uneven profile; VIQ ≥ PIQ; FSIQ varies from borderline to very high; practical sense impaired and out of proportion to IQ; may have adequate/superior abstract reasoning	Usually borderline to low-normal; auditory > visual; impaired concept formation, reasoning, problem solving, exploration of novelty	Precocious; high nonverbal (and possibly over-all); visual > auditory, often extreme discrepancy; excellent nonverbal problem-solving ability
Academic skills			
Reading; spelling	Precocious interest in letters and numbers; hyperlexia frequent early on	Reading decoding > comprehension; good, phonetically accurate spelling	Precocious interest in letters and numbers; early reading frequent
Mathematics	Variable, excellent in some; rote calculation may be outstanding	Remarkably poor arithmetic skills	Good to outstanding mathematical ability
Sociability	Impaired theory of mind, lack of social awareness; worse with peers than adults or babies	Sociable but impaired social judgment	Variable; some okay, others poor; not always responsive when called, etc.
Mood	Flat affect in some children; depression, bipolar disorder in some adolescents and adults	Tendency toward depression, especially in older children	No information

Key: NVLD = nonverbal learning disability; HFA = high-functioning autism; IQ = intelligence quotient; PIQ = performance IQ; VIQ = verbal IQ; FSIQ = full-scale IQ.

cents. Whereas papers on Asperger and NVLD syndromes were formal reports prepared by clinicians or researchers, the tabulated data from parent reports on the Einstein children were purely descriptive, without external validation.

Etiology and Gender

There is no information on the neurologic basis or etiology of Einstein syndrome, although information from the families points to a strong genetic influence. Multigenic influence is the leading causal hypothesis in AS, but this is not clearly the case in NVLD syndrome, especially not in the validation cases selected from the clinic. Although the male gender dominates in both the AS and Einstein samples, this is not the case in the syndrome of NVLD.

Neurologic Basis

Replicated morphometric studies in AS and HFA show larger than average mean brain volumes, with greater disparity in the white than the gray matter (Herbert et al., 2004). Most of the children who came to Dr. Rourke's consultation were not imaged. His second book described some conditions with clear white matter involvement like hydrocephalus, some leukodystrophies, and agenesis of the corpus callosum, as well as some selected genetic developmental conditions associated with the syndrome of NVLD such as Williams syndrome and the velo-cardio-facial and other syndromes in which pathology is not limited to the white matter. No information is available about the neurologic status of the Einstein children.

Motor Deficits

Some individuals in all three groups are described as clumsy, although this is by no means always the case. Clumsiness was mentioned by only 25% of the parents of Einstein children. Only in the syndrome of NVLD is there an indication that motor deficits may be asymmetrical and subtly worse on the left; Rourke (1989) stated that motor deficits may become more troublesome with age as the complexity of tasks requires ever-better visuospatial abilities. Impaired fine motor skill in some individuals with AS such as very large, delayed, and laborious handwriting (Asperger 1944/ 1991; Beversdorf et al., 2001) and difficulty learning to button or tie clothing or other items may reflect apraxia, which was interpreted by Mostofsky, Goldberg, Landa, and Denckla (2000) as deficient procedural learning. Fine motor skills are described as superior in some Einstein children. Impaired control of eye movements with difficulty inhibiting countersaccades (i.e., deliberately not looking at a particular target) has been found in some individuals with HFA (Minshew, Luna, & Sweeney, 1999). Gaze avoidance is well-known to characterize most individuals on the autism spectrum. A dramatic deficit in facial scanning (i.e., looking at the mouth rather than the eyes of the person speaking to them) has been shown to be one of the salient characteristics of AS (Klin, Jones, Schultz, Volkmar, & Cohen, 2002). Whether oculomotor abnormalities are an apraxia or the result of visuospatial or social deficits remains to be seen.

Visuospatial Deficits

The severe impairment of visuospatial-constructional skills that is one of the defining characteristics of the syndrome of NVLD distinguishes it from Einstein children, in whom this is an area of strength. These skills are variable in AS—excellent in some, average or poor in others. Many individuals with AS have a poor sense of interpersonal space (e.g., coming too close); again, whether this is because of social or visuospatial deficits is uncertain. The profound impairment of the ability to see the overall gestalt of a scene and the focus on detail characterizes some children with autism (Dakin & Frith, 2005), and is particularly salient in Williams syn-

drome, a prototypic exemplar of the syndrome of NVLD (Bellugi & St. George, 2001). It also characterizes many children with congenital or very early acquired focal lesions of the white matter (Nass & Trauner, 2004), which is one of the arguments for viewing the syndrome of developmental NVLD as a right hemispheric syndrome.

Somatosensory Deficits

Because Rourke (1989) used a standardized and thorough neuropsychologic battery on the children evaluated in his laboratory, he was able to detect deficits in two-point discrimination—especially in the left hand—in some children with the syndrome of NVLD, findings that support his right hemisphere surmise. He mentioned that the children may have had deficits in awareness of body scheme as well, also linked to right hemisphere function. This type of deficit does not appear to have been looked for systematically in individuals with AS, some of whom, like Temple Grandin (1995), report intolerance for some tactile stimuli. Parents of Einstein children seem not to have focused on cutaneous sensation.

Auditory Skills

What parents do focus on is their children's often superior ability and interest in music, a characteristic they share with other members of their families. Children with the syndrome of NVLD do not seem to have auditory perceptual problems, and those with Williams syndrome specifically have outstandingly acute hearing. An unusual number of individuals with AS and other ASDs have perfect pitch and exceptional memories for music, and some have musical gifts yet lack sensitivity to prosody (Heaton, 2003). Thus, it appears that auditory perception is largely unaffected in all three groups, which separates them from the many more severely affected individuals on the autism spectrum, some of whom are intolerant of sound and others who have much more difficulty processing information, in particular language, presented to the auditory rather than the visual channel.

Memory

Memory is an area of strength for all three groups. Some parents of Einstein children and children with AS state that their children have phenomenal memories for both visual and verbal material. Rourke's formal tests demonstrated strong rote—often verbatim—verbal memory in NVLD, but deficiencies in visual and tactile memory, especially on the left. Many children with AS and Einstein children have a precocious interest in letters and numbers, and there are a number of "calendar calculators" among those with AS. In contrast to the other two groups, those with NVLD continue to depend on rote learning and do not organize their memories into systems, which puts severe limits on their cognitive abilities.

Attention

A paradox for the parents of children with AS and other ASDs is their children's strong and prolonged attention to self-generated activities and their often marked deficit in the ability to pay attention jointly to a stimulus or an activity introduced by someone else (Mundy, Sigman, & Kasari, 1993). These characteristics may contribute to their rigidity and resistance to switching activities, and later to the obsessive-compulsive tendencies that some of them exhibit. The Einstein group is stated to have outstanding attention spans for what interests them. The NVLD group is described as having poor visual and tactile attention and as having particular difficulty paying attention and adapting to novel situations.

Language

By definition, expressive language is late to develop in the Einstein group and not delayed in the AS group. Speech may be somewhat delayed in some children with NVLD, but it later becomes one of their strengths. What they share with children who have AS is that a number of children in both groups have the semantic-pragmatic language disorder defined by Rapin and Allen (1998), the characteristics of which were considered for a long time to be *the* characteristics of high-functioning verbal children on the autism spectrum (Bishop, 1989). Such children have no deficit in expressive phonology or syntax; their semantic deficits include unusual word choices, impaired comprehension of discourse in the face of an unusually large vocabulary, and, especially, impaired comprehension of open-ended questions, which may give their language a tangential quality. The pragmatic deficits are grossly inadequate conversational skills and an inability to program coherent discourse, often compensated by the more or less appropriate use of memorized scripts (i.e., delayed echolalia, formulaic speech). Their prosody may be sing-song, their voices may be high-pitched, and their assertions may have the rising intonation of the prosodic contour of questions. The rhythm of their speech may be choppy, monotonous, or wooden (i.e., robotic). Descriptions of the speech of children with the syndrome of NVLD make it clear that some characteristics of their language fit this description.

It seems likely that there are several different reasons for the late speech of Einstein children. Some appear to have pure expressive deficits with adequate comprehension, whereas descriptions of others suggest that their comprehension is also deficient. As some of them continue to have poor verbal skills with inadequate phonology and syntax, they almost certainly have the mixed receptive/expressive lower-level language processing deficit—a deficit common in many children with frank autism, as well as in children without ASDs who have DLDs (Rapin, 1996; Rapin & Dunn, 2003), but not in those with either AS or the syndrome of

NVLD. Some parents of Einstein children believe their children chose not to speak because when language eventually started, it progressed rapidly and was fluent, a characteristic also reported by some parents of children with HFA (who by current criteria cannot be diagnosed with AS because of the delay in their speech). Because all young children on the autism spectrum have deficient comprehension of discourse, but not phonology in those with the semantic-pragmatic language disorder, I consider choosing not to speak as an explanation for late development of expressive language unconvincing.

Cognition

A hallmark of the children in all three groups is uneven cognitive abilities. On average the Einstein group is skewed toward children gifted in mathematics, chess, and other nonverbal reasoning skills. In contrast, the NVLD group has, on average, lower cognitive abilities, which their adequate or better verbal skills and sociability may mask early on. Later, however, their rote memory can carry them only so far in compensating for their limited reasoning and deficient visual/spatial abilities. Thus, their cognitive imitations tend to become more apparent as they mature.

The AS group is more varied. The AS label was arbitrarily limited to children having an IQ of 70 or better, which means that there are children with AS who possess borderline intelligence, but once again, they very likely have some areas of higher ability and others of frank deficiency. A significant percentage of them are of average overall intelligence, bright, or even highly gifted. In contrast to classic autism, where the prevalent pattern is that performance IQ (PIQ) is greater than verbal IQ (VIQ), children with AS are often stated to have a VIQ that is higher than or equal to their PIQ. This reverse pattern is not universal, considering

the adolescents and young adults Baron-Cohen, Wheelwright, Skinner, Martin, and Clubley (2001) identified among math finalists and Cambridge University students in physics, mathematics, and engineering; because most had not been identified in childhood, it is unlikely that they had spoken late, which qualifies them for a diagnosis of AS, HFA, or PDD-NOS. No doubt they had superior PIQs; all were in the hard sciences and none were in the humanities. I suspect that some of them were grown-up Einstein children, whose delay in early language was forgotten or had been ignored at the time in view of their exceptional abilities in other spheres.

Academic Skills

By definition, children with the syndrome of NVLD have academic difficulties despite early language, reading, and spelling acquisition. Mathematics, both arithmetic and geometry, may remain totally beyond them unless they can verbalize and learn the rules to apply. Their deficient reasoning ability, lack of curiosity, and difficulty dealing with novel situations progressively jeopardizes their academic success as educational demands escalate. Strong mathematical ability defines the Einstein group. Because most were described at preschool, there is limited information about other aspects of their academic careers; one can safely assume that at least those with strong cognitive abilities will encounter little or no difficulty in school. They may even excel, as is also the case for the children in the bright AS group, although their poor fit with the routine curriculum may make them "difficult" students. Less gifted children with AS may learn to read and calculate precociously, but their limited language comprehension means that they understand imperfectly what they read so fluently; consequently, the label of hyperlexia is an apt one for them and for some children with the syndrome of NVLD.

Poor handwriting is liable to create severe difficulty for all three groups, as they may be unable to finish assignments within a reasonable time frame.

Sociability

Very deficient social skills, a lack of insight into what others are thinking, or an inability to understand how their behavior may affect others are required for a diagnosis of AS (Baron-Cohen, Knickmeyer, & Belmonte, 2005). Individuals with these characteristics are often described as oblivious of others and severely lacking in empathy. However, the social deficits of some children with AS are subtle enough to remain undetected until the demands of middle childhood or adolescence bring them out. Still others who were quite impaired in early childhood seem to outgrow most of their childhood difficulties and function well as older children and adults. This resembles the trajectory of some of the Einstein children, although close reading of the vignettes in the Sowell books (1997, 2001) suggests that this is a sociably heterogeneous group of children, including some with typical social abilities and others who clearly meet the criteria for an ASD diagnosis. It seems likely that this variability was in part correlated with whether their late speaking was or was not associated with inadequate language comprehension, as children with pure expressive disorders are at extremely low or no risk for ASDs (Allen & Rapin, 1992). Young children with the syndrome of NVLD and some children with AS who have the semantic-pragmatic language deficit syndrome are often viewed as exceptionally sociable, in part because their large vocabularies, voluble scripted chatter, and intrusive questioning are interpreted as genuine friendliness and considered endearing; however, their peers and close family are rarely fooled. Rourke (1989) reported that the social deficits of children with the syndrome of NVLD tend to increase rather than improve as the children become older. Thus, sociability varies as a gradient across the three syndromes, but it does not necessarily follow the same trajectory.

Mood

As preschoolers, all of these children may seem happy and content, although those in Einstein and AS groups tended to engage in solitary activities and those in the NVLD group seek company. The parents of the Einstein children do not provide much information about their children's mood, presumably because it is not of concern. Individuals with AS may have a labile mood, and fierce temper tantrums may erupt when one attempts to intrude upon them or asks them to switch activities or give up a routine. These tantrums may persist, usually in muted form, into adulthood. Their affect is often perceived as flat, and some seem totally detached, yet they appear content despite lives that others would consider unacceptably monotonous and impoverished. According to Rourke (1989), children with the syndrome of NVLD tend to experience depression as they grow up. This is also the case in some older individuals with AS, some of whom may have bipolar comorbidity (DeLong & Dwyer, 1988).

CONCLUSION

Peas in a pod? Yes and no. Yes, in the sense that this review suggests to me that there are many areas of overlap between these syndromes carved out of a complex behavioral continuum defined on the basis of dimensionally defined characteristics. Yes, because each of the syndromes results from complex polygenic influences on brain development shaped by the differing life experiences of the individual child. (Children with the syndrome of NVLD who have defined biologic etiologies can be omitted here because they were selected a priori to have these etiologies, although their behavior is still under polygenic influence.) And yes, in the sense that some of the differences among these three disorders are due to the disparate selection criteria and interests of those who defined them, whose differing expertise and interests influenced and colored what they saw.

The answer is no, however, on the basis of other considerations. Children prototypic of these three syndromes differ in a number of ways. Language development comes to mind first, as well as visuospatial abilities, cognitive strengths and weaknesses, and, notably, social skills. Social skills are deficient by definition in people with AS, although subtly so in some individuals, and social skills do tend to improve with maturation so that ultimately the range and types of social deficits are extremely variable. Chatty children with the syndrome of NVLD appear to be at the other end of the spectrum of sociability compared with those in the AS and Einstein groups, although some experience increasing difficulty as they mature.

From a pragmatic point of view, the answer is no because telling parents what label to apply to their children will have a dramatic influence on what remedial resources society is willing to make available to them. In the United States, children on the autism spectrum receive the most intensive multidisciplinary evaluations and expensive interventions. In many cases, schools' resources are stretched to the breaking point because so many mildly affected children with AS and HFA are being identified in the hopes that early intervention will pay off and they will grow up to become self-supporting, successful members of society. But do all of them need every intervention available? Clearly no. All children require interventions that address their individual needs, regardless of the behavioral label, be it AS, syndrome of NVLD, and, yes, in some cases, Einstein syn-drome. These three syndromes bring into strong focus the fuzzy margins and elasticity of behaviorally defined diagnostic labels, their overlaps, and, by the same token, the fuzzy margins of typical development as well.

Circling back to the diagnostic boxes we as professionals created, this comparison has made it crystal clear to me, and I hope to the reader, that there are many individuals who do not fit our current boxes very well. Whether we decide to give them this—rather than that—label and to pigeonhole them into this or that box is largely a matter of expediency. We must be ready to discard our boxes as soon as we find that too many individuals do not fit comfortably in them. We start out with empirically defined diagnostic criteria, but this does not make the criteria true to nature. The patients are the data—and they are never wrong. It is we the professionals who may misinterpret what we see. As further observations and our understanding progress, we must be willing to change our classification criteria, however painful it may be to discard cherished categories. Classification schemes are hypotheses, and it is the nature of hypotheses to be disproved by further data. This review has shown that not one of the three diagnoses under consideration in this chapter is a well-shaped box or robust diagnosis. It is only until we know better that we should hold on to them, but with the clear understanding that their usefulness to us and to the children we serve is temporary.

REFERENCES

Allen, D.A. (1988). Autistic spectrum disorders: Clinical presentation in preschool children. *Journal of Child Neurology, 3,* s48–s56.

Allen, D.A., & Rapin, I. (1992). Autistic children are also dysphasic. In H. Naruse & E. Ornitz (Eds.), *Neurobiology of infantile autism* (pp. 73–80). Amsterdam, NL: Excerpta Medica.

American Psychiatric Association. (1987). *Diagnostic and statistical manual of mental disorders* (3rd ed., rev.). Washington, DC: Author.

American Psychiatric Association. (2000). *Diagnostic and statistical manual of mental disorders* (4th ed., text rev.) Washington, DC: Author.

Asperger, H. (1991). 'Autistic psychopathy' in childhood (U. Frith, Trans.). In U. Frith (Ed.), *Autism and Asperger syndrome* (pp. 37–92). Cambridge, United Kingdom: Cambridge University Press. (Original work published 1944)

Baron-Cohen, S., Knickmeyer, R.C., & Belmonte, M.K. (2005). Sex differences in the brain: Implications for explaining autism. *Science, 310,* 819–823.

Baron-Cohen, S., Leslie, A.M., & Frith, U. (1985). Does the autistic child have a "theory of mind"? *Cognition, 21,* 37–46.

Baron-Cohen, S., Wheelwright, S., Skinner, R., Martin, J., & Clubley, E. (2001). The Autism-Spectrum quotient (AQ): Evidence from Asperger syndrome/high-functioning autism, males and females, scientists, and mathematicians. *Journal of Autism and Developmental Disorders, 31,* 5–17.

Bellugi, U., Lichtenberger, L., Mills, D., Galaburda, A., & Korenberg, J.R. (1999). Bridging cognition, the brain, and molecular genetics: Evidence from Williams syndrome. *Trends in Neurosciences, 22,* 197–207.

Bellugi, U., & St. George, M. (2001). *Journey from cognition to brain to gene: Perspectives from Williams syndrome.* Cambridge, MA: MIT Press.

Beversdorf, D.Q., Anderson, J.M., Manning, S.E., Anderson, S.L., Nordgren, R.E., Felopulos, G.J., et al. (2001). Brief report: Macrographia in high-functioning adults with autism spectrum disorder. *Journal of Autism and Developmental Disorders, 31,* 97–101.

Bishop, D.V.M. (1989). Autism, Asperger's syndrome, and semantic-pragmatic disorder: Where are the boundaries? *British Journal of Disorders of Communication, 24,* 107–121.

Bishop, D.V.M., & Adams, C. (1990). A prospective study of the relationship between specific language impairment, phonological disorders, and reading retardation. *Journal of Child Psychology and Psychiatry and Allied Disciplines, 31,* 1027–1050.

Bryant, J. (1993). *The opening door.* Cherry Gardens, South Australia: Author.

Cassidy, S.B., Dykens, E., & Williams, C.A. (2000). Prader-Willi and Angelman syndromes: Sister imprinted disorders. *American Journal of Medical Genetics, 97,* 136–146.

Chapman, R.S., & Hesketh, L.J. (2000). Behavioral phenotype of individuals with Down syndrome. *Mental Retardation and Developmental Disabilities Research Reviews, 6,* 84–95.

Cockayne, E.A. (1936). Dwarfism with retinal atrophy and deafness. *Archives of Disease in Childhood, 11,* 1–8.

Curatolo, P. (2003). *Tuberous sclerosis complex: From basic science to clinical phenotypes.* London: Mac Keith Press.

Dakin, S., & Frith, U. (2005). Vagaries of visual perception in autism. *Neuron, 48,* 497–507.

DeLong, R., & Dwyer, J.T. (1988). Correlation of family history with specific autistic subgroups: Asperger's syndrome and bipolar affective illness. *Journal of Autism and Developmental Disorders, 18,* 593–600.

Fisher, S.E., Vargha-Khadem, F., Watkins, K.E., Monaco, A.P., & Pembrey, M.E. (1998). Localisation of a gene implicated in a severe speech and language disorder. *Nature Genetics, 18,* 168–170.

Gillberg, C. (2002). *A guide to Asperger syndrome.* Cambridge, United Kingdom: Cambridge University Press.

Grandin, T. (1995). *Thinking in pictures and other reports from my life with autism.* New York: Doubleday.

Hagerman, P.J., & Hagerman, R.J. (2004a). Fragile X-associated tremor/ataxia syndrome (FXTAS). *Mental Retardation and Developmental Disabilities Research Reviews, 10,* 25–30.

Hagerman, P.J., & Hagerman, R.J. (2004b). The fragile-X premutation: A maturing perspective. *American Journal of Human Genetics, 74,* 805–816.

Harmon, A. (2004, April 29). Answer, but no cure, for a social disorder that isolates many. *The New York Times.*

Heaton, P. (2003). Pitch memory, labeling, and disembedding in autism. *Journal of Child Psychology and Psychiatry and Allied Disciplines, 44,* 543–551.

Herbert, M.R., Ziegler, D.A., Makris, N., Filipek, P.A., Kemper, T.L., Normandin, J.J., et al. (2004). Localization of white matter volume increase in autism and developmental language disorder. *Annals of Neurology, 55,* 530–540.

Klin, A., Jones, W., Schultz, R., Volkmar, F., & Cohen, D. (2002). Visual fixation patterns during viewing of naturalistic social situations as predictors of social competence in individuals with autism. *Archives of General Psychiatry, 59,* 809–816.

Klin, A., Volkmar, F.R., Sparrow, S.S., Cichetti, D.V., & Rourke, B.P. (1995). Validity and neuropsychological characterization of Asperger syndrome: Convergence with nonverbal learning disabilities syndrome. *Journal of Child Psychology and Psychiatry and Allied Disciplines, 36,* 1127–1140.

Kraemer, H.C. (1992a). How many raters? Toward the most reliable diagnostic consensus. *Statistics in Medicine, 11,* 317–331.

Kraemer, H.C. (1992b). Measurement of reliability for categorical data in medical research. *Statistical Methods in Medical Research, 1,* 183–199.

Lai, C.S., Gerrelli, D., Monaco, A.P., Fisher, S.E., & Copp, A.J. (2003). FOXP2 expression during brain development coincides with adult sites of pathology in a severe speech and language disorder. *Brain, 126,* 2455–2462.

Landgren, M., Pettersson, R., Kjellman, B., & Gillberg, C. (1996). ADHD, DAMP, and other neurodevelopmental/psychiatric disorders in 6-year-old children: Epidemiology and comorbidity. *Developmental Medicine and Child Neurology, 38,* 891–906.

Liegeois, F., Baldeweg, T., Connelly, A., Gadian, D.G., Mishkin, M., & Vargha-Khadem, F. (2003). Language fMRI abnormalities associated with FOXP2 gene mutation. *Natural Neuroscience, 6,* 1230–1237.

Macdermot, K.D., Bonora, E., Sykes, N., Coupe, A.M., Lai, C.S., Vernes, S.C., et al. (2005). Identification of FOXP2 truncation as a novel cause of developmental speech and language deficits. *American Journal of Human Genetics, 76,* 1074–1080.

Mehler, M.F., & Mattick, J.S. (2007). Noncoding RNAs and RNA editing in brain development, functional diversification, and neurological disease. *Physiological Reviews, 87*(3), 799–823.

Minshew, N.J., Luna, B., & Sweeney, J.A. (1999). Oculomotor evidence for neocortical systems but not cerebellar dysfunction in autism. *Neurology, 52,* 917–922.

Mostofsky, S.H., Goldberg, M.C., Landa, R.J., & Denckla, M.B. (2000). Evidence for a deficit in procedural learning in children and adolescents with autism: Implications for cerebellar

contribution. *Journal of the International Neuropsychological Society, 6,* 752–759.

Mundy, P., Sigman, M., & Kasari, C. (1993). The theory of mind and joint-attention deficits in autism. In S. Baron-Cohen, H. Tager-Flusberg, & D.J. Cohen (Eds.), *Understanding other minds: Perspectives from autism* (pp. 181–203). Oxford, United Kingdom: Oxford University Press.

Nance, M.A., & Berry, S.A. (1992). Cockayne syndrome: Review of 140 cases. *American Journal of Medical Genetics, 42,* 68–84.

Nass, R., & Gutman, R. (1997). Boys with Asperger's disorder, exceptional verbal intelligence, tics, and clumsiness. *Developmental Medicine and Child Neurology, 39,* 691–695.

Nass, R.D., & Trauner, D. (2004). Social and affective impairments are important to recovery after acquired stroke in childhood. *CNS Spectrums, 9,* 420–434.

Rapin, I. (1996). Practitioner review: Developmental language disorders: A clinical update. *Journal of Child Psychology and Psychiatry and Allied Disciplines, 37,* 643–655.

Rapin, I. (2002). Diagnostic dilemmas in developmental disabilities: Fuzzy margins at the edges of normality. An essay prompted by Thomas Sowell's new book: The Einstein syndrome. *Journal of Autism and Developmental Disorders, 32,* 49–57.

Rapin, I., & Allen, D.A. (1998). The semantic-pragmatic deficit disorder: Classification issues. *International Journal of Language and Communication Disorders, 33,* 82–87.

Rapin, I., & Dunn, M. (2003). Update on the language disorders of individuals on the autistic spectrum. *Brain & Development, 25,* 166–172.

Rourke, B.P. (1989). *Nonverbal learning disabilities: The syndrome and the model.* New York: Guilford Press.

Rourke, B.P. (Ed.). (1995). *Syndrome of nonverbal learning disabilities: Neurodevelopmental manifestations.* New York: Guilford Press.

Shaywitz, B.A., Fletcher, J.M., & Shaywitz, S.E. (1995). Defining and classifying learning disabilities and attention-deficit/hyperactivity disorder. *Journal of Child Neurology, 10,* S50–S57.

Shaywitz, S.E. (2003). *Overcoming dyslexia: A new and complete science-based program for overcoming reading problems at any level.* New York: Alfred A. Knopf.

Shprintzen, R.J., Higgins, A.M., Antshel, K., Fremont, W., Roizen, N., & Kates, W. (2005).

Velo-cardio-facial syndrome. *Current Opinions in Pediatrics, 17,* 725–730.

Sowell, T. (1997). *Late-talking children.* New York: Basic Books.

Sowell, T. (2001). *The Einstein syndrome: Bright children who talk late.* New York: Basic Books.

Stevenson, J., & Richman, N. (1976). The prevalence of language delay in a population of 3-year-old children and its association with general retardation. *Developmental Medicine and Child Neurology, 18,* 431–441.

Tager-Flusberg, H. (2003). Language impairments in children with complex neurodevelopmental disorders: The case of autism. In Y. Levy & J. Schaeffer (Eds.), *Language competence across populations: Toward a definition of specific language impairment* (pp. 297–321). Mahwah, NJ: Lawrence Erlbaum Associates.

Vargha-Khadem, F., Watkins, K.E., Price, C.J., Ashburner, J., Alcock, K.J., Connelly, A., et al. (1998). Neural basis of an inherited speech and language disorder. *Proceedings of the National Academy of Sciences of the United States of America, 95,* 12695–12700.

Weintraub, S., & Mesulam, M.M. (1983). Developmental learning disabilities of the right hemisphere. Emotional, interpersonal, and cognitive components. *Archives of Neurology, 40,* 463–468.

Wing, L. (1991). The relationship between Asperger's syndrome and Kanner's autism. In U. Frith (Ed.), *Autism and Asperger syndrome* (pp. 93–121). Cambridge, United Kingdom: Cambridge University Press.

Zoghbi, H.Y. (2003). Postnatal neurodevelopmental disorders: Meeting at the synapse? *Science, 302,* 826–830.

4

Developmental Regression, Autism, and Epilepsy

John F. Mantovani

Loss of neurological abilities may occur in children, as in adults, from acquired neurological insults or from genetic, metabolic, or neurodegenerative disorders. In children, however, both isolated language loss and global developmental regression occur in the absence of such disorders, specifically in children with autism spectrum disorders (ASDs) and in those with rare epileptic encephalopathies such as Landau-Kleffner syndrome (LKS) (Mantovani, 2000). Affected children vary in their preexisting developmental status, as well as in their ages and patterns of regression, which can either be limited to language (i.e., language regression [LR]) or can affect development more broadly with the loss of communication, social interaction, appropriate interests, and behavioral responses leading to ASDs (Shinnar et al., 2001).

Because the loss of single words or broader communication abilities does not occur in typically developing children or those with the common forms of developmental language disorder (DLD), regression serves as a useful clinical marker for ASDs and epileptic encephalopathies (Rapin, 1996). Not surprisingly, this clinical overlap has raised questions of a possible relationship between these conditions, including concerns that autistic regression (AR) might, in fact, result from an epileptic encephalopathy (Nass & Petrucha, 1990). This chapter reviews current information regarding the complex interrelationships among ASDs, epilepsy, and electroencephalographic findings, particularly as they pertain to AR in young children.

LANGUAGE/AUTISTIC REGRESSION

Developmental regression is a complex phenomenon that is well-described but poorly understood. Research has tended to divide affected children into two groups—those with isolated LR and those with AR. Loss of single words, which occurs in both groups, is the most commonly recognized form of regression. In reports of children referred to neurologists for developmental evaluation, a minority (15%–30%) are noted to have isolated loss of verbal language, some of whom have the uncommon pattern of developmental verbal auditory agnosia (Rapin, 1996; Wilson, Djukic, Dharmani, & Rapin, 2003). Studies have also described several distinctions between those with isolated LR and those with AR, including more prevalent epilepsy in older children with isolated LR and more frequent global AR in those with onset under 24 months of age (Shinnar et al., 2001; Wilson et al., 2003). Isolated language loss in children older than 3 years also occurs in the LKS, which is discussed in the next section. Certain triggering events (i.e., illness, physical or emotional trauma, seizures) may contribute to the occurrence of language regression in some children with LR, and it has been suggested that the regression in these situations may be more rapid (Wilson et al., 2003). Although language regression is usually monophasic, affected children rarely recover fully, and they typically suffer serious long-term impairments and functional limitations.

The majority of children with reported language regression also regress in social and behavioral areas. Following regression, these individuals meet the diagnostic criteria for ASDs and are indistinguishable from those with nonregressive forms of ASD (Rogers, 2004). Although ASDs may present with atypical social and communication development beginning in infancy, or with initially appropriate development followed by a plateau and failure to progress normally, the most striking pattern is typical or nearly typical development followed by a relatively abrupt regression of language and broader interactive skills between 12 and 24 months of age (Rogers & DiLalla, 1990). Initially described in 1985, this pattern has been confirmed in many additional studies (Kurita, 1985). AR is found in one third to one half of children with ASDs (Maestro et al., 2005; Rogers, 2004). Studies using blinded reviews of birthday and home videotapes and follow-up telephone interviews have validated the prevalence of AR, as well as the reliability and consistency of caretakers' reports in this regard (Luyster et al., 2005; Werner, Dawson, & Munson, 2005). Recent studies using adaptations of the Autism Diagnosis Interview–Revised (ADI-R; Lord, Shulman, & DiLavore, 2004) have also confirmed that nonlanguage and global regression occur more commonly than isolated language loss. In addition, they have identified the presence of atypical development preceding regression in a significant number of children with AR (Goldberg et al., 2003).

Children with AR usually experience the regression between 18 and 24 months, although it also occurs in younger and older children. Despite two decades of study, the pathophysiology of AR is unknown and has engendered considerable research, including evaluation of a possible relationship to epilepsy (Ballaban-Gil & Tuchman, 2000).

SEIZURES, ELECTROENCEPHALOGRAPHS, AND EPILEPTIC ENCEPHALOPATHY

Seizures occur in 3%–5% of children, but they are much more frequent in children with neurodevelopmental disabilities in whom the prevalence is 30%–50% (Arzimanoglou, Guerrini, & Aicardi, 2004). A seizure has two components—a pathophysiological mechanism, in which cerebral neurons produce abnormal synchronous depolarizing discharges, and a resultant clinical event, including altered consciousness, perception, motor activity, or sensory function. Seizures result from genetic, structural, metabolic, and toxic conditions that affect brain formation or function. The condition of recurrent, unprovoked seizures (excluding febrile seizures and those due to acute trauma, infection, or metabolic disturbance) is termed *epilepsy*. The electroencephalogram (EEG) is a diagnostic instrument that permits the recording of spontaneous brain electrical activity from electrodes that are usually placed on the scalp. Specific EEG patterns (i.e., spikes, sharp waves, spike waves) are known to predispose to and be associated with epilepsy. These EEG abnormalities are therefore termed *epileptiform*. Seizures are classified as *generalized* or *partial* based on their site of origin and the location and extent of abnormal brain activity using clinical and EEG criteria.

During seizures, excessively synchronized neuronal activity produces sustained epileptiform activity on the EEG and coincident clinical symptomatology, which typically lasts for several minutes and is followed by a more prolonged postictal recovery phase. Identical epileptiform discharges lasting fractions of seconds also occur as interictal epileptiform discharges (IEDs) and by definition are clinically silent. Although IEDs occur frequently in children with neurodevelopmental impairments, they are also found in 2%–3% of typically developing school children and up to 30% of healthy adult volunteers in overnight recordings (Beun, Van Emde Boas, & Dekker, 1998). Epileptiform EEGs show spikes or spike wave discharges that are highly associated with but not specific for clinical epilepsy.

The relationship of epilepsies and developmental impairments is also complex, but the concept that developmental regression may result from the pathophysiological disturbance associated with certain types of epilepsy is well-accepted. Such conditions, termed epileptic encephalopathies, are individually rare disorders in which developmental regression is associated with dramatic epileptiform patterns on EEGs and often with clinical epilepsy (Dulac, 2001). Electrical status epilepticus in slow-wave sleep (ESES)—also termed *continuous spike waves* during slow-wave sleep (CSWS) partial epilepsy due to structural lesions or tumors, infantile spasms, and other infantile myoclonic epilepsies including Lennox-Gastaut syndrome—are well-described epileptic encephalopathies.

ESES is particularly relevant in this context and is an age-specific clinical syndrome diagnosed on the basis of characteristic EEG patterns occurring during the slow-wave portions of sleep (Tassinari et al., 2000). Initially described in 1971, ESES is now defined by the presence on EEG of continuous spike wave discharge in more than 85% of recorded non-REM sleep. This pattern is highly associated with marked cognitive and behavioral regression. It occurs in children with a variety of known central nervous system (CNS) disorders as well as in previously typically developing children. ESES is the characteristic EEG finding in cases of LKS.

LKS is a rare but well-known epileptic encephalopathy in which previously typically developing children, usually between the ages of 3 and 8 years, experience relatively isolated speech and language regression (i.e., verbal auditory agnosia, expressive

aphasia/oral-motor dyspraxia) and exhibit variable behavioral abnormalities coincident with severely epileptiform EEGs and/or clinical seizures (Robinson, R.O., Baird, Robinson, G., & Simonoff, 2001). In LKS, the characteristic epileptiform EEG activity overlies the eloquent, perisylvian centrotemporal cortex, and in many cases, is markedly activated during slow-wave sleep, thereby conforming to the designation of ESES.

Based on long-standing observations and clinical experience, it seems highly probable that continuous epileptiform discharges and/or ESES are pathophysiologically important in the developmental disruption that occurs in epileptic encephalopathies. Experimental studies on the mechanisms by which epileptiform discharge disrupts function are limited, but they suggest that activation of inhibitory neuronal networks in the region of spike wave discharge and connections through thalamocortical projections may disrupt the neural mechanisms required to initiate and sustain neurodevelopmental functions (Tharp, 2004).

EPILEPSY AND AUTISM SPECTRUM DISORDERS

There is a clear relationship between epilepsy and ASDs. In fact, the frequency of seizures in those with ASDs was important in the initial suggestion that ASDs might result from brain dysfunction rather than maladaptive parenting. Seizures occur in 20%–30% of individuals with ASDs, with the highest prevalence in individuals with the most cognitive and motor impairments. Seizures typically begin before the age of 5 years or after puberty, and then increase in prevalence with age (Tuchman & Rapin, 2002). In addition, individuals with ASDs who do not have clinical seizures have a high frequency of epileptiform EEGs (15%–60%), the prevalence of which is directly related to the patient age and intelligence quotient (IQ) score, as well as the number, recording characteristics, and duration of the EEGs (Trevathan, 2004).

All seizure types occur in ASDs, including complex-partial and secondarily generalized, atypical absence, myoclonic, and generalized tonic-clonic. Similarly, various patterns of EEG abnormalities, including focal and multifocal epileptiform activity with predominant central-temporal or frontal focality, have also been described (Levisohn, 2004). Importantly, ESES has not been reported with any significant frequency in the population with ASDs.

The evaluation and treatment of epilepsy in those with ASDs is similar to that in others with the condition, although the clinical challenge of distinguishing behavioral staring and/or repetitive mannerisms from seizures increases the complexity of clinical diagnosis. In addition, the practical difficulty of obtaining good quality EEGs often requires the use of prolonged studies with overnight video-EEG telemetry. Most individuals with isolated ASDs and epilepsy achieve seizure control with the usual antiepileptic drugs (AEDs), although medications without prominent cognitive slowing or sedating side effects are preferable. Even then, behavioral reactions and other negative effects are not unusual.

In any event, the critical issue concerning the relationship of ASDs to epilepsy is related less to the diagnosis and management of seizures than to the possibility that epileptiform abnormalities might be instrumental in the disruption of neuropsychological processes related to autistic regression (i.e., the possibility that AR may result from an epileptic encephalopathy).

LANGUAGE/AUTISTIC REGRESSION AND EPILEPTIC ENCEPHALOPATHY

The unknown pathogenesis of regression in children with AR and the increased frequency of epilepsy and epileptiform EEGs in ASDs, as well as some similarities between AR and LKS, have raised concerns that

regression in ASDs may relate to an epileptic encephalopathy. The possible relationship of AR to LKS or LKS-variants has been a confusing area of neurology and developmental medicine (Mantovani, 2000; Trevathan, 2004). Fortunately, a recent series of studies has begun to clarify some of the issues pertaining to language regression, seizures, and epileptiform EEGs. The key points of analysis relate to the type and age of regression, as well as to the cooccurrence of epilepsy or epileptiform EEGs during sleep.

Initially, Rapin and her group (Wilson et al., 2003) reviewed their experience between 1988 and 1996 in the evaluation of 196 children with a history of language regression. Their results showed that nearly one quarter of the children had experienced isolated language regression, whereas approximately three quarters developed ASDs and met criteria for AR. The prevalence of clinical seizures in this population was 15%, and the overall developmental prognosis was found to be poor. An important observation was the tendency for the children with older onset of regression (> 24 months) to have isolated LR more often than AR.

These preliminary results, although published later, led to a collaborative prospective study in four major medical centers between 1996 and 1998 (Shinnar et al., 2001). In this study, 177 children were evaluated for loss of verbal language minimally defined as three single words. The mean age of the children with language regression was 23 months, and 88% of the children were diagnosed with either definite or suspected ASDs. Analysis of the data showed that more than 90% of the children younger than 36 months of age who had regressed were in the ASD group. Full AR was also more common in those without clinical seizures. In the older group (i.e., regression after 36 months), only 58% were diagnosed with ASDs, whereas 42% had isolated LR and also a significantly higher prevalence of seizures.

A third study from this group focused on EEG results in a subgroup of 149 of the children reported in the two previous studies by reviewing the medical records and EEG findings (McVicar et al., 2005). All had experienced language regression and had been evaluated between 1992 and 2004 with overnight EEGs. Epileptiform abnormalities were found in 37% and seizures in 15% of the total group, but segregation by isolated LR and AR was informative. In this study, 46 children (31%) had isolated language regression, 56% of whom had epileptiform EEGs and 33% had seizures. In comparison, 28% of the 103 children with AR had epileptiform EEGs and only 8% had seizures. These differences in EEG results and prevalence of epilepsy were highly significant on statistical analysis, indicating that the age of regression is an important variable with respect to the cooccurrence of epilepsy and epileptiform EEG patterns.

Recent noteworthy studies from Europe and the United States provide further data on this topic. Canitano, Luchetti, and Zappella (2005) reported on 46 children with ASDs and intellectual disability (ID) who had daytime sleep EEGs. They noted epileptiform EEGs in 35% of their group of whom one third had epilepsy. Of the 24 children (52%) who had AR, 9 had epileptiform EEGs, which was not statistically different from the EEG results in the children without a history of AR. The authors concluded that there was no difference in the regression rate between patients with and without EEG abnormalities.

Baird, Robinson, Boyd, and Charman (2006) reviewed daytime sleep EEG results in 64 children with ASDs evaluated at their center. Thirty-nine (61%) of these children had experienced AR, almost all had the onset of regression before 25 months of age, and slightly more than half had evidence of preexisting developmental abnormalities before the regression. Twenty of the 64 children had epileptiform EEGs, 15 of whom had experienced regression and 5 of whom

had not. Of the 44 patients without epileptiform EEGs, 24 had regressed and 15 had not. Neither difference was statistically significant. The EEG abnormalities in this study were predominantly over the frontal and temporal regions, and none of the children had ESES. The authors' conclusions supported the view that epileptiform discharges occurring during sleep are not causally related to autism or AR.

Chez et al. (2006) reported a large retrospective study of EEG results in a series of nearly 900 children with ASDs who had overnight ambulatory EEGs between 1996 and 2005. They found sleep-activated epileptiform activity in 61%, with the most frequent abnormalities localized over the temporal regions—the right slightly more than the left. These authors confirmed the lack of correlation between EEG abnormalities and regression. This group also recommended treatment with divalproex for epileptiform EEG findings and reported EEG improvements following this therapy. This controversial position is not supported by most other authors or prior trials (Aldenkamp & Arends, 2004; Baird, Robinson, Boyd, & Charman, 2006; Mantovani, 2000; Ronen et al., 2000; Tharp, 2004). The authors also failed to provide any data regarding the developmental effects of such treatment to support their recommendations.

Most recently, Trevathan et al. (2006) reported their data on 121 children who had 24-hour video EEGs following referral for evaluation of possible ESES or sleep-activated epileptiform activity (SAEA) between 1995 and 2005. Sixty-six of these children were diagnosed with ASDs, 56 had language, autistic, or cognitive-behavioral regression, and 13 had global AR. In this study, 33 (i.e., 58%) of those with isolated LR had sleep-activated epileptiform activity and 11 (i.e., 33%) had ESES. Isolated language regression was strongly associated with ESES, and no child with AR presented with that pattern.

Overall, these studies supported the existence of two groups of children with developmental regression—younger children who are more likely to have AR but less likely to have seizures/epileptiform EEGs and older children who are more likely to have both isolated LR and clinical and EEG features related to epilepsy. Consequently, the much larger group of children with regression before the age of 3 years who manifest the broader AR profile appear very unlikely to have an epileptic encephalopathy. It is not clear what determines the differences in the prevalence of epileptiform features between the age groups, and whether it is the earlier age of onset or distinct pathophysiologies remains unknown.

There are additional observations from multiple studies that also argue against a causal relationship between AR and epileptic encephalopathy. These include the lack of clinical seizures or EEG abnormalities in the majority of children with AR (Baird et al., 2006; Canitano et al., 2005; ; Levisohn, 2004; McVicar et al., 2005; Trevathan, 2004), the lack of clinical distinction between children with ASDs who do and do not experience regression (Baird et al., 2006; Canitano et al., 2005; Chez et al., 2006; Shinnar et al., 2001), and the extremely low prevalence of EEG patterns characteristic of epileptic encephalopathies in those children with ASDs with abnormal EEGs (Baird et al., 2006; Canitano et al., 2005; Chez et al., 2006; Trevathan et al., 2006).

CONCLUSION

There is no current evidence to support a causal relationship between ASDs and EEG abnormalities or epilepsy. Data on the relationship between epilepsy and regression indicate that the vast majority of children with AR do not have an epileptic encephalopathy. Nonetheless, it is not possible to completely exclude the possibility that an epileptic encephalopathy may underlie the process in an individual child. It is therefore important to be sensitive to the possibility of occult seizures and ESES whenever regression occurs. Although all children with AR do not require an overnight EEG, children with isolated language regression after the age of 24 months and those who experience global regression after the age of 36 months are most likely to have seizures and epileptiform EEGs. This is the group that should be studied most aggressively with EEGs because they are more likely to benefit from antiepileptic medication if frequent epileptiform patterns are found.

In view of the increased prevalence of epilepsy in ASDs, clinicians are also well-advised to maintain a high index of suspicion for the role of seizures in transient alterations of behavior among children with ASDs and to use EEGs selectively in these situations. The most recent review of the evidence relating to screening EEGs for children with ASDs found insufficient evidence to recommend for or against this practice (Kagan-Kushnir, Roberts, & Snead, 2005). Additional research to establish evidence-based criteria for diagnostic testing and specific therapies is needed.

Because there is little evidence to support an epileptic process as the cause of AR, clinicians and researchers are faced with the need to continue the search for etiological explanations and the neurobiological basis of regressive ASDs. Additional studies to define the pathophysiology of regression remain a priority and have great potential to enlarge our understanding of the complex interrelationships between normal and pathological influences on children's development. There is still much to be done.

REFERENCES

Aldenkamp, A., & Arends, J. (2004). Effects of epileptiform EEG discharges on cognitive function: Is the concept of transient cognitive impairment still valid? *Epilepsy Behavior, 5,* S25–S34.

Arzimanoglou, A., Guerrini, R., & Aicardi, J. (2004). *Aicardi's epilepsy in children* (3rd ed.) Philadelphia: Lippincott, Williams, & Wilkins.

Baird, G., Robinson, R.O., Boyd, S., & Charman, T. (2006). Sleep electroencephalograms in young children with autism with and without regression. *Developmental Medicine and Child Neurology, 48,* 604–608.

Ballaban-Gil, K., & Tuchman, R. (2000). Epilepsy and epileptiform EEG: Association with autism and language disorders. *MRDD Research Reviews, 6,* 300–308.

Beun, A.M., Van Emde Boas, W., & Dekker, E. (1998). Sharp transients in the sleep EEG of healthy adults: A possible pitfall in the diagnostic assessment of seizure disorders. *Electroencephalography and Clinical Neurophysiology, 106,* 44–51.

Canitano, R., Luchetti, A., & Zappella, M. (2005). Epilepsy, electroencephalographic abnormalities, and regression in children with autism. *Journal of Child Neurology, 20,* 27–31.

Chez, M.G., Chang, M., Krasne, V., Coughlan, C., Kominsky, M., & Schwartz, A. (2006). Frequency of epileptiform EEG abnormalities in a sequential screening of autistic patients with no known clinical epilepsy from 1996–2005. *Epilepsy Behavior, 8,* 267–271.

Dulac, O. (2001). Epileptic encephalopathy. *Epilepsia, 42*(Suppl. 3), 23–26.

Goldberg, W.A., Osann, K., Filipek, P.A., Laulhere, T., Jarvis, K., Modahl, C., et al. (2003). Language and other regression: Assessment and timing. *Journal of Autism and Developmental Disorders, 33,* 607–616.

Kagan-Kushnir, T., Roberts, W., & Snead, C.O. (2005). Screening electro-encephalograms in autism spectrum disorders: Evidence-based guidelines. *Journal of Child Neurology, 20,* 197–206.

Kurita, H. (1985). Infantile autism with speech loss before the age of thirty months. *Journal of the American Academy of Child and Adolescent Psychiatry, 24,* 191–196.

Levisohn, P. (2004). Electroencephalography findings in autism: Similarities and differences from Landau-Kleffner syndrome. *Seminars in Pediatric Neurology, 11,* 218–224.

Lord, C., Shulman, C., & DiLavore, P. (2004). Regression and word loss in autistic spectrum disorders. *Journal of Child Psychology and Psychiatry, 45,* 936–955.

Luyster, R., Richler, J., Risi, S., Hsu, W.I., Dawson, G., Bernier, R., et al. (2005). Early regression in social communication in autism spectrum disorders: A CPEA study. *Developmental Neuropsychology, 27,* 311–336.

Maestro, S., Muratori, F., Cesari, A., Cavallero, M.C., Paziente, A., Pecini, C., et al. (2005). Course of autism signs in the first year of life. *Psychopathology, 38,* 26–31.

Mantovani, J.F. (2000). Autistic regression and Landau-Kleffner syndrome: Progress or confusion? *Developmental Medicine and Child Neurology, 42,* 349–353.

McVicar, K.A., Ballaban-Gil, K., Rapin, I., Moshe, S.L., & Shinnar, S. (2005). Epileptiform EEG abnormalities in children with language regression. *Neurology, 65,* 129–131.

Nass, R., & Petrucha, D. (1990). Acquired aphasia with convulsive disorder: A pervasive developmental disorder variant. *Journal of Child Neurology, 5,* 327–328.

Rapin, I. (1996). Developmental language disorders: A clinical update. *Journal of Child Psychology and Psychiatry, 37,* 643–655.

Robinson, R.O., Baird, G., Robinson, G., & Simonoff, E. (2001). Landau-Kleffner syndrome: Course and correlates with outcome. *Developmental Medicine and Child Neurology, 43,* 243–247.

Rogers, S.J. (2004). Developmental regression in autism spectrum disorders. *MRDD Research Reviews, 10,* 139–143.

Rogers, S.J., & DiLalla, D. (1990). Age of symptom onset in young children with pervasive developmental disorders. *Journal of the American Academy of Child and Adolescent Psychiatry, 29,* 863–872.

Ronen, G.M., Richards, J.E., Cunningham, C., Second, M., & Rosenbloom, D. (2000). Can sodium valproate improve learning in children with epileptiform bursts but without clinical seizures? *Developmental Medicine and Child Neurology, 42,* 751–755.

Shinnar, S., Rapin, I., Arnold, S., Tuchman, R.F., Shulman, K., Ballaban-Gil, M., et al. (2001). Language regression in childhood. *Pediatric Neurology, 24,* 185–191.

Tassinari, C.A., Rubboli, G., Volpi, L., Meletti, G., d'Orsi, M., Franca, A.R., et al. (2000). Encephalopathy with electrical status epilepticus during slow wave sleep or ESES syndrome including acquired aphasia. *Clinical Neurophysiology, 111*(Suppl. 2), S94–S102.

Tharp, B.R. (2004). Epileptic encephalopathies and their relationship to developmental disorders: Do spikes cause autism? *MRDD Research Reviews, 10*, 132–134.

Trevathan, E. (2004). Seizures and epilepsy among children with language regression and autism spectrum disorders. *Journal of Child Neurology, 19*(Suppl. 1), S49–S57.

Trevathan, E., Ekinci, O., Reed, N., Zempel, J., Thio, L.L., Wong, M., et al. (2006). Isolated language regression is strongly associated with electrographic status epilepticus in sleep (Abstract). *Annals of Neurology, 60,* S138.

Tuchman, R., & Rapin, I. (2002). Epilepsy in autism. *Lancet Neurology, 1*, 352–358.

Werner, E., Dawson, G., & Munson, J. (2005). Validation of the phenomenon of autistic regression using home videotapes. *Archives of General Psychiatry, 62*, 889–895.

Wilson, S., Djukic, A., Dharmani, C., & Rapin, I. (2003). Clinical characteristics of language regression in children. *Developmental Medicine and Child Neurology, 45*, 508–514.

5

A Neurodevelopmental Perspective on Developmental Language Disorders

Bruce K. Shapiro

Neurodevelopmental disabilities are a group of chronic brain disorders that have their onset in childhood and have a high likelihood of limiting adult function. They are functional descriptors not tied to etiology or mechanism. There are no biologic markers for neurodevelopmental disorders. With the exception of intellectual disability (ID), the severity of these disorders is not specified beyond having a high likelihood of limiting adult function. Consequently, neurodevelopmental disorders are behavioral phenotypes that represent the final common pathways of multiple etiologies and mechanisms. The categorization of neurodevelopmental disorders may be useful for determining etiology, developing interventions, planning management strategies or required supports, or providing a prognosis for the future.

Neurodevelopmental disabilities constitute a spectrum of brain dysfunction. They occur, multiply, and commonly exhibit comorbidities. Neurodevelopmental disabilities are all associated with deficits in adaptive behavior. They are lifelong disorders that evolve over time and show continuing impairments, even in the absence of obvious limitations. Despite the potential uses, the constructs of neurodevelopmental disabilities are limited by the discriminative abilities of the neurodevelopmental diagnoses.

Neurodevelopmental diagnoses are dimensional. Examples of dimensional diagnoses are anemia or hypertension. These diagnoses do not have sharp boundaries in biology but instead are defined by convention. Similarly, the border between typical development and neurodevelopmental disability is indistinct. Defining what constitutes impairment in the typically developing population is an issue of heated debate. Distinguishing impairment from lack of perfection is not simple.

The borders of the various neurodevelopmental disorders are debated as well. This is more complex than hypertension or anemia because the defining characteristics are not universally accepted. They change with maturation, and multiple dimensions are addressed simultaneously. It is understandable why novices complain, "It seems that every child has everything." Figure 5.1 demonstrates the overlaps that may result from dimensional diagnoses. Some clinicians deal with the overlaps by trying to include everything in one diagnosis and exclude functionally important diagnoses. Others develop endless lists of diagnoses that may be overwhelming to parents.

Typical presentations are distinctive. Hearing loss is a sensory impairment. ID is a general cognitive impairment. Autism spectrum disorders (ASDs) have deviant language, social deficits, and stereotypies. Receptive-expressive language disorders (RELDs) demonstrate discrepant development affecting a focused area. Blending occurs at the margins of these disorders, and the distinctiveness of the disorders dimin-

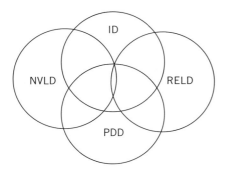

Figure 5.1. Dimensional diagnoses: Overlapping syndromes. (*Key:* ID = intellectual disability; NVLD = nonverbal learning disorder; PDD = pervasive developmental disability; RELD = receptive-expressive language disorder.)

ishes. Children with RELDs have been shown to have deficits in socialization (Bartak, Rutter, & Cox, 1975), nonverbal intelligence (Silva, 1987), and motor areas (Powell & Bishop, 1992). ID is associated with deficits in socialization and deviancies in language (Rondal, 1987). Hearing loss may be mistaken for any of the other disorders.

The validity of the specific neurodevelopmental diagnoses has been questioned (McArthur, Hogben, Edwards, Heath, & Mengler, 2000; Rispens & van Yperen, 1997). A number of questions must be answered to establish the validity of a diagnosis. Are the diagnoses unique? Are the diagnoses reliable? Do the diagnoses provide information about etiology or mechanism? Are overlaps the result of comorbidity or differing aspects of a single disorder? Are the defining characteristics unique or the consequence of a child's performance on a test? Does asynchronous development (i.e., dissociation) define a unique disorder? How do the defining characteristics change with maturation? For example, do ASDs manifest themselves the same way in a 2-year-old as in a 9-year-old? If an adult is literate, can he or she be diagnosed as having a specific reading disability?

Neurodevelopmental diagnosis is a useful, albeit imperfect, clinical approach to

chronic encephalopathy. Future studies that relate the biologic underpinnings and functional impairments will allow classification that is independent of functional abilities, behavioral phenotype, and maturation; improve understanding of the full extent of the disorders; and elevate intervention from empiricism. Pending future developments, studies that better quantify behavior and serve to develop a consensus that will lead to reliable diagnoses are crucial. In addition, studies that address outcome will illuminate the utility of the construct. This chapter brings together a group of studies that focus on the outcomes of developmental language disorders (DLDs) that present in preschool children and tries to place the diagnosis of DLD into a developmental context.

CLINICAL CONSIDERATIONS

The development of language is amazing. Infants advance from grunts and sputters to words in the first year of life. The second year of life marks an explosion in language abilities, with children showing a 50-fold increase in vocabulary size. By the age of 3 years, children have substantial communicative abilities.

At a fundamental level, language is not just the number of words a child possesses. Language is a symbol system that represents objects, actions, ideas, and emotions. It may be expressed in various ways, not all of which are spoken. Language conveys thought and offers a bridge to another mind.

The acquisition of language skills is not random. Even in the "prelinguistic" phase, language achievement is ordered and sequential. The ordered quality of language achievement allows the assignation of a functional age to a child's abilities. Functional age is the age that a typically developing child usually performs a task. The relationship between functional age and chronological age can be expressed as a developmental quotient.

Most DLDs in preschool children are recognized because these children evidence too few words for their chronological age. Not all children with too few words have language delays. Some children with severe speech impairments may have sound approximations that are not understandable as words. Although these children may have sufficient language, the inability to understand their utterances as words may result in their mistakenly being penalized on test measures and identified as having language delays. Children with selective mutism use normal language in some situations but not in others. Often, they are manifesting anxiety disorders, but approximately 20% have co-existing language disorders. Other forms of DLDs that affect pragmatics or figurative language also may be seen, but they present at an older age.

The sequential nature of language development underlies its ability to predict later development. Even mild delays in language development, not to the level of disorders, were associated with poorer outcomes. Klackenberg (1980) followed a cohort of 212 children who were recruited at birth and followed annually through age 20 years. Children who had language delays at age 3 years (speaking single words only or elementary sentences that seldom exceeded three words or speaking a few longer utterances interspersed with jargon) demonstrated significant differences in intellectual, scholastic, and social areas throughout the course of the study.

Despite the association of too few words with DLDs, there is no universally accepted quantitative definition of language delay. For example, for many research studies, delay is a rate of language acquisition of less than 85% (i.e., 1.0 standard deviation below the mean). For the Early Intervention Program for Infants and Toddlers (Part C of the Individuals with Disabilities Education Act [IDEA]), delay is a rate of language acquisition of less than 75%. Older studies focused

on rates of language acquisition of less than 70% (i.e., −2.0 standard deviations) to be consistent with the definition of ID. Each of these definitions may be justified on the basis of the size of the population served, the severity of the disorder, the objectives of the authors, availability of treatment services, and associated findings.

Language delays are the most frequent presentations of developmental dysfunction in preschool children. Language delay is the final pathway through which neurodevelopmental dysfunction is expressed. It is a symptom, not a diagnosis. Although delay brings children to attention, it is dissociation that allows for early diagnosis. *Dissociation* refers to asynchronous development. Table 5.1 lists the differential diagnosis of language delay and the associated dissociation patterns.

In addition to delay and dissociation, language disorders may violate developmental sequences. *Deviance* is the term used to describe nonsequential development. It is commonly expressed as an uncoupling of typical language milestone associations. One example is found in children who have a vocabulary of 100 words but do not use sentences. Another is seen in children who have many words but use them in stereotypic fashions. Yet another is noted when children's expressive language exceeds their receptive language. On further review, deviance is often associated with echolalia, programmed speech, word phrases (e.g., *hot dog*), or mistaking jargon for words.

RELD is a specific developmental disorder that affects language abilities. It is distinguished from the more global delays seen in ID or ASDs. The diagnosis requires that the language abilities are significantly discrepant from the child's other cognitive abilities. The difficulty with this diagnosis is that there is no "gold standard." Just as there is no universal agreement about the definition of delay, there is also no universal classification system for DLDs. The

Table 5.1.   The differential diagnosis of language delay and the associated dissociation patterns

Disorder	Gross motor	Fine motor/ problem solving	Expressive language	Receptive language	Personal	Social
Intellectual disability	Typical to mild impairment	Decreased	Decreased	Decreased	Decreased	Decreased
Selective mutism	Typical	Typical	Typical in some settings	Typical	Typical	Typical
Hearing impairment	Typical	Typical	Decreased	Decreased	Typical	Decreased
Expressive language disorder	Typical	Typical	Decreased	Typical	Typical	Typical
Receptive language disorder	Typical	Typical	Decreased	Decreased	Typical	Decreased
Autism spectrum disorders	Typical to mild impairment	Typical	Typical to decreased	Decreased	Decreased	Decreased

type of language disability, degree of discrepancy, comparison to cognitive abilities, and severity of functional impairments are some of the criteria used to define the diagnosis.

Some classifications focus on global language skills. Early studies separated speech from language abilities. Other classification schemas distinguish disorders that affect expressive language from those that affect understanding and expression.

Discrepancy models have been employed to group DLDs. These models compare language abilities to the child's nonverbal intelligence quotient (IQ) score. A series of arguments that have been employed against the use of discrepancy definitions in specific learning disabilities (SLDs) may be relevant to DLDs. The use of nonverbal IQ as a measure of potential in children with delayed language development has not been established. Nonverbal IQ, although relatively unaffected in groups of children with DLDs, may not be predictive for individual children, nor may it be independent of language abilities. It may be deflated in children with language disorders because the task may require language abilities to understand the instructions or mediate the solution to the task. Evaluation of

language abilities in preschool children requires a sampling of a wide range of behaviors, but most instruments are limited in scope. Discrepancies may be blunted by comorbid conditions, poor test performance because of anxiety, environmental exposure, or effective therapy. The use of a discrepancy model also allows for average function to be deemed "disordered" in the face of advanced function in other areas.

Still others classify based on components of language, syntax, semantics, and pragmatics. Most language tests used in preschool children do not address all the components of language. The formal evaluation of pragmatic skills in preschool children is still evolving.

Others attempted to classify based on more fundamental abilities. Classification based on perceptual characteristics such as auditory processing, speech discrimination, short-term verbal memory, and syntactic skills has been proposed. Table 5.2 lists some classification systems for RELDs.

At a fundamental level, the present classifications of DLDs are preliminary. No classification has been validated. Distinctive mechanisms of dysfunction (i.e., neuropsychology, genetic studies, or neuroimaging), responses to therapy, or prognoses must be

Table 5.2.   Classifications of receptive-expressive language disorders (RELDs)

Type	Subgroups	Definitions
Discrepancy		
American Psychiatric Association (2000)	Expressive language disorder	1. Scores on standardized tests substantially below those obtained from standardized measures of both nonverbal and receptive language development 2. Difficulties with expressive language are functionally impairing 3. Does not meet criteria for RELD or pervasive developmental disorder (PDD) 4. If coexistent intellectual disability (ID), speech-motor or sensory deficit, or environmental deprivation, the language difficulties are in excess of those usually associated with these problems
	Mixed RELD	1. Scores on standardized tests of receptive and expressive language development substantially below those obtained from standardized measures of nonverbal intellectual capacity 2. Difficulties with expressive and receptive language are functionally impairing 3. Does not meet criteria for PDD 4. If coexistent ID, speech-motor or sensory deficit, or environmental deprivation, the language difficulties are in excess of those usually associated with these problems
Kamhi (1998) Hall & Aram (1996)	Specific language impairment	1. Language delay in the presence of nonverbal cognitive abilities within one standard deviation of the mean (intelligence quotient > 85) 2. Excludes phonological disorders (variable degree of delay)
Language usage		
Rapin (1996b) Bishop & Rosenbloom (1987)	Mixed RELD	Verbal auditory agnosia: profoundly impaired comprehension deficit because of very deficient phonologic decoding with resultant severe expressive deficit Phonologic/syntactic disorder: comprehension equal to or better than production that is impoverished with short, often ungrammatical utterances, impaired phonology, and a limited vocabulary
	Expressive disorders	Verbal dyspraxia: extremely dysfluent subtype with sparse output and very poor phonology Speech programming deficit disorder: fluent subtype with jargon
	Higher-order processing deficits	Lexical deficit disorders: severe word finding deficits and comprehension difficulty for connected speech Semantic pragmatic deficit disorder: verbosity with comprehension deficits for connected speech; inadequate conversational skills

Processing deficits
(c.f., Haynes & Naidoo, 1991; Rapin & Allen, 1983)
		Processing deficits have been noted in the following domains:
		    Auditory processing
		    Speech discrimination
		    Short-term verbal memory
		    Syntactic skills
		    Language decoding

demonstrated before one classification can be endorsed over the others.

LANGUAGE DISORDERS

Delayed acquisition of language milestones is common, although this is more often seen in boys. Approximately 3%–5% of preschool children evidence delayed milestone acquisition (Stevenson, 1984).

The prevalence of DLDs varies by age. At 24 months 9%–17% of children evidence expressive language delay (i.e., less than 30 words, no word combinations at 24 months). In 3-year-olds, the prevalence of specific language delay not associated with general ID is 5.7/1,000 (Stevenson & Richman, 1976). Among kindergarten children, the prevalence of speech language impairment is 6%–8% (Tomblin et al., 1997). The prevalence of speech language disorders in school-age children decreases after 10 years.

Language disorders are fairly stable across time. In a study of 857 children who had language assessments at 3, 5, and 7 years of age, language disorder at any point in time was highly predictive of later language delay. Three-year-old function predicted functions at 5 and 7 years with 8.7%–79.2% of children exhibiting later delays. Between 17.6% and 52.9% of children identified as having language delays at age 5 also had language delays at age 7. Generalized language delays were more predictive than specific deficits in comprehension or expression. Almost 80% of 3-year-old children with generalized language delays maintained that classification at ages 5 and 7 (Silva, McGee, & Williams, 1983).

Generalized language disorders are associated with higher degrees of persistence than specific disorders of comprehension or expression (Silva et al., 1983). They also have substantially increased cognitive, behavioral, and academic comorbidity (Silva, 1987). Specific expressive language disorders that occur in early childhood are thought to have minimal developmental consequences, and some have questioned the need for therapeutic intervention (Whitehurst & Fischel, 1994). By contrast, expressive disorders that persist to later ages have substantial developmental consequences (Beitchman, Wilson, Brownlie, Walters, & Lancee, 1996a, 1996b).

OUTCOMES

The outcomes of interest for preschool language disorders are later functions in communicative, cognitive, academic, behavioral, social, and motor spheres.

Communicative Outcomes

Almost all children with preschool language disorders ultimately communicate effectively. Many resolve their language delays by age 5½ (Bishop & Edmundson, 1987). The best predictor of resolution was the ability to verbally relay a story that was constructed from pictures. Most children with language delay will acquire the language characteristics of adults by middle childhood (Stevenson, 1984). Persisting language impairments may be noted when children with language disorders are compared to controls on later testing (Hall & Tomblin, 1978; Rescorla, Roberts, & Dahlsgaard, 1997; Scarborough & Dobrich, 1990). However, the functional import of these comparative impairments remains to be established, and consistent patterns of language development that predict persistence of language disorders have not been identified.

Cognitive Outcomes

The relationship between language and cognition is complex. Does cognition grow out of language or is language a symbolic outgrowth of the way we think? Do language and cognition modify each other?

There is a close relationship between language function and cognition. Language is the best predictor of future intelligence, and delayed language development is a powerful risk factor for cognitive dysfunction. Of 3-year-old children with generalized language disorders, 75% had intellectual delays (Stanford Binet Intelligence Scales IQ < 76) at age 5 (Silva, 1980). Of the total group of 5-year-old children with intellectual delays, 84% had generalized language delay at age 3 (Silva, 1980).

Follow-up studies note that children with language disorders are three to six times more likely than controls to have impairments on nonverbal IQ measures; 21% to 37% of children with preschool language disorders had low Performance IQs on the Wechsler Intelligence Scale for Children–Revised (WISC-R) (Silva, 1987). Possible explanations for these findings include

1. Measurement of preschool nonverbal skills and school-age performance IQ assess different skills.

2. The WISC-R performance subscales (i.e., picture arrangement, picture completion, object assembly) may require language strategies for optimal performance.

3. Language and cognition subsume similar processes.

4. A cognitive plateau is seen in children with language disorders.

The long-term studies of cognitive function support a temporal relationship between preschool language disorders and later impairment on IQ tests. Aram, Ekelman, and Nation (1984) followed a group of children with preschool language disorders into adolescence and found that almost half of the children had verbal IQs of less than 80 and 20% had WISC-R Full Scale IQs in the deficient range. This study, as is true of most follow-up studies, suffers from a selected clinical population, incomplete follow-up, and a single outcome point. There are, however, several studies that support this finding (Felsenfeld, Broen, & McGue, 1994; Stern, Connell, Lee, & Greenwood, 1995;

Stothard, Snowling, Bishop, Chipchase, & Kaplan, 1998). Finally, the deceleration of cognitive trajectories has been noted in children with reading disabilities (Stanovich, 1988). Long-term longitudinal follow-up of a large nonpreferred population that had comprehensive evaluations as preschool children and periodic evaluations—including IQ and other cognitive factors that are thought not to be language-based—through adolescence is required to confirm the findings of deceleration of cognitive trajectories in children with preschool language disorders, as well as to determine the reasons for the observation.

Academic Outcomes

Preschool language disorders are powerful predictors of academic underachievement. In one follow-up study, two thirds of children recognized as having language disorders at age 5 years were in classes for students with learning disabilities or ID by age 9 (Wolpaw, Nation, & Aram, 1977). Another group that followed a cohort of children with preschool language disorders from age 5 to age 9 found that 75% had persistent oral language and naming difficulties, 60% were at the beginning stages of reading acquisition, and only 5% were reading at grade level (Strominger & Bashir, 1977). Others found a more positive outcome and reported that children with speech-language delays who resolved their disorder by age 5½ exhibited later reading abilities at age 8 that were not significantly depressed relative to controls (Bishop & Adams, 1990).

The discrepant findings may be the result of differing definitions, measures, or interventions. Alternatively the differences may result from differing populations that are defined by persistence of substantial language difficulties through the sixth year. Although it is usually thought that children who are diagnosed as language disordered at an earlier age have more guarded prognoses, it may be that early intervention strategies have resulted in identifying a large group of children who have transient developmental syndromes that resolve early and have a very different outcome from children who have persisting language disorders. For example, isolated expressive language delays are common between 18 and 27 months and usually resolve by the age of 3 years without significant developmental consequences (Paul, Murray, Clancy, & Andrews, 1997; Whitehurst & Fischel, 1994).

Bishop and Adams (1990) expressed optimism for children who showed early resolution of their language disorders, but the optimistic outcome noted at age 8 was not continued into adolescence. Further follow-up showed that the children in the early resolution group were not completely unscathed as they approached adulthood. Children whose language problems had resolved by age 5½ did not differ from age-matched controls on tests of vocabulary or language comprehension skills, but they did perform worse on tests of phonological processing and literacy skill. Children with persisting difficulties at age 5½ had significant impairments in all aspects of spoken and written language functioning and fell further behind their peer group in vocabulary growth over time (Stothard et al., 1998). In a companion article, Snowling studied 56 adolescents who had specific language impairment as preschoolers and did not evidence a general delay at age 4 years (Snowling, Bishop, & Stothard, 2000). It was found that 35% had reading skills in the normal range and that isolated impairments in expressive phonology were associated with particularly good outcome. It was also noted that the rate of specific reading delays increased between ages 8½ and 15 years, and difficulties with reading accuracy were seen in all children with specific language impairments independent of the age of resolution. The authors noted the interactive nature of reading development and posited that language difficulties outside of the phonological domain prevented top down compensations as the range of written vocabulary increased and the texts became more demanding linguistically.

The relationship between DLDs and academic underachievement does not imply that specific reading disability is a less severe form of specific language impairment. The onset of later reading difficulties in adolescents with specific language impairment supports the separateness of the disorders. In addition, one study assessed 110 children with a specific reading disability and 102 children with a specific language impairment and found that 53% of the children could be equally classified as having a specific reading disability or a specific language impairment; 51% of the children with specific language impairment had a reading disability; and 55% of the children with specific reading disabilities had impaired oral language (McArthur et al., 2000). Although there was a clear overlap in diagnoses, there were also separate syndromes in approximately half of the cases. The previously outlined longitudinal findings emphasize the need for continuing follow-up of children with preschool language disorders so that necessary interventions may be applied (Bashir & Scavuzzo, 1992).

Behavioral Outcomes

Behavioral disturbances often accompany DLDs. Preschool children with language disorders have increased rates of the full spectrum of behavioral disturbance. Hyperactivity, anxiety, and affective disorders are much more common in preschoolers with language disorders than in typically developing children. Most commonly, preschool children evidence adjustment reactions that result from their inability to comply with the demands of certain situations. This behavior is mistakenly called oppositional defiant disorder (ODD), but the key differentiation is that these children are unable to meet the expectations, as opposed to being unwilling to do so.

Language delay is a predictor of persistence of hyperactivity in preschool children (Palfrey, Levine, Walker, & Sullivan, 1985). Approximately two thirds of children with language disorders have psychiatric diagnoses, most commonly attention-deficit/hyperactivity disorder (Cantwell, Baker, & Mattison, 1981). Another study of 99 children found that 11% of 4-year-old children with DLDs had Child Behavior Checklist scores in the clinical range (total scores), versus 2% in controls (Benasich, Curtis, & Tallal, 1993). On follow-up at 8 years of age, psychopathology scores were in the clinical range for 32% of the children with DLDs. Neither the degree of early language impairment nor the amount of language improvement predicted 8-year behavioral or emotional status.

DLDs are common in children who are seen in mental health clinics. Cohen, Davine, Horodezky, Lipsett, and Isaacson (1993) studied 399 children consecutively referred to three mental health centers and found that 53% had DLDs. The behavior disturbance often masked the language disorder. Of the children with DLDs, almost half were undiagnosed.

Longitudinal studies tend to support the associations of DLDs and behavioral disturbance. Beitchman and colleagues (1996a) enrolled 169 subjects recruited from 1,665 kindergarten children and followed the cohort until age 19. The 7-year follow-up studied 124 children and occurred when they were 12.5 years old. The authors noted that children with pervasive language problems performed less well on linguistic, cognitive, and academic measures (Beitchman et al., 1996a). They also noted that children with receptive or pervasive language problems demonstrated greater behavioral disturbance than children without such impairment. This was true even after controlling for initial behavior status. Isolated articulation disorders improved with time (Beitchman et al., 1996b).

In a review of the nature of the relationship between language impairment and psychiatric disorder, Rutter and Lord (1987) noted five relationships that address the causality of behavior and language disorders. First, the psychiatric disorder caused the language problem. This was exemplified by elective mutism. Second, the language problem resulted in a psychiatric disorder, as was noted in adjustment disorders. Third, the association between the language and psychiatric disorders was not causal but rather both problems were possible aspects of another underlying problem, as in the case of autism. Fourth, the language delay and the psychiatric problem arose from different causal processes that stemmed from a broader risk situation. In these situations, the language delay and the psychiatric disorder do not reflect the same underlying problem because the risk mechanisms differ. An example may be poverty where the language delay may be familial, and thus the behavioral disturbance may result from poor role models. Fifth, there is evidence of multiple interconnected causal processes, as exemplified by ID. Children with ID frequently exhibit behavioral disturbances and have delays in their language development. This schema is useful for thinking about the relationships of language and the other outcomes.

Social Outcomes

The relationships between preschool language disorders and social outcomes are difficult to establish. In contrast to the other outcomes, there are no long-term longitudinal studies that address social outcomes of children with preschool language disorders. In addition, social outcomes lack a uniform definition. Depending on the setting, social outcomes may refer to adaptive behavior, play, employment, or maladaptive behavior (e.g., behavioral disorders, emotional disorders, criminality). Each of these constructs is large and can be subdivided.

Social outcomes are more likely than the other outcomes to be affected by the environment. Lack of opportunity imposed by segregated school settings that remove children from the mainstream may impede social development. Similarly, diminished language abilities may cause children with DLDs to be teased by other children in certain social situations.

Parental stress, negatively expressed emotion, peer rejection, or temperamental characteristics may lower self-esteem. The result may adversely influence attempts to establish social relationships.

Attempting to study social outcomes in children with DLDs may be impossible because of the overlap between pragmatics and socialization. Poor pragmatic abilities are associated with more difficulty establishing friendships and consequent difficulties establishing social competence. Finally, children who have disordered language and impaired social skills are likely to be grouped within the autism spectrum.

A cross-sectional study found that when compared with typically developing peers, late-talking toddlers (i.e., 21–31 months of age) rated higher in depression and withdrawal and lower in social relatedness, pretend play and imitation, and compliance on the Infant-Toddler Social and Emotional Assessment, as well as more depressed and withdrawn on the Child Behavior Checklist. Observation indicated that late talkers were more serious, more depressed and withdrawn, and less interested in play; they also scored lower on the socialization domain of the Vineland Adaptive Behavior Scales (Irwin, Carter, & Briggs-Gowan, 2002).

One longitudinal long-term study followed children whose language disorder was diagnosed at 7 years of age—therefore a bias toward more severe disorders—and a comparison group of children with autism into early adult life. The children with language impairments were less impaired in their social use of language than the children with autism, but they still showed a number of atypical features in this domain. Qualitative differences noted in the language group were a decreased amount of conversational speech, limited flexibility, problems in reporting past events, and general conversational skills. Early language abilities, IQ, or sociability were not related to adult language outcomes in the language group (Mawhood, Howland, & Rutter, 2000).

The groups also had social, behavioral, and psychiatric outcomes assessed (Howlin, Mawhood, & Rutter, 2000). The children with language impairments experienced problems in social relationships, jobs, and independence. Many still lived with their parents (65%), and few had close friends (26.3%) or permanent jobs (35%). On a composite measure, based on linguistic and social competence and the presence or absence of autistic behaviors, 10% of the children in the language group were assessed as having severe social difficulties, 65% had moderate social problems, and 25% were rated as being typical or near typical. Regression analysis showed little relationship between measures of childhood function and adult outcome in the group of children with language impairments.

Motor Outcomes

First impressions would question the rationale for looking at motor disorders in children with DLDs. If the disorder is thought to be specific and related to language, a child's motor development should be typical. However, as previously noted, brain dysfunction in childhood has diffuse manifestations. Speech difficulties may be the oral manifestation of a more generalized motor coordination disorder. Although the mechanism for the motor dysfunction is unknown, there is a close association between DLDs and motor dysfunction.

In a longitudinal study of children with developmental speech and language disorders, poor gross motor coordination was noted in almost half (46%) and poor or delayed fine motor abilities were noted in almost two thirds (61%) (Paul, Cohen, & Caparulo, 1983). In a study of students with language impairments at the Dawn House School, 36% had deficits in gross motor performance, 17% in fine motor, and 20% in oral-motor, whereas 21% demonstrated constructional difficulties (Mellor, 1991). Hypotonia and limb apraxia were the most common neurologic findings in a study of preschoolers with language impairment (Rapin, 1996a).

Another study compared 4- to 7-year-old children with DLDs to those with typical development on a series of motor activities (Owen & McKinlay, 1997). The children with developmental speech and language disorders were significantly slower than controls on three of four motor tasks. The differences in time performance on peg boards, bead threading, and button tests diminished as the children aged.

The motor difficulties were functionally significant. In a study of 96 2½-year-old children, those with language impairment had significantly more difficulty copying four figures (i.e., vertical line, horizontal line, circle, and cross) than typically developing children (Moore & Law, 1990). This difficulty was related to impaired language expression and comprehension. Copying was also poorer for the index subjects than their performance on two other nonverbal tests. Longitudinal studies are lacking that would link the motor difficulties to poor handwriting or problems with complex motor tasks such as skipping or shoe tying.

SPECULATION

Preschool language disorders change. Some delays improve, only to reemerge when the demands of a situation approximate mature function. Some evolve into other neurodevelopmental diagnoses. Is it justifiable to subdivide preschool developmental dysfunction into diagnoses? If preschool language disorders are the prediagnostic manifesta-

tions of developmental dysfunction, would it be reasonable to defer diagnosis until the syndrome was clarified? ID is a diagnosis that often is deferred until at least age 3 years. This deferral does not preclude the application of therapeutic services but permits the clinician to be more secure in his or her diagnosis and prognosis.

At a more fundamental level lies the question of whether preschool language disorders form a valid construct. Substantial evidence supports the view that preschool language disorders are heterogeneous. They are not unique in their phenotype. The defining characteristics are not generally accepted. They overlap with other disorders. The associated problems with academics, cognition, movement, and socialization are variable and cannot be attributed to a single mechanism. The long-term outcomes vary widely. Confronting this evidence would lead some to conclude that preschool language disorders are heterogeneous, whereas others would question whether they form a valid construct.

The final area for further discussion is therapy. Given that almost all children with preschool language disorders speak, a number of questions are appropriate. Are the therapies currently being used more effective than maturation alone? Can groups for whom therapy is irrelevant because of the poor outcome and groups for whom therapy is unnecessary because of the good outcome be distinguished from groups that benefit from therapy? Can early intervention influence the expression of the later deficits in cognition, academics, and socialization?

CONCLUSION

Language delay is the most common presenting symptom for developmental disorders in preschool children. The underlying diagnosis is a major determinant of the outcomes of language delay (i.e., ID, ASDs, RELDs—expressive or mixed). Other factors that relate to outcomes are severity, age of diagnosis, age of resolution, type of delay (i.e., expressive versus generalized), nonverbal intelligence, family history, and associated dysfunctions.

The developmental disorders are points on a continuum of language dysfunction. There is substantial overlap among syndromes. All diagnoses exhibit aspects of other diagnoses. There are no pure syndromes.

Many practitioners mistakenly view preschool language disorders as benign because of their favorable communicative outcomes. However, preschool language disorders are important markers for later developmental dysfunction. Cognitive, behavioral, and academic associations have been well established. Deficits in nonlanguage areas are common. Many children with preschool language disorders experience academic difficulties as they age. As such, preschool language disorders may be viewed as way stations on the highway of developmental dysfunction.

▉ REFERENCES

American Psychiatric Association. (2000). *Diagnostic and statistical manual of mental disorders* (4th ed., text rev.). Washington, DC: Author.

Aram, D.M., Ekelman, B.L., & Nation, J.E. (1984). Preschoolers with language disorders: 10 years later. *Journal of Speech and Hearing Disorders, 27,* 232–244.

Bartak, L., Rutter, M., & Cox, A. (1975). A comparative study of infantile autism and specific developmental receptive language disorder: I. The children. *British Journal of Psychiatry, 126,* 127–145.

Bashir, A.S., & Scavuzzo, A. (1992). Children with language disorders: Natural history and academic success. *Journal of Learning Disabilities, 25,* 53–65.

Beitchman, J.H., Wilson, B., Brownlie, E.B., Walters, H., & Lancee, W. (1996a). Long-term consistency in speech/language profiles: I. Developmental and academic outcomes. *Journal of the American Academy of Child and Adolescent Psychiatry, 35,* 804–814.

Beitchman, J.H., Wilson, B., Brownlie, E.B., Walters, H., & Lancee, W. (1996b). Long-term consistency in speech/language profiles: II. Behavioral, emotional, and social outcomes. *Journal of the American Academy of Child and Adolescent Psychiatry, 35,* 815–825.

Benasich, A.A., Curtis, S., & Tallal, P. (1993). Language, learning, and behavioral disturbances in childhood: A longitudinal perspective. *Journal of the American Academy of Child and Adolescent Psychiatry, 32,* 585–594.

Bishop, D.V.M., & Adams, C. (1990). A prospective study of the relationship between specific language impairment, phonological disorders and reading retardation. *Journal of Child Psychology and Psychiatry, 31,* 1027–1050.

Bishop, D.V.M., & Edmundson, A. (1987). Language-impaired 4-year-olds: Distinguishing transient from persistent impairment. *Journal of Speech and Hearing Disorders, 52,* 156–173.

Bishop, D., & Rosenbloom, L. (1987). Childhood language disorders: Classification and overview. *Clinics in Developmental Medicine* (Serial No. 101/102).

Cantwell, D.P., Baker, L., & Mattison, R. (1981). Prevalence, type, and correlates of psychiatric diagnoses in 200 children with communication disorders. *Journal of Developmental and Behavioral Pediatrics, 2,* 131–136.

Cohen, N.J., Davine, M., Horodezky, N., Lipsett, L., & Isaacson, L. (1993). Unsuspected language impairments in psychiatrically disturbed children: Prevalence and language and behavioral characteristics. *Journal of the American Academy of Child and Adolescent Psychiatry, 32,* 595–603.

Felsenfeld, S., Broen, P.A., & McGue, M. (1994). A 28-year follow-up of adults with a history of moderate phonological disorder: Educational and occupational results. *Journal of Speech and Hearing Research, 37,* 1341–1353.

Hall, N., & Aram, D.M. (1996). Classification of developmental language disorders (DLDs). In I. Rapin (Ed.), *Preschool Children with Inadequate Communication* (pp. 10–20). London: Mac Keith Press.

Hall, P.K., & Tomblin, J.B. (1978). A follow-up study of children with articulation and language disorders. *Journal of Speech and Hearing Disorders, 43,* 227–241.

Haynes, C., & Naidoo, S. (1991). Children with specific speech and language impairment. *Clinics in Developmental Medicine* (Serial No. 119).

Howlin, P., Mawhood, L., & Rutter, M. (2000). Autism and developmental receptive language disorder—comparative follow-up in early adult life: II. Social, behavioural, and psychiatric outcomes. *Journal of Child Psychology and Psychiatry, 41,* 561–578.

Irwin, J.R., Carter, A.S., & Briggs-Gowan, M.J. (2002). The social-emotional development of "late-talking" toddlers. *Journal of the American Academy of Child and Adolescent Psychiatry, 41*(11), 1324–1332.

Kamhi, A.G. (1998). Trying to make sense of developmental language disorders. *Language, Speech and Hearing Services in Schools, 29,* 35–44.

Klackenberg, G. (1980). What happens to children with retarded speech at age 3? *Acta Paediatrica Scandinavica, 69,* 681–685.

Mawhood, L., Howlin, P., & Rutter, M. (2000). Autism and developmental receptive language disorder—comparative follow-up in early adult life. 1. Cognitive and language outcomes. *Journal of Child Psychology and Psychiatry, 41,* 547–559.

McArthur, G.M., Hogben, J.H., Edwards, V.T., Heath, S.M., & Mengler, E.D. (2000). On the "Specifics" of specific reading disability and specific speech language impairment. *Journal of Child Psychology and Psychiatry, 41,* 869–874.

Mellor, D.H. (1991). Neurologic correlates of language impairment. *Clinics in Developmental Medicine* (Serial No. 119).

Moore, V., & Law, J. (1990). Copying ability of preschool children with delayed language development. *Developmental Medicine and Child Neurology 32,* 249–257.

Owen, S.E., & McKinlay, I.A. (1997). Motor difficulties in children with developmental disorders of speech and language. *Child Care Health and Development, 23*(4), 315–325.

Palfrey, J.S., Levine, M.D., Walker, D.K., & Sullivan, M. (1985). The emergence of attention deficits in early childhood: A prospective study. *Journal of Developmental and Behavioral Pediatrics, 6,* 339–348.

Paul, R., Cohen, D.J., & Caparulo, B.K. (1983). A longitudinal study of patients with severe developmental disorders of language learning. *Journal of the American Academy of Child and Adolescent Psychiatry, 22,* 525–534.

Paul, R., Murray, C., Clancy, K., & Andrews, D. (1997). Reading and metaphonological outcomes in late talkers. *Journal of Speech, Language, and Hearing Research, 40,* 1037–1047.

Powell, R.P., & Bishop, D.V.M. (1992). Clumsiness and perceptual problems in children with specific language impairment. *Developmental Medicine and Child Neurology, 34,* 755–765.

Rapin, I. (1996a). Neurological examination. In I. Rapin (Ed.), *Preschool children with inadequate communication* (pp. 98–122). London: Mac Keith Press.

Rapin, I. (1996b). Practitioner review: Developmental language disorders: A clinical update. *Journal of Child Psychology and Psychiatry, 37,* 643–655.

Rapin, I., & Allen D. (1983). Developmental language disorders: Nosologic considerations. In U. Kirk (Ed.), *Neuropsychology of language, reading, and spelling* (pp. 155–184). San Diego: Academic Press.

Rescorla, L., Roberts, J., & Dahlsgaard, K. (1997). Late talkers at 2: Outcome at age 3. *Journal of Speech, Language, and Hearing Research, 40,* 556–566.

Rispens, J., & van Yperen, T.A. (1997). How specific are "Specific Developmental Disorders"? The relevance of the concept of specific developmental disorders for the classification of childhood developmental disorders. *Journal of Child Psychology and Psychiatry, 38*(3), 351–363.

Rondal, J. (1987). Language development and mental retardation. In W. Yule & M. Rutter (Eds.), *Language development and disorders* (pp. 248–261). Philadelphia: Lippincott Williams & Wilkins.

Rutter, M., & Lord, C. (1987). Language disorders associated with psychiatric disturbance. *Clinics in Developmental Medicine* (Serial No. 101/102).

Scarborough, H.S., & Dobrich, W. (1990). Development of children with early language delay. *Journal of Speech and Hearing Research, 33,* 70–83.

Silva, P. (1980). The prevalence, stability, and significance of developmental language delay in preschool children. *Developmental Medicine and Child Neurology, 22,* 768–777.

Silva, P. (1987). Epidemiology, longitudinal course, and some associated factors: An update. *Clinics in Developmental Medicine* (Serial No. 101/102).

Silva, P., McGee, R., & Williams, S.M. (1983). Developmental language delay from three to seven years and its significance for low intelligence and reading difficulties at age seven.

Developmental Medicine and Child Neurology, 25, 783–793.

Snowling, M., Bishop, D.V.M., & Stothard, S.E. (2000). Is preschool language impairment a risk factor for dyslexia in adolescence? *Journal of Child Psychology and Psychiatry, 41*(5), 587–600.

Stanovich, K.E. (1988). Explaining the differences between the dyslexic and the garden-variety poor reader: The phonological-core variable-difference model. *Journal of Learning Disabilities, 21,* 590–604.

Stern, L.M., Connell, T.M., Lee, M., & Greenwood, G. (1995). The Adelaide preschool language unit: Results of follow-up. *Journal of Pediatrics and Child Health, 31,* 207–212.

Stevenson, J. (1984). Predictive value of speech and language screening. *Developmental Medicine and Child Neurology, 26,* 528–538.

Stevenson, J., & Richman, N. (1976). The prevalence of language delay in population of three year old children and its association with general retardation. *Developmental Medicine and Child Neurology, 18,* 431–441.

Stothard, S.E., Snowling, M.J., Bishop, D.V.M., Chipchase, B.B., & Kaplan, C.A. (1998). Language-Impaired preschoolers: A follow-up into adolescence. *Journal of Speech, Language, and Hearing Research, 41,* 407–418.

Strominger, A.Z., & Bashir, A.S. (1977, November). *A nine year follow-up of language disordered children.* Paper presented at the meeting of the American Speech-Language-Hearing Association, Chicago.

Tomblin, J.B., Records, N.L., Buckwalter, P., Zhang, X., Smith, E., & O'Brien, M. (1997). Prevalence of specific language impairment in kindergarten children. *Journal of Speech, Hearing, and Language, 40,* 1245–1260.

Whitehurst, G.J., & Fischel, J.E. (1994). Practitioner review: Early developmental language delay: What, if anything, should the clinician do about it? *Journal of Child Psychology and Psychiatry, 35*(4), 613–648.

Wolpaw, T., Nation, J.E., & Aram, D.M. (1977). Developmental language disorders: A follow-up study. *Illinois Speech and Hearing Journal, 12,* 14–18.

6

Discourse Skills of Individuals with Higher-Functioning Autism or Asperger Syndrome

Janet E. Turner

Children diagnosed with autism spectrum disorders (ASDs), including the original diagnostic group (Kanner, 1943), possess affective, cognitive, and communicative skills that have a marked impact on their lives. Modest improvements have been reported over the life course of individuals with ASDs, but functional deficits remain, leading to the characterization of ASDs as lifelong disorders (Seltzer, Shattuck, Abbeduto, & Greenberg, 2004; Sigman, 1994). Social and language deficits, which are at the heart of ASDs, include the inability to understand, respond to, and share other's feelings (Howlin, 2004; Rogers, 2000). Social and communicative skills are directly related to clinical outcomes for individuals with ASDs (Volden, Magill-Evans, Goulden, & Clarke, 2006). Review of discourse-level language skills in more cognitively capable individuals with ASDs provides a more sensitive index of their abilities than the administration of standardized tests (Volkmar, Lord, Bailey, Schultz, & Klin, 2004).

This chapter focuses on social and communication skills of children with high-functioning autism (HFA) or Asperger syndrome (AS). These areas are particularly problematic, even when children meet early linguistic milestones (Volkmar et al., 1996). Children and adolescents with HFA or AS may actually experience greater social penalties than individuals with more severe cognitive and linguistic deficits because they appear to be capable and yet they struggle to use language effectively (Volden, 2004). The chapter offers reviews of recent research in children's use of nonliteral language and conversational discourse and concludes with comments about assessment and treatment practices.

AUTISM SPECTRUM DIAGNOSES

Consistent and accurate application of diagnostic labels is beneficial for clinical and research purposes, as it allows comparisons over time, across patient populations, and between biological and behavioral data. Fitting clinical evidence into meaningful diagnostic categories can be challenging. Factors complicating the use of diagnostic terms include the trend toward earlier diagnosis, a broad range of severity, the presence of coexisting conditions, the developmental trajectory of disorders over time, sensitivity of evaluation instruments, heterogeneity of the disorder, and individual variability (Volkmar et al., 2004).

The author acknowledges the assistance of Wendy Jennejahn, M.S., CCC-SLP, Manager, Speech-Language Outpatient Program, Kennedy Krieger Institute.

With the fairly recent broadening of the criteria for diagnosing ASDs to include individuals with milder cognitive and language disorders, new criteria were needed for differentiating subtype profiles. Age of onset of word and phrase speech serves as such a criterion.

Although it is useful for differentiating some pervasive developmental disorders (PDDs), inclusion of these criteria in AS diagnosis may allow for more overlap between HFA and AS (Klin, Pauls, Schultz, & Volkmar, 2005). It is interesting to note that, although the term *HFA* appears frequently in literature, it is not an official diagnosis. HFA is actually a hybrid between a formal clinical diagnosis (i.e., autism) and descriptive terminology (i.e., high functioning, in which IQ scores fall in the ≥ 70 range). Many of the studies summarized in this chapter combine these two diagnostic labels because differences between individuals who are given each of these labels are minimal or absent. Future research will likely help describe critical diagnostic features and determine how distinct these categories are.

Ambiguity in criteria for diagnosis can result in poor interrater reliability, as was found in a study conducted to distinguish autism from other PDDs (Volkmar et al., 1994). A review of the ways in which the diagnosis of pervasive developmental disorder-not otherwise specified (PDD-NOS) is applied revealed that the population who received this diagnosis did have "diverse clinical and heterogeneous features," partly due to the tendency to offer "this diagnosis for lack of a better clinical definition" (Walker et al., 2004, p. 178).

The movement toward increased specificity in diagnostic terminology for research purposes has markedly constrained diagnosis of AS (Klin et al., 2005). The definition of AS "as a condition in which there is no clinically significant delay in expressive or receptive language development" does not mesh with "clinical experience and research

[in] that such individuals do usually show problems in language use and discourse" (Adams, Green, Gilchrest, & Cox, 2002, p. 680). To cope with these constraints, practitioners and researchers have modified diagnostic criteria to improve their usefulness. A review of three approaches for categorizing ASD diagnoses resulted in 56% of the individuals studied qualifying for at least two different diagnoses on the basis of the guidelines used (Klin et al., 2005).

Currently, researchers take care to report the criteria they used for ascribing subjects to diagnostic categories and employ multiple measures to confirm the appropriateness of the diagnosis. Caution is still needed when making comparisons across patient populations and research studies.

PRAGMATICS

The study of language is generally divided into five components: phonology (i.e., the study of the sounds of a language system), semantics (i.e., the way meaning is used in language), morphology (i.e., the way units of meaning combine in words), syntax (i.e., rules for combining words into sentences), and pragmatics (i.e., context-bound, functional language use). With its emphasis on function, pragmatics entails all of the other components of language. In the broadest sense, children whose phonological, semantic, or syntactic language difficulties are severe enough to compromise function experience, in some form, a pragmatic language disorder.

Pragmatic language disorders are a hallmark of ASDs (Landa, 2000; Ozonoff & Miller, 1996; Tager-Flusberg, 1981). Controversy has been reported "over whether PLI [pragmatic language impairment] and autism are one and the same thing," (Norbury & Bishop, 2002, p. 232). Yet, difficulties with social and discourse-level language have been reported in children diagnosed with attention disorders (Flory et al., 2006; Humphries, Koltun, Malone,

& Roberts, 1994), learning disabilities (Loveland, Fletcher, & Bailey, 1990; Vallance & Wintre, 1997), cerebral palsy (Pennington, Goldbart, & Marshall, 2004), fetal alcohol spectrum disorders (O'Malley & Nanson, 2002), and traumatic brain injury (Body & Parker, 2005; Chapman et al., 2001; Ewing-Cobbs, Brookshire, Scott, & Fletcher, 1998; McDonald, 1993). Careful review of patterns in these nonmutually exclusive groups may reveal core features to which pragmatic language disorders can be linked, such as the reported link between the attention disorders and social language difficulties experienced by children with neurofibromatosis (Barton & North, 2004).

Poor pragmatic language skills affect every facet of people's lives, from their ability to form and maintain relationships to their academic and vocational success. Pragmatic language deficits can occur in the presence of other strong language and cognitive skills, as happens in higher-functioning individuals with ASDs. A look at the processes involved in creating pragmatic language illustrates why language interaction proves so challenging to this population.

The following description of pragmatics captures the "on line" adjustments people must make based on information they distill from the interaction. Levinson (1983) explained this process by observing

> The point is that we can compute out of sequences of utterances, taken together with background assumptions about language usage, highly detailed inferences about the nature of the assumptions participants are making, and the purposes for which utterances are being used. In order to participate in ordinary language usage, one must be able to make such calculations, both in production and in interpretation. This ability is independent of idiosyncratic beliefs, feelings, and usages (although it may refer to those shared by the participants), and it is based for the most part on quite regular and relatively abstract principles. Pragmatics can be taken to be the description of this ability. (p. 53)

Consideration of functional language skills is essential in assessment and treatment of language disorders, particularly for individuals who do not communicate well in "real-life" situations, despite having better cognitive and linguistic skills. Children and adolescents who have HFA or AS fit this pattern, as they may obtain good scores on standardized language tests, but they have less than adequate functional language skills (Landa, 2000; Minshew, Goldstein, & Siegel, 1997). Their strong performance on standardized tests can result from the structure present in the formal tests and testing conditions. In other words, the tightly controlled context and content can offer enough support for higher-functioning children and adolescents to perform better on standardized tests than they can in functional communication settings. Observation and assessment of discourse-level language provides a means for tapping into the communication skills people use in naturally occurring functional communication settings.

DISCOURSE

Discourse can be informally described as connected stretches of spoken or written text. Linking sentences can create new meaning that did not exist in either sentence alone, hence resulting in a speaker's need to sift through several possible meanings to determine which was intended in a given setting (Schiffrin, Tannen, & Hamilton, 2001). For example, adjacent signs at a college football stadium illustrate how placing two bits of text side by side can create a new meaning. The first sign reads, "Fans, please line up here." The second reads, "Students, please line up here," with an arrow pointing in the opposite direction.

At the interpersonal level, discourse involves a dynamic process in which the speaker or writer attempts to accomplish a communication goal by addressing the needs of the listener or reader, as well as the needs dictated by the context. Thus, discourse analysis looks at "what people using language are doing, and . . . [accounts] for the linguistic features in the discourse as the means employed in what they are doing" (Brown & Yule, 1983, p. 26).

Like other components of language, pragmatics and discourse are rule-governed and context dependent. In fact, the orderly nature of discourse makes it "describable in terms of its structure and function" (Johnstone, 2001, p. 638). Listeners attribute meaning to execution and violation of discourse rules (Grice, 1975). As intricate and subtle as the rules for discourse may seem, exposure to meaningful language in context is sufficient to start typically developing infants along the path for successful use of different types of discourse (Ervin-Tripp & Mitchell-Kernan, 1977; Nelson, 1993).

GENERAL OBSERVATIONS

Results from many of the studies of individuals with HFA or AS reported in this chapter reveal a surprising paradox. On many tasks, children and adolescents with HFA or AS can function like their age-matched, IQ-matched, or language-matched peers but exhibit marked deficits in other skills. These contrasts can occur in the same domain. For example, strengths in structural aspects of language coexist with marked deficits in pragmatic language skills in higher-functioning individuals with ASDs (Volkmar, Klin, Schultz, Rubin, & Bronen, 2000). Gaps in skill can be difficult to detect or understand in light of notable strengths. It is essential for children with HFA or AS, their families, and the professionals who work with them to appreciate that the children's performance can vary by task and situational demands. Capturing these patterns of strength and need is critical, given the implications for assessment and treatment.

Of course, factors outside the language domain also affect performance of language tasks. Although it is beyond the scope of this

chapter to address, it is worth mentioning that children with ASD diagnoses function differently or have difficulty with attention, executive function, working memory, information processing, emotional status, and sensory and motor skills (Anzalone & Williamson, 2000; Jansiewicz et al., 2006; Kenworthy et al., 2005; Minshew et al., 1997). Execution of everyday tasks requires integration of skills across domains, such as the combined attention, motor, language, and perspective-taking skills needed for written language tasks. When task demands are high in other areas of dysfunction, language skills can be further compromised—and vice versa. In other words, overall demand is a factor affecting performance in language and other domains.

NONLITERAL LANGUAGE

Individuals with HFA or AS have difficulty interpreting nonliteral language. Combined with skills needed for literal language comprehension and production, interpretation of nonliteral language may require resolution of incongruities, reference to social contexts, re-formulation of ideas, and perspective-taking. The following sections discuss the nonliteral language skills of humor, irony, inferencing, and figurative language.

Humor

Humor serves many purposes in human interactions: communication, cohesion within groups, stress management, and emotional release. Appreciation of humor often involves the resolution of an incongruity. Accurate interpretation of humor can hinge on "a variety of cognitive functions, including problem solving, memory and mental flexibility, abstract reasoning, and imagination. . . . [In addition, it] also requires an affective response and needs to be placed in a social context" (Lyons & Fitzgerald, 2004, p. 523). The inability to detect humor or share it with others can affect one's development of relationships and limit one's opportunities for social exchange and learning (Reddy, Williams, & Vaughan, 2002).

In one study of the appreciation of humor, performance of preschool children diagnosed with ASDs was contrasted with performance of children diagnosed with Down syndrome (Reddy et al., 2002). The children with Down syndrome served as an interesting contrast, given their relative strengths in areas where children with ASDs struggle (e.g., semantics, social language skills) (Chapman, 1999). Results of this study with preschool children were also interesting in light of known difficulties that school-age children and adults with ASD diagnoses experience using humor.

Study subjects with autism diagnoses according to the *Diagnostic and Statistical Manual of Mental Disorders, Fourth Edition* (*DSM-IV*; American Psychiatric Association, 1994) and *International Classification of Diseases, Tenth Revision (ICD-10)* criteria ($n = 19$, mean age = 49.6 months) were matched to children diagnosed with Down syndrome ($n = 16$, mean age = 41.3 months) on the basis of nonverbal mental age. Although the groups had similar overall developmental scores, the children with ASDs had significantly lower verbal mental age and significantly higher chronological age than the children with Down syndrome. In the initial home visit, parents participated in an interview and received training for focused observations. A follow-up home visit included videotaping of sessions of spontaneous play and play with toys. Data from parent interviews were coded, as were episodes of children's laughter captured on videotape. Instances of laughter were coded for duration, the person who initiated it, the type and direction of the child's response, and any social-contextual characteristics (Reddy et al., 2002).

Analysis of videotaped results revealed that laughter occurred often in homes of children in both clinical groups with no significant difference in frequency of occurrence (Reddy et al., 2002). Significant differences did exist regarding the referent of laughter. Children in the ASD group had more instances of laughter with nonshared content; shared laughter at an external target was virtually nonexistent in children with ASDs. None of the children with ASDs laughed in response to socially inappropriate acts, in contrast to half of the children with Down syndrome who did. Fewer parents of children with ASDs reported that their children laughed when shown funny faces. Responses to funny faces were not related to developmental age in children with ASDs, although they were in the children with Down syndrome. All but one of the parents of children with ASDs spontaneously reported that their children "laughed at strange or odd things, at odd times or at incomprehensible or inappropriate stimuli" (Reddy et al., 2002, p. 228), an observation none of the parents of the children with Down syndrome made.

Although the most frequent response to laughter of others in both groups was no reaction, children with ASDs responded significantly less often than children with Down syndrome. Less laughter was directed toward children in the ASD group by people in the room during taping than to children in the Down syndrome group. Instances of children "clowning" (i.e., trying to elicit laughter from others) occurred less often and were simpler in form for the children diagnosed with ASDs.

Differences were observed in patterns of teasing (i.e., playfully trying to provoke others) with parents and children across the two groups. Parental teasing of children occurred significantly less often in the ASD group. Most parents of children with ASDs reported that they did not tease their children; some did so only through simple visually based play. Parents of the children with ASDs reported concern that their children would not understand the teasing or would respond negatively to it. A few children in the ASD group continued teasing younger siblings even when signs of distress were present, a behavior not observed in children with Down syndrome (Reddy et al., 2002).

In summary, results showed that the young children diagnosed with ASDs engaged in laughter as often as the children with Down syndrome, whose social skills are considered a strength. Parents of the children with ASDs experienced their children's emotional responsiveness, although to a lesser degree than the parents of the children diagnosed with Down syndrome (Reddy, et al, 2002).

In a study of comprehension of humor, eight adolescents (chronological age: 11–17 years) with parent-reported HFA or AS diagnoses were age- and gender-matched to peers who had no history of cognitive or language problems. Humor was assessed through cartoon and joke tasks. In the cartoon task, examiners asked the ASD and control group members to complete a two-panel captioned cartoon of the character Garfield with a third panel that revealed the correct funny ending (Emerich, Creaghead, Grether, Murray, & Grasha, 2003). Modeled after previous studies (Bihrle, Brownell, Powelson, & Gardner, 1986; Ozonoff & Miller, 1996), the array of five choices depicted 1) a funny, correct answer that was surprising and coherent with the story, 2) a straightforward coherent ending that lacked surprise or humor, 3) a surprising and humorous ending that lacked coherence, 4) a surprising ending without humor that was only associated with the story, and 5) a neutral ending that was surprising but not humorous or coherent with the story. The joke task paralleled the cartoon task, in which adolescents were shown and read the body of the joke. Adolescents were asked to choose the correct funny answer from an array of five choices that were parallel to the options in the cartoon condition.

Results of this humor appreciation task revealed that subjects with ASDs made significantly more errors on the joke task than

their typically developing peers (Emerich et al., 2003). No significant difference was present relative to the category of response chosen for the joke task. For the HFA or AS adolescent group, better performance on the cartoon task than the joke task was attributed to a higher degree of abstraction present in the joke task.

For the cartoon task, the subjects with HFA or AS chose the straightforward ending most often and the surprising and humorous but unrelated ending least often. The authors suggested that the adolescents with HFA or AS preferred the straightforward ending and the humorous noncoherent ending because neither condition required that they rethink the initial information once they heard the punch line—a reference to the two-stage model of humor processing proposed by Suls (1972). Specifically, straightforward endings required no revision of the initial conclusion because of their coherence with prior story information; humorous endings were simply funny by themselves (Emerich et al., 2003). These results were consistent with an earlier study of high-functioning adults with diagnoses of autism (Ozonoff & Miller, 1996). Results of the adolescent study may be constrained by the small sample size, heterogeneity of ASDs, and the limited use of formal diagnostic measures to characterize the subject pool beyond single-word vocabulary.

Some parallels exist between patterns of performance described for interpretation and use of humor in preschool children diagnosed with ASDs and adolescents or adults with ASDs. For example, individuals with ASDs do engage in humor across the age span, although on a simpler level than peers. Factors that appear to affect their ability to interpret humor include demands in the areas of affect, interpersonal engagement, linguistic or cognitive flexibility, and the degree to which social and contextual cues affect meaning. Many high-functioning adults who have AS use and understand verbal humor "but the quality seems to be of a more cognitive nature, based on linguistic and logical principles and motivated by obsessional characteristics" (Lyons & Fitzgerald, 2004, p. 528).

Also noteworthy are the similarities between the performance of individuals with HFA and adults who have sustained unilateral right hemisphere damage. These similarities occur in their clinical presentation to tasks involving humor or inferencing, as well as in communication style (Ozonoff & Miller, 1996). The brain's right hemisphere appears to have "a specificity of function and localization related to humor" (Shammi & Stuss, 1999, p. 663). Tasks needed for interpretation of humor that appear to be associated with the right frontal lobe include integration of information, interpretation of current experiences in light of past ones (i.e., episodic retrieval), and emotional responsiveness. Data pointing toward a right frontal lobe focus for humor appreciation do not preclude critical roles played by the left hemisphere and the role of distributed processing across brain hemispheres (Shammi & Stuss, 1999).

Irony

Interpreting or using ironic remarks also involves recognition of an incongruity. Ironic remarks can be used to convey an opposite meaning from the literal one. Irony may also result from opposition between what is said and the context in which it is said. Interpreting irony requires mental representation skills because "the listener needs to understand not only that the speaker does not mean exactly what she/he said, but also that she/he does not expect to be taken literally" (Wang, Lee, Sigman, & Dapretto, 2006, p. 932).

One study evaluated how well two different theoretical constructs could be used to predict difficulties individuals with ASDs experience interpreting nonliteral language (Martin & McDonald, 2004). The theory of mind construct involves the ability to

interpret mental states, a skill used to understand and predict behaviors in others (Baron-Cohen, 1989; Miller, 2006). The weak central coherence construct suggests "a processing bias for featural and local information, and relative failure to extract gist or 'see the big picture' in everyday life" (Happe & Frith, 2006, p. 6). Using the theory of mind construct, Martin and McDonald (2004) anticipated that significant associations would occur between social inference and pragmatic language ability in the absence of a strong association with general inferencing ability. Using the weak central coherence construct, the authors anticipated significant associations between the subjects' "ability to organize perceptual details into a meaningful whole" and their "ability to make pragmatic inferences" (Martin & McDonald, 2004, p. 315).

Study subjects ($n = 14$, mean age 19.76 years) all met the *DSM-IV* criteria for AS. The control subjects ($n = 24$, mean age 19.75 years) were freshman psychology students. A significant difference in verbal IQ scores between the AS and control groups was handled statistically during analysis.

Pairs of tasks were presented to subjects to allow for comparisons. Example paired tasks included timed assembly of meaningful versus nonmeaningful puzzles, repetition of meaningful versus nonsense word lists, and a local-global task requiring memory of a large letter made of small letters that matched or differed from it. Results were reviewed in light of predictions about performance made on the basis of the theoretical constructs.

Results revealed that subjects used a local processing approach in a puzzle assembly task based on their completion of meaningful and nonmeaningful puzzles in the same amount of time. In other words, study subjects obtained no apparent benefit from the contextual cue of a meaningful image on the surface of one puzzle in the pair. No evidence of a local processing approach was present in paired sentence recall or the local-global letter recall task. The authors reported that their results did not support the weak central coherence construct. They found no relationship between these results and performance on the pragmatic interpretation task, nor did they find an association with theory of mind (Martin & McDonald, 2004).

A significant association existed for subjects with AS between their ability to interpret nonliteral utterances and second order theory of mind reasoning (i.e., the ability to infer the beliefs someone has about another person's beliefs). Because the subjects with AS achieved ceiling-level performance with first order theory of mind tasks (i.e., inference about another person's beliefs), no association was found there. Evidence of mental inferencing difficulty absent difficulty with nonmental inferencing was taken to indicate "a domain specific impairment in autism that is related to social functioning and the comprehension and use of social linguistic devices" (Martin & McDonald, 2004, p. 325).

Limitations of the study included the small sample size, assessment of weak central coherence only in the visuospatial domain, and some possible task constraints (e.g., differences in complexity between visual and verbal stimuli, the possible confounding effect of verbal instructions), as well as general issues like the heterogeneity of ASDs and potential differences individuals with ASDs may have in processing information presented in different ways and in different contexts. (See Baron-Cohen, 1989; Happe & Frith, 2006; and Miller, 2006 for complete reviews of weak central coherence- and theory of mind-based tasks, outcomes, and implications.)

Behavioral and neuroimaging (fMRI) findings from a recent study on the interpretation of irony provided interesting insights into the profiles of children diagnosed with AS or ASDs (Wang et al., 2006). Eighteen males age 7.4–16.9 years served as subjects for this study. Prior clinical ASD

diagnoses were confirmed with the Autism Diagnostic Interview–Revised (ADI-R; Rutter, LeCouteur, & Lord, 2003) and the Autism Diagnostic Observation Schedule–Generic (ADOS-G; Lord et al., 2000). The control group did not differ from the ASD group by age or IQ. All subjects for this study had verbal IQ scores of 70 or better on formal IQ tests.

Tasks involved presenting adolescents in both groups with a brief description of a scenario and then asking them to determine whether the speaker was being ironic or sincere. The three test conditions included 1) the provision of prosodic cues in the speaker's voice paired with contextual cues present in the short description, 2) prosodic cues only, or 3) contextual cues only. As expected, the typically developing children were significantly more accurate than the children with ASDs at interpreting irony in the conditions where contextual cues were available. Surprisingly, performance between groups did not differ when only prosodic cues were available. These results illustrate the lack of benefit that children with ASD diagnoses drew from contextual cues in the interpretation of meaning and intention in the speaker's remarks (Wang et al., 2006).

The neuroimaging results from this study revealed that adolescents with ASDs recruited prefrontal and temporal regions to a greater degree than the typically developing children (Wang et al., 2006). These differences were stimulus dependent. When only contextual cues were available, adolescents in the ASD group increased recruitment of the right inferior frontal gyrus (IFG). Greater activity was present in bilateral IFG regions for adolescents with ASDs than for controls when both contextual and prosodic cues were present. With only prosodic cues available, adolescents with ASDs recruited bilateral temporal regions more heavily than did controls. The latter finding is consistent with previous research showing that the activated temporal regions are part of an affective prosody processing frontotemporal network. Adolescents with ASDs whose social and communicative skills were stronger showed greater activity in the right temporal pole, an area activated during familiar face and voice recognition, as well as during retrieval of emotional and semantic content (Wang et al., 2006).

Increased recruitment of brain regions by children with ASDs may reflect the additional effort needed to complete the task and use of compensatory strategies (i.e., verbal reasoning to supplement interpretation of communicative intent). The authors thought the absence of significant group differences in the activation of the medial prefrontal cortex (MPFC) may have been due to differences in task presentation from some other studies (e.g., requirement that subjects make explicit judgment about intent). Results suggest that high-functioning children who have ASDs bring some skills to judgment tasks like this, given their ability to perform like their typically developing peers in the interpretation of irony when contextual cues were absent, although some differences were present (Wang et al., 2006).

Inferencing

Typically developing toddlers acquire words quickly and efficiently at a rate of a new word every 2 hours for 2-year-olds (Pinker, 1999). Part of children's word learning involves mapping labels onto objects or actions in the environment. When there is ambiguity regarding a label's referent, children need to use some strategy for identifying it. One way a child can resolve the ambiguity is to determine the speaker's intention, a skill children this age can successfully use (Bloom, 2000). Given the observation that 2-year-olds with autism map new words onto objects in their gaze rather than objects targeted by adult gaze (Baron-Cohen, Baldwin, & Crowson, 1997), questions have been raised about the skills

needed for word learning and the kinds of strategies children employ in this process.

Two experiments were set up to evaluate word mapping skills in children diagnosed with autism ($n = 18$, mean age 7.8 years) and a group of typically developing toddlers ($n = 20$, mean age 23.8 months) (Preissler & Carey, 2005). Children in the experimental group met *DSM-IV* criteria for autism (e.g., a mean IQ score of 62 [range: 37–90]). Half of the children diagnosed with ASDs were nonverbal. Test sessions took place in the children's homes and were videotaped for later analysis.

Two conditions for new object labeling were presented. In both of the conditions, the experimenter and the child each held a novel object. In the first condition, the experimenter and the child both looked at the child's object as the experimenter offered a novel label for the object. In the second condition, they each looked at their own objects when the experimenter produced the novel label. At the conclusion of each task condition, the experimenter placed all of the objects into a bag and asked the child to retrieve one, using the new object label. In the coordinated gaze condition, the children with ASDs selected the appropriate object with 67% accuracy, performance not statistically different than the preschool control group's accuracy of 85% (Preissler & Carey, 2005).

In the discrepant gaze naming condition, performance of children with ASDs differed significantly from that of the children in the preschool control group, both in accuracy (39% for ASD group versus 80% for control group) and in instances in which the child looked up at the experimenter's eyes (17% of ASD group versus 95% of control group). Comparison of the children's performance across the two task conditions revealed strategies that they employed to determine label referent. Some children consistently paired the new word with the object in their gaze (39% in ASD group versus 15% in control group); others always selected the object in the speaker's gaze (28% in ASD group versus 70% in control group); and fewer children consistently chose the most novel object (11% in ASD group versus 15% in control group). A subset of children in the ASD group chose the object in the speaker's hands in the coordinated gaze condition and their own object in the discrepant gaze condition (22%)—an opposite pattern not seen in the toddler control group. Results of this portion of the study confirmed earlier findings and showed that typically developing children "actively use the gaze of an adult speaker to determine the referent of a novel word," but children with ASDs do not; instead, they often map novel words onto objects of their own interest (Preissler & Carey, 2005, p. B18).

A second experiment was conducted to determine whether children's knowledge of a label for one object affects how they map a label to another object. Subjects for this study included the same group of children with ASDs and a new group of typically developing toddlers (mean age 24.0 months). Test stimuli included line drawings and objects that their parents confirmed as novel or familiar. In test conditions, a familiar labeled object or picture was paired with an unfamiliar counterpart (i.e., an unlabeled object or picture). Children in both groups achieved a high rate of accuracy in mapping the novel name onto the novel object or picture. Performance did not differ across groups, nor did it differ on the basis of whether the stimuli were objects or pictures. Results of this pair of experiments showed that inferencing skills may not be required for word mapping. Under certain task conditions, children simply pair a new label with the unnamed object or picture. Typically developing children do, however, appear to be more aware of and guided by a speaker's intentions than children with ASDs (Preissler & Carey, 2005).

The ability to draw accurate inferences plays a role in discourse-level language tasks in which older children also engage. In a task that required inferencing, story comprehension and story recall skills were measured in a group of children (chronological age: 6–10 years, nonverbal scaled scores ≥ 80). Children in the study were recruited for four groups: specific language impairment ($n = 16$), pragmatic language impairment ($n = 24$), children with HFA ($n = 10$), and a control group ($n = 18$). The authors acknowledged the challenges and controversies associated with "differential diagnosis of subgroups of both language impairment subtypes and pervasive developmental disorders" (Norbury & Bishop, 2002, p. 231) linked to assigning children to these diagnostic groups. Several tools were used for assigning group placement and measuring children's performance. One instrument, the Children's Communication Checklist (CCC; Bishop, 1998), was described as a tool for assessing pragmatic language impairment. The CCC consists of two scales to assess language form (i.e., speech and syntax), two scales to "assess nonlinguistic aspects of behaviour associated with autism (social relationships, interests)," and five scales that form the "pragmatic composite" (Norbury & Bishop, 2002, p. 234).

The inferencing task for this study was based on previous work by Cain and Oakhill (1999). In the current study, stories of approximately 150 words in length were read aloud to avoid disadvantaging poor readers. After hearing each story, the children were asked two literal questions, two questions that required text-connecting inferences (i.e., integrate information across sentences to link concepts), and two questions that required gap-filling inferences (i.e., integrate personal knowledge with text). When children did not respond accurately, a graded prompt sequence was used to try to elicit the correct response: 1) reread the relevant paragraph, 2) reread the relevant sentence, and 3) ask a targeted question to help the child make the connection. The amount of prompting needed to achieve a correct response was documented.

After the children answered questions about the final story, they were asked to recall it, at which time they were provided with general prompts to elicit their responses.

Results revealed that children in the control group answered literal and inference-based questions better than children in the three clinical groups. Children with HFA had significantly more difficulty with inferencing than did children with pragmatic or specific language impairments. This difficulty could not be explained on the basis of their language skills (Norbury & Bishop, 2002). This outcome is in keeping with previous research with older children in conditions where the stories were less natural. Some of the success children with pragmatic language impairment had in interpreting inferences was attributed to task artifacts (e.g., responding to some questions without needing to draw an inference, whether inferences required judgments of mental state).

All of the children in the study demonstrated skill in making inferences. Error analysis revealed that the most common type of incorrect response involved making inferences that did not relate to the story context. This error pattern occurred across groups, causing the authors to note that explanations for this error pattern need not entail theoretical constructs that are typically ascribed to children with ASD diagnoses. Possible explanations included poor story recall and difficulty suppressing a natural response based on personal experiences that could conflict with story information (Norbury & Bishop, 2002).

Not surprisingly, story recall was more tightly linked to receptive rather than expressive language skill, but performance on language tests did not distinguish children who could make appropriate inferences from those who could not. Children's digit recall and story recall skills were correlated, but performance on digit recall tasks did not fully account for performance on story recall tasks (Norbury & Bishop, 2002).

Story comprehension abilities correlated significantly with story recall. This correlation held when age, digit recall, and receptive language skills were factored out. This finding adds credence to the belief that children actively construct mental representations while listening to stories that facilitate comprehension and then recall of the stories, although the effect could be in the opposite direction, in which good recall aids comprehension (Norbury & Bishop, 2002).

The authors noted that the pragmatic language group did not appear to be cohesive, given the amount of within-group variability (Norbury & Bishop, 2002). Decisions about child placement in groups could have contributed to this variability, which may also have been true of the use of the CCC, with its emphasis on characteristics of autism, to sort children with specific language impairment (i.e., higher scores on the CCC) from children with pragmatic language impairment (i.e., lower scores on the CCC).

Another study included a series of questions designed to see whether children with HFA or AS could make some of the pragmatic inferences needed for successful communication (Dennis, Lazenby, & Lockyer, 2001). In this study, children who met *DSM-IV* criteria for a diagnosis of autism ($n = 4$) or AS ($n = 4$) were age-matched to three separate control groups of typically developing peers ($n = 8$ children each). All children fell into the 9–10-year age range. Children in the HFA and AS group had mean verbal IQ scores of 93.5 (range 71–146).

No significant differences were found between children in the HFA and AS group and the matched control groups in recognizing and describing different meanings of ambiguous sentences. No between-group differences were observed on a presupposition task (Dennis et al., 2001).

Significant differences, however, were found between the HFA and AS group and the control groups on several other tasks. Group differences occurred where pragmatic inferences involving implication (i.e., offer yes/no/maybe response about the truth of statements based on semantic or syntactic information). Children in a control group performed significantly better than children in the HFA and AS group in drawing inferences about familiar social scripts, interpretation, and definition of figurative language, as well as in their ability to create sentences to describe what someone in a particular communication context might have said. The latter three tasks and the ambiguity task, in which no significant between-group difference was found, comprise the Test of Language Competence–Extended Edition (Wiig & Secord, 1985).

Results of this study support observations from previous research showing that children with HFA and AS have some linguistic flexibility (e.g., interpreting multiple-meaning words and sentences), but they cannot draw other inferences that are essential for successful communication interaction. In this study, children with HFA appeared to "make inferences from text to fixed knowledge more readily than from text to local sentence context" (Dennis et al., 2001, p. 5). The HFA and AS children's stronger performance on ambiguity tasks than on metaphor tasks was interpreted as indicating that the intentionality of an utterance was challenging to interpret, as opposed to the fact that multiple meanings were possible. Despite some successes in inferential tasks, the authors concluded that children with HFA or AS "often fail to make inferences that are the basis of successful social communication . . . those that elaborate meaning for the listener or signal awareness of intentions" (Dennis et al., 2001, p. 53).

Figurative Language: Idioms and Metaphors

Children with HFA and AS have difficulty interpreting and using figurative language to a degree that cannot be accounted for by deficits in cognition or other areas of language. Idioms occur frequently in language, so difficulty understanding and using them can compromise communication and learning. As with other aspects of nonliteral language, contextual cues assist with interpretation of figurative language, as does recognition that the speaker does not intend the remarks to be taken literally. Interpretation of idioms is easier for typically developing children when the idioms are familiar or their meaning is transparent (Nippold & Rudzinski, 1993), but mastery of the skills needed for understanding idioms continues into adolescence and adulthood (Nippold & Duthie, 2003).

A systematic review of idiom comprehension was conducted across clinical groups to discern patterns of performance and to see what relationships exist between idiom comprehension and other cognitive and language skills (Norbury, 2004). Establishment of diagnostic boundaries was challenging for this study, as had been the case for others. Through clinician report and results of standardized and informal assessment, children were grouped according to presence or absence of ASD features and presence or absence of language impairment as measured by standardized tests. The two-stage decision tree resulted in the establishment of four clinical groups of children—1) language impaired without autistic features ($n = 29$), 2) pragmatically impaired without autistic features ($n = 6$), 3) ASD with language impairment ($n = 29$), and 4) ASD without language impairment ($n = 29$)—as well as one control group ($n = 39$). Mean age across groups ranged from 11.12 (control group) to 12.23 (children with ASD and language impairment). Mean IQ scores across groups ranged from 97.59 (language impaired group without autistic features) to 108.31 (ASD without language impairment).

Children were asked to define idioms to measure their understanding of them. Offering definitions can be challenging for children with language impairments, but conducting the task in this way eliminated the reading burden of a multiple-choice task and allowed for a review of the literal level of the children's responses.

In this study, children defined opaque idioms more successfully than transparent ones when nested in context or provided in isolation. This result differed from previous research findings. Factors that may have affected children's performance included disadvantages to expressively language impaired children (given task demands for explanation) and to children with weaker literacy skills (given the likelihood that typically developing children learn many idioms through reading).

Results indicated that context provided cues about idiom interpretation to the children with language and communication impairments. Structural language impairments reduced the children's ability to interpret idioms. Children with ASD features who did not have structural language deficits used contextual cues as well as their peers. Notably, "language ability was one of the most significant predictors of idiom understanding" (Norbury, 2004, p. 1188). Memory for the story also affected the children's performance. Results from theory of mind tasks did not account for idiom comprehension abilities after language ability was considered. Several explanations were offered for the inability of theory of mind results to account for idiom comprehension apart from language. The author noted that the theory of mind tasks and language tasks might have employed overlapping skill sets, that mental state judgments were not needed for the interpretation of the idioms, or that higher-functioning children might apply learned strategies to interpret idioms.

In summary, sentence processing skills predicted idiom comprehension better than semantic skills or the presence of ASD features (Norbury, 2004). Results of this study did not offer strong support for the weak central coherence theory. Not using contextual cues could have stemmed from deficits

in language, memory, or attention skills, as well as the inability to integrate information to recognize global meaning. Correlations existed between the theory of mind task and idiom comprehension, but other variables could have accounted for this outcome.

CONVERSATION: STRUCTURE AND FUNCTION

Conversational skill is essential for human interaction. Typically developing children learn the basic turn-taking and topic management skills necessary for conversational interaction during their preschool years (McTear, 1985). By contrast, these skills remain challenging for individuals with ASDs in later childhood (Kelley, Paul, Fein, & Naigles, 2006). Speakers who lack the language, social, or cognitive skills to adjust to audience, situational, and task demands risk being misunderstood or judged as inappropriate or rude (Volden et al., 2006). Conversational interaction serves as a means for establishing peer relationships.

Typically developing adolescents interact with their peers largely through conversations. As a result, successful conversational interactions "may contribute to an adolescent's sense of social success, affecting his or her willingness to engage in future social interactions" (Turkstra, Ciccia, & Seaton, 2003, p. 118).

Analysis of extemporaneous conversations in peer dyads revealed that typically developing adolescents asked and answered questions and offered contingent responses frequently (Turkstra et al., 2003). High frequency nonverbal behaviors included nodding and neutral or positive facial expressions. Nonverbal back-channel responses serve to engage the speaker, hand the conversational turn back, and sustain the interaction. Typically developing adolescents "rarely showed negative emotions, turned away from each other, repeated or completed partners' utterances, asked for clarification or confirmation or information, gave non-contingent responses, or failed to answer questions" (Turkstra et al., 2003, p. 122). In opposite-sex dyads, participants used less eye contact, but smiled, nodded, and chimed in more frequently than in same-sex dyads (Turkstra, 2001).

The above description of typically developing adolescents' conversational interactions serves as a template of the skills that adolescents with HFA and AS must employ to converse successfully with their peers who do not have ASDs. Unfortunately, in their struggles to communicate, adolescents with HFA or AS often exhibit the behaviors rarely seen in typical peer conversational dyads. In fact, adolescents with HFA or AS can have naïve impressions about the concept of friendship, and thus they may have an inaccurate interpretation of peer feedback regarding the ways their verbal and nonverbal actions are received (Howlin, 2004).

Audience Adaptation

Changes in an audience or conversational partner alter the demands on both speakers. Children who have language impairments tend to play with younger peers who match their level of language skill. They also select adults as conversational partners because most adults have the ability to overcome problems and sustain the interaction. Children with ASDs were found to respond more positively to adults than to other children, perhaps as a way of getting their needs met (Jackson et al., 2003).

As with other studies conducted with high-functioning children who have HFA and AS, the 8- to 11-year-old children (VIQ 70–140) in this study of affect marking in family dialogue at the dinner table matched their typically developing peers in some skill areas, but showed deficits in others (Muller & Schuler, 2006). The children with HFA or AS marked affect verbally by stating a feeling or preference proportionally more often than their typically developing peers. Their

repertoire of affect words was larger, although some were used in an idiosyncratic or less conventional way. Negative affective terms were more intense than their peers' negative terms (e.g., "nasty," "pathetic"). Children with HFA or AS stated or elicited causal explanations of affect more frequently than typically developing peers.

These findings, which seem to indicate competence, may actually be an attempt to develop a collaborative narrative "with parents or other individuals, to generate a more comprehensive understanding of certain events or situations and the causal forces/motivations underlying them" (Muller & Schuler, 2006, p. 1097). Other explanations for proportionally more verbal marking of affect and comments about causal issues include weak judgment about socially appropriate remarks, difficulty inhibiting positive and negative affect remarks, or the parents' focus on affect in dinnertime discussions due to the child's history of difficulty in this area (Muller & Schuler, 2006).

Knowledge and Use of Scripts

Scripts can be defined as "general expectations about nature and sequence of component activities" that individuals formulate through their experience with events that are similar (Volden & Johnston, 1999). Knowledge of familiar scripts creates predictability regarding those events and results in some predictability about the language that will be paired with them.

Higher-functioning children (6–16 years of age) diagnosed with ASDs were stratified into higher developmental (i.e., language age of 96+months) and lower developmental groups. Then, these groups were matched to two control groups, one on the basis of the children's language age and the other on their nonverbal cognitive abilities. Tasks assessed the children's ability to cite elements in common scripts, predict next steps in videotapes of people executing the scripts, and recognize violations in drawings of the event sequence in the scripts (Volden & Johnston, 1999).

Results showed that children with ASDs included fewer elements in their scripts than matched control subjects. Children with ASDs demonstrated script knowledge, however, as they included more than half of the core script elements. In addition, children with ASD diagnoses predicted the elements of scripts that they had omitted, which suggested better knowledge of the overall scripts than they had conveyed in the earlier expressive task. All but the children with ASDs in the lower developmental group recognized violations in script sequence, where the combination of ASDs and weaker developmental skills likely constrained their completion of this metacogntive task (Volden & Johnston, 1999). While findings from this study confirmed differences in the performances of higher-functioning children diagnosed with ASDs and peers matched on the basis of language age or nonverbal cognitive abilities, it also illustrated "knowledge of everyday scripts [that] is somewhat surprising given the inappropriate behavior often displayed by people with autism in situations that would ordinarily be scripted" (Volden & Johnston, 1999, p. 209).

Structure of Conversation

Conversations are developed jointly by the participants "on line" during the interaction. Through this process, "the development of coherent dialogue" takes place (McTear, 1985, p. 127). As a discourse structure, conversations are rule-governed, but no set patterns exist for the way any specific conversation will take shape. One can "think of a conversation as a uniquely human and extraordinarily important way by which separate minds are able to influence and be influenced by each other, managing to some extent, and always imperfectly, to bridge the gap between them, not by constructing any

kind of lasting object but through a constant interplay of constantly changing ideas" (Chafe, 2001, p. 686).

Turn-Taking

Conversational partners typically work together to construct the turn-taking exchanges that occur within their dialogue. Overlaps of conversational turns are not random; they generally occur at phrase or sentence endings, where the conversational partner anticipated an opening to take a turn at a possible juncture point. Pauses in conversation can be divided into grammatical pauses (i.e., between phrases) or nongrammatical pauses (i.e., within a phrase), where the former seems to indicate linguistic (i.e., syntactic) choices and the latter the cognitive load on the speaker (Thurber & Tager-Flusberg, 1993). Gaps in turn-taking, also called switching pauses (Thurber & Tager-Flusberg, 1993), occur while conversational partners are exchanging speaking roles. Extended gaps signal awkwardness in conversation (McTear, 1985).

Turn-taking can take on different characteristics in conversations with individuals who have HFA or AS. Turn exchanges of both partners are shaped by difficulties of the partner with HFA or AS, so the exchanges may not be as "clean" or as easily accomplished. For example, overlaps may occur as a result of a delay in the completion of an utterance or the need to revise or repair earlier remarks (Dobbinson, Perkins, & Boucher, 1998). This effect may be especially visible in the dynamic interplay of exchanging conversational turns (Garcia-Perez, Lee, & Hobson, 2006).

People with HFA or AS have sometimes been described as dominating conversations. This issue was addressed in a study by Adams et al. (2002). The boys in this study ($n = 19$, age range 11–19 years, nonverbal IQ ≥ 70) who met *ICD-10* criteria for diagnoses of AS were age- and IQ-matched with a clinical group of boys who met *ICD-10* criteria for conduct disorder. Analysis of two conversational sections of the Autism Diagnostic Observational Schedule (ADOS; Lord et al., 1989) served as part of the data for AS subjects in this study. Conversational analysis revealed that the boys with AS initiated exchanges more often than the boys with conduct disorder, but group data did not indicate that the children in the AS group dominated the conversation. Analysis of response patterns revealed that three boys in the AS group were quite talkative, with an outlier score well outside the interquartile range for the rest of their group. Their talkative style was restricted to socioemotional topics, "suggesting that the variations between individuals and contexts are sufficient to make the task of pinpointing the exact conversational strategies and strengths of individuals with AS very difficult" (Adams et al., 2002, p. 687). This analysis supports the perception that individuals with AS are heterogeneous with respect to conversational skills. Some of the boys with AS presented with "extreme patterns of conversational behavior"; others did not differ from their peers with conduct disorder, nor did they appear to differ from typically developing peers on the conversational skills analyzed for this study (Adams et al., 2002).

Topic Management: Initiation, Maintenance, and Closure

A topic can be described as discourse produced by one or more speakers who talk about "the same thing" (Chafe, 2001, p. 674) or simply "what a conversation was 'about'" (Brown & Yule, 1983, p. 73). The informal sense of what qualifies as a conversational topic suffices for participating in interactions, but it masks the complexities of topic that conversational participants manage in dynamic interactions. Topics can occur in single or multiple utterances. Topic-related turns may appear contiguously or resurface periodically in conversations and be carried by one or more speakers.

In conversations, topics operate on more than one level and then tend to progress somewhat sequentially. Several basic (i.e., utterance-level) topics may nest under a higher order supertopic (Chafe, 2001). For example, friends' conversation about the utterance-level topics of car problems and high gas prices could be linked under the supertopic of "the hazards of commuting."

Topic changes may be marked explicitly (e.g., "Let me tell you about . . .") or shift direction gradually over the course of several utterances. Speakers signal topic shifts by changing message content and prosodic features, as well as by leaving longer pauses. Conversational partners' linguistic actions can introduce, maintain, or change topics. Conversational topics are not preplanned; they are developed collaboratively during the interaction (Brown & Yule, 1983; McTear, 1985).

Typical speakers use many discourse devices to manage topics in conversations. Individuals with ASDs often initiate topic changes abruptly without negotiation, which may reflect a lack of awareness, an inability to handle subtle variables, or the individual's desire to return to a preferred topic (Dobbinson et al., 1998). As a result, circular patterns of topic movement can occur in conversations with individuals who have ASDs. Off-topic or noncontingent remarks can derail conversational interactions. A relationship has been found to exist between children's difficulty sustaining conversational topics and the severity of their ASD symptomatology (Hale & Tager-Flusberg, 2005).

Development of conversational topics requires elaboration or the addition of new information. Conversational partners of individuals with HFA or AS may be put in the position of having to ask questions to elicit new information. If this cycle repeats, the partner without HFA or AS may eventually abandon the task, resulting in the termination of a topic or the conversation (Dobbinson et al., 1998).

Topic content can affect how successfully high-functioning children with ASD diagnoses participate in interactions. Children with AS had significantly more difficulty conversing with adults when topics of conversation involved emotional content (Adams et al., 2002). Clinical experience suggests that high-functioning individuals with ASDs may experience or report boundaries for emotional content of topics differently than their conversational partners without ASDs. For example, one young man declined to "disclose personal information to someone I hardly know" when asked to describe his class schedule at school, then spontaneously reported that children at school frequently teased him because of the size of his head. Topics with emotional content may also require the use of subjective language (to offer opinions), instead of objective language (to cite facts). The same young man knew details about many different car models but could not offer an opinion about which he liked best, nor did he like classes taught through discussion where students offered their viewpoints on different topics.

Communication Breakdowns and Repairs

Communication breakdowns are common in conversations between capable language users. Familiar examples include "where a listener has failed to hear or understand part or the whole of a preceding utterance and uses the next turn to make a request for clarification . . ." (McTear, 1985, p. 50). In conversations between mature communicators, these breakdown–repair exchanges are barely noticeable because the misunderstandings are quickly resolved, allowing the conversation to continue after the brief detour. The ease with which able communicators repair communication breakdowns belies the difficulty involved in the task.

Resolving communication breakdowns is a multistep process that requires strong language and attentional skills, paired with the ability to take the listener's perspective into account. Steps include detecting the breakdown, determining possible reasons for it, and initiating a repair attempt, or responding to a partner's request to address the problem and evaluating the effectiveness of the repair to resolve the miscommunication (Brinton & Fujiki, 1989). Complexity is added by the interactional nature of the communication repair process, in which either partner can complete any of the steps and feedback is needed to see if the attempt was successful. Signals of the need for communication repairs and the repairs themselves vary by type and in the degree of specificity (e.g., "What?" versus "I didn't hear you."). Children's use of communication repairs, like other language skills, follows a developmental sequence, with simple repetitions of the original message appearing first developmentally, followed by attempts to modify the message for the listener or context (Golinkoff, 1986).

Children with deficient language and social skills encounter more frequent communication breakdowns. Unrepaired communication breakdowns can terminate interactions. Resolving breakdowns is essential "to persevere in communication exchanges" (Meaden, Halle, Watkins, & Chadsey, 2006, p. 57) and can be done even with limited expressive language abilities (Keen, 2004).

Environmental factors affect strategies that children use in communication repairs. In one-on-one interactions with an adult in their homes, two young children diagnosed with limited expressive language and ASDs altered the quantity and type of communication repair strategies they used based on the ongoing activity and the way the communication breakdown was signaled (Meaden et al., 2006). Specifically, they attempted communication repairs most often when the adult explicitly signaled the breakdown with a request for clarification (e.g., "What?"), in contrast to no adult response or a wrong response. The children repaired roughly 70% of the breakdowns in structured sessions. The authors hypothesized that the children's differential responses indicated awareness of the features of the tasks, the success of their previous repair attempts, and the ways in which the breakdowns were signaled (Meaden et al., 2006).

Although there were differences from peers individually matched by language skills, high-functioning school-age children with ASDs (i.e., diagnosed with PDD-NOS by *DSM-IV* criteria) showed some surprising parallels to controls in their responses to a series of three sequential requests for clarification (Volden, 2004). After engaging children in conversation on topics of interest, an unfamiliar adult requested clarification using three sequential requests. The initial request for clarification was always neutral (e.g., "What?"), as was the second request (e.g., "I don't understand."). The third request was a semistructured request (e.g., "Tell me another way."). Children's verbal and nonverbal responses to these stacked requests for clarification were coded by type according to guidelines developed by Brinton, Fujiki, Winkler, and Loeb (1986). Verbal response types included repetition, revision (i.e., the use of a different form with the same content), cue (i.e., the addition of new information), metacomments (e.g., remarks about one's inability to complete the communication repair), or inappropriate responses (e.g., no response, off-topic responses, attempts to discontinue). Nonverbal responses requesting clarification included gestures when they appeared as an attempt to clarify the message and suprasegmental changes (e.g., increases in vocal volume, word emphasis, greater precision in speaking, slower speech).

Children in both groups modified the type of repair strategy they used as the adult produced successive requests for clarification. For both groups, the children decreased the average number of repetitions they used and increased the average number of cues they provided to the listener across successive attempts to repair the breakdown. The children's revisions showed their continued attempts to resolve the assumed misunderstanding and their awareness that the repair had not been accomplished yet, a pattern that "should be taken as an awareness of listener difficulty and an acknowledgment of speaker responsibility for repair" (Volden, 2004, p. 184). The mean number of metacomments (i.e., about the interaction itself) increased most sharply for both groups after the third request. Children's gestures increased after the second request for clarification.

It is interesting to note that the number of inappropriate responses (e.g., off-topic responses, odd answers, attempts to discontinue the interaction) increased between the second and third requests, when children in both groups may have given up or tried to opt out of the interaction. The children with ASDs produced significantly more inappropriate responses than their language-matched peers. This difference was attributed to possible subtle language disorders not captured on the standardized language tests used for matching controls, as well as related cognitive and social skills likely required by this task (Volden, 2004). Although children with HFA or AS have many of the constituent skills necessary for engaging others in conversation, impairments in these skill areas "may present the most significant barrier to full participation in daily social life" that adolescents can experience (Turkstra et al., 2003, p. 118).

ASSESSMENT

Individuals who have HFA or AS have many strengths that can mask their areas of deficiency and result in inappropriate educational programming (Volkmar et al., 2000). Assessment practices require ecological validity (Landa, 2000)—that is, a measure of language that represents a realistic picture of the children's ability to meet the demands placed on them in social and academic settings. While acknowledging that "some aspects of extemporaneous socializing may always escape laboratory measurement" (Turkstra et al., 2003, p. 124), reasonable attempts should be made in assessment practices to mirror the type of tasks and levels of difficulty children will encounter.

Global scores of performance may mask important strengths and needs in the children's performance of discrete tasks. Global measures of performance should be paired with reviews of discrete measures to avoid neutralizing variability in skills that can affect function and provide useful information for treatment planning (Kelley et al., 2006). Rigid use of standardized tests and adherence to cutoff scores may serve a purpose for some research activities, but this approach could result in a marked under-referral of children with HFA or AS for clinical services.

Assessment practices also need to be "fine grained," given the specific nature of cognitive and linguistic differences and deficits experienced by children with HFA or AS. Pairing quantitative assessment with qualitative assessment offsets disadvantages of reliance on either type of instrument. Informal assessment and structured observation should assist in determining what discourse level knowledge (e.g., scripts) children with ASDs have, as their inability to display certain behaviors may not represent a complete lack of understanding of the features involved (Volden & Johnston, 1999).

Analysis of error patterns during formal assessment, ongoing treatment, and day-to-day interaction can help determine strategies children use to tackle the tasks they face. Error analysis can reveal patterns of performance that even high-functioning children with ASDs who process the world differently and have concomitant language

disorders cannot report. Extension testing and dynamic assessment practices can afford evaluators insights about premises children with ASDs hold or strategies they use linguistically. Replacement of an ineffective strategy could result in a more significant change than training skills one by one. A simple example of strategic teaching illustrates this point. One child's difficulty getting to specific rooms in a large building related to the fact that he did not realize that the first numeral of a room number generally identified the floor on which the room was located (Howlin, 2004).

Assessment of pragmatic language skills at the discourse level is critical. Pragmatic language is context bound. Capable speakers reflect awareness of changes in context, task, and audience by altering their communication. Assessment of pragmatic language skills requires documentation of contextual features, which when varied, may alter a child's success in interaction.

Use of a structured system for collection, analysis, or rating of observational data could serve as a useful probe during treatment or in conducting a comparison of skills across settings. An example observational rating scale for conversational behaviors in individuals who have ASD diagnoses includes the following areas: atypical intonation (including limited or atypical intonation), semantic drift (disengagement or topic switching), receptive interactivity (absent, delayed, or minimal response), perseveration (not attending to a topic or situation change), and pedantic speech (more detailed, technical, or specific information than needed) (de Villiers, Fine, Ginsberg, Vacarella, & Szatmari, 2006). Strengths of this scale include its basis in analysis of conversational data and the good interrater reliability obtained. Potential drawbacks include small sample size, the absence of a control group, and the semi-structured conversational format that resembled a clinical interview, as opposed to spontaneous conversation.

Knowledge of the verbal and nonverbal skills that typically developing children use in social engagement is critical for setting realistic targets. Adult expectations of how typically developing children and adolescents interact may not parallel what actually happens in natural interactions (Rogers, 2000). Assessment of the skills adolescents with ASDs exhibit in these "natural" settings may be equally important, as the adolescent–adult conversational dyads conducted in evaluation sessions may not be as challenging as peer interactions and thus may not reveal potential difficulties (Turkstra, 2001).

Assessment should be a part of any ongoing treatment program. Ideally, the child, family, educators, and medical and therapeutic professionals should participate in program development and monitoring activities. Collaboration among these critical players increases the likelihood that treatment goals and strategies will be meaningful and adapted to each child's unique skills and needs. Generalization is also more likely when opportunities for using new skills are available across settings.

TREATMENT

Treatment outcomes for children with ASDs vary widely. Encouragingly, research has shown that children "are responsive to a wide variety of interventions aimed at increasing their social engagement with others, both adults and typical peers" (Rogers, 2000, p. 406). Variables known to have a positive effect on treatment outcomes include the early onset of treatment, higher verbal and IQ scores prior to the start of treatment, and the intensity and duration of behavioral and educational programming (Howlin, 2004; Kelley et al., 2006). Individuals with ASD diagnoses may be more successful in meeting the long-term outcome of integration into adult life if they are able to develop skills and interests that they can leverage for obtaining employ-

ment and making interpersonal connections (Howlin, 2004).

Several treatment strategies have promise in improving social skills of individuals with ASDs. These strategies nest under critical targeted areas that are difficult for people with ASDs. Goals include increasing social motivation, increasing social initiations, improving appropriate social responding, reducing interfering behaviors, and promoting skill generalization (White, Keonig, & Scahill, 2006). Given some strong cognitive and language skills, individuals with HFA or AS may be able to learn new skills in clinical settings, but generalization to novel settings is essential for improved functioning. Generalization continues to be challenging for individuals with ASDs (Barry et al., 2003; White et al., 2006).

As is true for assessment, treatment planning should be sensitive to the children's overall level of functioning, as well as the variability in their skills. Knowledge of an individual's developmental level paired with understanding of his or her ASD diagnosis predicts outcomes better than does the ASD label alone (Landa, 2000; Volden & Johnston, 1999). Treatment approaches for individuals with HFA or AS may need to be adapted, if they were aimed at the level predicted by their better language skills (structure and form) without sufficient accommodation for their weaker social language skills (Volkmar et al., 2000). Fortunately, stronger structural language skills can be used to foster development of weaker language skills in individuals with ASDs. For example, stronger "verbal skills can be used to teach problem-solving techniques that can be generalized from one situation to another" (Volkmar et al., 2000, p. 266).

Typically developing children generally do not need to be explicitly taught the rules for social interaction and subtle language use because they abstract those rules from exposure to different social language experiences. The same cannot be said for children with HFA and AS. Inclusive school placements with typically developing peers offer more social opportunities, but "physical integration does not necessarily foster social integration" for children with ASDs without direct instruction (Rogers, 2000, p. 406).

The rule-governed nature of communication interactions makes it possible to teach children with ASDs explicit social language rules, almost as if they were learning a foreign language. This "very explicit verbal approach" can include teaching "a set of rules to use to identify contextual cues such as location, facial expressions, body proximity, and gesture to facilitate more appropriate comments, topic initiations, and social inferences" (Volkmar et al., 2000, p. 266).

The number of critical verbal and nonverbal cues, along with the quick pace of interactions, can make it difficult to illustrate the process. "Freezing" the moments of interaction through videotape allows individuals with ASDs to attend to different cues on sequential playbacks, practice new skills, and see what other options might have been possible within that particular context (LeBlanc et al., 2003; Nikopoulos & Keenan, 2007). Sufficient and appropriate training opportunities are needed, however, to allow children to generalize these skills to nonclinical environments (LeBlanc et al., 2003). Helping children create stories about social situations they encounter and working with them to devise responses appropriate for those settings have helped to decrease inappropriate behaviors and to increase use of appropriate social skills (Scattone, Tingstrom, & Wilczynski, 2006).

Types of discourse (e.g., conversation, narration, event description, classroom discourse) serve as broad frameworks within which language and other segments of discourse with unique features can be nested (e.g., a story about recent trip nested in a conversation). Because each of these types

of discourse has some unique features (i.e., in turn-taking and management of topics), training in the use of discourse skills should be adapted accordingly.

Explicit teaching about conversational interactions can target particular areas of deficit. Areas to target should be chosen on the basis of potential for functional gain, in light of what patterns of performance currently interfere the most with interaction and what skills and strategies are realistic for the individual's cognitive-communicative repertoire. General options include direct instruction with the individual (e.g., teach how to track markers of topic change), teaching a mature conversational partner strategies to assist the individual (e.g., illustrate ways of marking topic change more explicitly), and adaptation of the communication situation (e.g., offer communication opportunities in familiar settings with preferred topics). Some example skill areas to address follow.

Children and adults who have ASDs often miss subtle but critical cues in social interactions, particularly when additional layers of complexity are present. Typically functioning adults can point out salient aspects of communication situations that they use for interpreting messages that are implied, incongruous, or have missing or conflicting sources of information. Guiding a person with an ASD through the process of interpreting a message like this in context illustrates the process itself and eases high-level language comprehension (Wang et al., 2006).

In the studies surveyed here, children with ASDs often attempted to repair communication breakdowns but needed assistance in doing so. Adult conversational partners can offer explicit feedback to signal communication breakdowns in conversation and indicate how to complete the repair (e.g., "I don't know Sam. Who is Sam?"). When communication breakdowns can be repaired, conversations last longer. Having a conversational partner who can "encourage responsiveness to children's communicative attempts" is helpful (Meaden et al., 2006, p. 67).

Interactions that require drawing inferences about emotional reactions can prove challenging for individuals with ASDs. Individuals with ASDs may benefit from having a conversational partner make explicit statements about subtle emotional reactions that they did not notice or interpret correctly. Following a hierarchy of cues to which typical adults attend illustrates how they use verbal, nonverbal, and contextual cues to interpret messages within communicative interactions. An adult might point out something about a person, then offer normative information (i.e., what people usually experience in situations like this), and finally provide information about the physical or social situation (Gnepp, Klayman, & Trabasso, 1982). For example, an adult might explain a child's reaction to having to share a new toy at a family gathering to a young child with HFA or AS by walking him through these steps (i.e., noting the peer's facial expression, labeling the probable emotions, and stating in simple language why the peer finds the request difficult in this context).

As previously noted, task difficulty can be altered with changes to language and social demands, as well as demands in related areas (e.g., attention, executive function, memory, emotional sensory, motor). Decreases in demands present in related areas can ease children's difficulty in conquering tasks that are linguistically and socially challenging. Easing language and social demands can also give children more resources for tackling tasks that challenge them in other ways. Decreasing complexity in related areas may be useful when children are learning new strategies.

CONCLUSION

Individuals with HFA and AS have many strengths, including skills in structural aspects of language. Despite many good cog-

nitive and language skills, their difficulties with social language often surface as problems interpreting and using discourse level language skills. Difficulties in these areas persist over time but do respond to strategic intervention. This chapter has reviewed research regarding an individual's skill in understanding and using nonliteral language and conversational discourse and has discussed assessment and treatment practices. Future research will guide the evaluation of existing treatment paradigms and foster the development of new methods. With their relatively stronger cognitive and language skills, children and adolescents with HFA and AS are likely to receive good benefit from these treatment and research endeavors.

REFERENCES

Adams, C., Green, J., Gilchrest, A., & Cox, A. (2002). Conversational behavior of children with Asperger syndrome and conduct disorder. *Journal of Child Psychology and Psychiatry, 43,* 679–690.

American Psychiatric Association. (1994). *Diagnostic and statistical manual of mental disorders* (4th ed.). Washington, DC: Author.

Anzalone, M.E., & Williamson, G.G. (2000). Sensory processing and motor performance in autism spectrum disorders. In A.M. Wetherby & B.M. Prizant (Eds.), *Communication and language intervention series: Vol. 9. Autism spectrum disorders: A transactional developmental perspective* (pp. 143–166). Baltimore: Paul H. Brookes Publishing Co.

Baron-Cohen, S. (1989). The autistic child's theory of mind: A case of specific developmental delay. *Journal of Child Psychology and Psychiatry and Allied Disciplines, 30,* 285–297.

Baron-Cohen, S., Baldwin, D.A., & Crowson, M. (1997). Do children with autism use the speaker's direction of gaze strategy to crack the code of language? *Child Development, 68,* 48–57.

Barry, T., Grofer Klinger, L., Lee, J., Palardy, N., Gilmore, T., & Bodin, S.D. (2003). Examining the effectiveness of an outpatient clinic-based social skills group for high-functioning children with autism. *Journal of Autism and Developmental Disorders, 33,* 685–701.

Barton, B., & North, K. (2004). Social skills of children with neurofibromatosis type 1. *Developmental Medicine and Child Neurology, 46,* 553–563.

Bihrle, A.M., Brownell, H.H., Powelson, J.A., & Gardner, H. (1986). Comprehension of humorous and nonhumorous materials by left and right brain-damaged patients. *Brain and Cognition, 5,* 399–411.

Bishop, D.V.M. (1998). Development of the Children's Communication Checklist (CCC): A method for assessing qualitative aspects of communicative impairment in children. *Journal of Child Psychology and Psychiatry, 39,* 879–891.

Bloom, P. (2000). *How children learn the meanings of words.* Cambridge, MA: MIT Press.

Body, R., & Parker, M. (2005). Topic repetitiveness after traumatic brain injury: An emergent, jointly managed behaviour. *Clinical Linguistics and Phonetics, 19,* 379–392.

Brinton, B., & Fujiki, M. (1989). *Conversational management with language-impaired children: Pragmatic assessment and intervention.* Rockville, MD: Aspen Publications.

Brinton, B., Fujiki, M., Winkler, E., & Loeb, D. (1986). Responses to requests for clarification in linguistically normal and language-impaired children. *Journal of Speech and Hearing Disorders, 51,* 370–378.

Brown, G., & Yule, G. (1983). *Discourse analysis.* New York: Cambridge University Press.

Cain, K., & Oakhill, J.V. (1999). Inference making ability and its relation to comprehension failure in young children. *Reading and Writing, 11,* 489–503.

Chafe, W. (2001). The analysis of discourse flow. In D. Schiffrin, D. Tannen, & H.E. Hamilton (Eds.), *The handbook of discourse analysis* (pp. 673–687). Malden, MA: Blackwell Publishing.

Chapman, R.S. (1999). Language development in children and adolescents with Down syndrome. In J.F. Miller, M. Leddy, & L.A. Leavitt (Eds.), *Improving the communication of people with Down syndrome* (pp. 41–60). Baltimore: Paul H. Brookes Publishing Co.

Chapman, S.B., McKinnon, L., Levin, H.S., Song, J., Meier, M.C., & Chiu, S. (2001). Longitudinal outcome of verbal discourse in children with traumatic brain injury: Three-year follow-up. *Journal of Head Trauma Rehabilitation, 16,* 441–455.

Dennis, M., Lazenby, A.L., & Lockyer, L. (2001). Inferential language in high-functioning children with autism. *Journal of Autism and Developmental Disorders, 31,* 47–54.

de Villiers, J., Fine, J., Ginsberg, G., Vacarella, L., & Szatmari, P. (2006). Brief report: Scale for rating conversational impairment in autism spectrum disorder. *Journal of Autism and Developmental Disorders.* [ePub ahead of print] DOI: 10.1007/s10803-006-0264-1.

Dobbinson, S., Perkins, M.R., & Boucher, J. (1998). Structural patterns in conversations with a woman who has autism. *Journal of Communication Disorders, 31,* 113–134.

Emerich, D.M., Creaghead, N.A., Grether, S.M., Murray, D., & Grasha, C. (2003). The comprehension of humorous materials by adolescents with high-functioning autism and Asperger's syndrome. *Journal of Autism and Developmental Disorders, 33,* 253–257.

Ervin-Tripp, S., & Mitchell-Kernan, C. (1977). Introduction. In S. Ervin-Tripp & C. Mitchell-Kernan (Eds.), *Children's discourse. Language, thought, and culture: Advances in the study of cognition* (pp. 1–23). San Diego: Academic Press.

Ewing-Cobbs, L., Brookshire, B., Scott, M.A., & Fletcher, J.M. (1998). Children's narratives following traumatic brain injury: Linguistic structure, cohesion, and thematic recall. *Brain and Language, 61,* 395–419.

Flory, K., Milich, R., Lorch, E.P., Hayden, A.N., Strange, C., & Welsh, R. (2006). Online story comprehension among children with ADHD: Which core deficits are involved? *Journal of Abnormal Child Psychology, 34,* 853–865.

Garcia-Perez, R.M., Lee, A., & Hobson, R.P. (2006). On intersubjective engagement in autism: A controlled study of nonverbal aspects of conversation. *Journal of Autism and Developmental Disorders* [ePub ahead of print] DOI: 10.1007/s10803-006-0276-x.

Gnepp, J., Klayman, J., & Trabasso, T. (1982). A hierarchy of information sources for inferring emotional reactions. *Journal of Experimental Child Psychology, 33,* 111–123.

Golinkoff, R.M. (1986). I beg your pardon?: The preverbal negotiation of failed messages. *Child Language, 13,* 455–476.

Grice, P. (1975). Logic and conversation. In P. Cole & J. Morgan (Eds.), *Syntax and semantics: Speech acts* (pp. 41–58). San Diego: Academic Press.

Hale, C., & Tager-Flusberg, H. (2005). Brief report: The relationship between discourse deficits and autism symptomatology. *Journal of Autism and Developmental Disorders, 35*, 519–524.

Happe, F., & Frith, U. (2006). The Weak Coherence Account: Detail-focused cognitive style in autism spectrum disorders. *Journal of Autism and Developmental Disorders, 36*, 5–25.

Howlin, P. (2004). *Autism and Asperger syndrome: Preparing for adulthood* (2nd ed.). New York: Routledge.

Humphries, T., Koltun, H., Malone, M., & Roberts, W. (1994). Teacher-identified oral language difficulties among boys with attention problems. *Journal of Developmental Behavioral Pediatrics, 15*, 92–98.

Jackson, C.T., Fein, D., Wolf, J., Jones, G., Hauck, M., Waterhouse, L., et al. (2003). Responses and sustained interactions in children with mental retardation and autism. *Journal of Autism and Developmental Disorders, 33*, 115–121.

Jansiewicz, E.M., Goldberg, M.C., Newschaffer, C.J., Denckla, M.B., Landa, R., & Mostofsky, S.H. (2006). Motor signs distinguish children with high-functioning autism and Asperger's syndrome from controls. *Journal of Autism and Developmental Disorders, 36*, 613–621.

Johnstone, B. (2001). Discourse analysis and narrative. In D. Schiffrin, D. Tannen, & H.E. Hamilton (Eds.), *The handbook of discourse analysis* (pp. 635–649). Malden, MA: Blackwell Publishing.

Kanner, L. (1943). Autistic disturbances of affective content. *Nervous Child, 2*, 227–250.

Keen, D. (2004). The use of nonverbal repair strategies by children with autism. *Research in Developmental Disabilities, 26*, 243–254.

Kelley, E., Paul, J.J., Fein, D., & Naigles, L.R. (2006). Residual language deficits in optimal outcome children with a history of autism. *Journal of Autism and Developmental Disorders, 36*, 807–828.

Kenworthy, L.E., Black, D.O., Wallace, G.L., Ahluvalia, T., Wagner, A.E., & Sirian, L.M. (2005). Disorganization: The forgotten executive dysfunction in high-functioning autism (HFA) spectrum disorders. *Developmental Neuropsychology, 28*, 809–827.

Klin, A., Pauls, D., Schultz, R., & Volkmar, F. (2005). Three diagnostic approaches to Asperger syndrome: Implications for research.

Journal of Autism and Developmental Disorders, 35, 221–234.

Landa, R. (2000). Social language use in Asperger syndrome and high-functioning autism. In A. Klin, F. Volkmar, & S. Sparrow (Eds.), *Asperger syndrome* (pp. 125–158). New York: Guilford Press.

LeBlanc, L.A., Coates, A.M., Daneshvar, S., Charlop-Christy, H., Morris, C., & Lancaster, B.M. (2003). Using video modeling and reinforcement to teach perspective-taking skills to children with autism. *Journal of Applied Behavior Analysis, 36*, 253–257.

Levinson, S.C. (1983). *Pragmatics*. New York: Cambridge University Press.

Lord, C., Risi, S., Lambrect, L., Cook, Jr., E.H., Leventhal, B.L., DiLavore, P.C., et al. (2000). The Autism Diagnostic Observation Schedule–Generic: A standard measure of social and communication deficits associated with the spectrum of autism. *Journal of Autism and Developmental Disorders, 30*(3), 205–223.

Lord, C., Rutter, M., Goode, S., Heemsbergen, J., Jordan, H., Mawhood, L., et al. (1989). Autism Diagnostic Observation Schedule: A standardized observation of communicative and social behaviour. *Journal of Autism and Developmental Disorders, 19*, 185–212.

Loveland, K.A., Fletcher, J.M., & Bailey, V. (1990). Verbal and nonverbal communication of events in learning-disability subtypes. *Journal of Clinical Experimental Neuropsychology, 12*, 433–447.

Lyons, V., & Fitzgerald, M. (2004). Humor in autism and Asperger syndrome. *Journal of Autism and Developmental Disorders, 34*, 521–531.

Martin, I., & McDonald, S. (2004). An exploration of causes of nonliteral language problems in individuals with Asperger syndrome. *Journal of Autism and Developmental Disorders, 43*, 311–328.

McDonald, S. (1993). Pragmatic language skills after closed head injury: Ability to meet the informational needs of the listener. *Brain and Language, 44*, 28–46.

McTear, M. (1985). *Children's conversations*. New York: Basil Blackwell.

Meaden, H., Halle, J.W., Watkins, R.V., & Chadsey, J.G. (2006). Examining communication repairs of two young children with autism spectrum disorder: The influence of environment. *American Journal of Speech-Language Pathology, 15,* 57–71.

Miller, C.A. (2006). Developmental relationships between language and theory of mind. *American Journal of Speech-Language Pathology, 15,* 142–154.

Minshew, N.J., Goldstein, G., & Siegel, D.J. (1997). Neuropsychological functioning in autism: Profile of a complex information processing disorder. *Journal of the International Neuropsychological Society, 3,* 303–316.

Muller, E., & Schuler, A. (2006). Verbal marking of affect by children with Asperger Syndrome and high functioning autism during spontaneous interactions with family members. *Journal of Autism and Developmental Disorders, 36,* 1089–1100.

Nelson, N.W. (1993). *Childhood language disorders in context: Infancy through adolescence.* New York: Macmillan.

Nikopoulos, C., & Keenan, M. (2007). Using video modeling to teach complex social sequences to children with autism. *Journal of Autism and Developmental Disorders, 37,* 678–693.

Nippold, M.A., & Duthie, J.K. (2003). Mental imagery and idiom comprehension: A comparison of school-age children and adults. *Journal of Speech, Language, and Hearing Research, 46,* 788–799.

Nippold, M.A., & Rudzinski, M. (1993). Familiarity and transparency in idiom explanation: A developmental study of children and adolescents. *Journal of Speech and Hearing Research, 36,* 728–737.

Norbury, C.F. (2004). Factors supporting idiom comprehension in children with communication disorders. *Journal of Speech, Language, and Hearing Disorders, 47,* 1179–1193.

Norbury, C.F., & Bishop, D.V.M. (2002). Inferential processing and story recall in children with communication problems: A comparison of specific language impairment, pragmatic language impairment, and high-functioning autism. *International Journal of Language and Communication Disorders, 37,* 227–251.

O'Malley, K.D., & Nanson, J. (2002). Clinical implications of a link between fetal alcohol spectrum disorder and attention-deficit/hyperactivity disorder. *Canadian Journal of Psychiatry, 47,* 349–354.

Ozonoff, S., & Miller, J. (1996). An exploration of right hemisphere contributions to the pragmatic impairments of autism. *Brain and Language, 52,* 411–434.

Pennington, L., Goldbart, J., & Marshall, J. (2004). Interaction training for conversational partners of children with cerebral palsy: A systematic review. *International Journal of Language and Communication Disorders, 39,* 151–170.

Pinker, S. (1999). *Words and rules: The ingredients of language.* New York: HarperCollins.

Preissler, M.A., & Carey, S. (2005). The role of inferences about referential intent in word learning: Evidence from autism. *Cognition, 97,* B13–B23.

Reddy, V., Williams, E., & Vaughan, A. (2002). Sharing humor and laughter in autism and Down's syndrome. *British Journal of Psychology, 93,* 219–242.

Rogers, S.J. (2000). Interventions that facilitate socialization in children with autism. *Journal of Autism and Developmental Disorders, 30,* 399–409.

Rutter, M., LeCouteur, A., & Lord, C. (2003) *Autism Diagnostic Interview–Revised (ADI-R).* Los Angeles: Western Psychological Services.

Scattone, D., Tingstrom, D., & Wilczynski, S. (2006). Increasing appropriate social interactions of children with autism spectrum disorders using Social Stories™. *Focus on Autism and Other Developmental Disabilities, 21*(4), 211–222.

Schiffrin, D., Tannen, D., & Hamilton, H.E. (2001). Introduction. In D. Schiffrin, D. Tannen, & H.E. Hamilton (Eds.), *The handbook of discourse analysis* (pp. 1–10). New York: Blackwell Publishing.

Seltzer, M.M., Shattuck, P., Abbeduto, L., & Greenberg, J.S. (2004). Trajectory of development in adolescents and adults with autism. *Mental Retardation and Developmental Disabilities Research Reviews, 10,* 234–247.

Shammi, P., & Stuss, D.T. (1999). Humour appreciation: A role of the right frontal lobe. *Brain, 122,* 657–666.

Sigman, M. (1994). What are the core deficits in autism? In S.H. Broman & J. Grafman (Eds.), *Atypical cognitive deficits in developmental disorders: Implications for brain function* (pp. 139–157). Mahwah, NJ: Lawrence Erlbaum Associates.

Suls, J.M. (1972). A two-stage model for the appreciation of jokes and cartoons: An information processing analysis. In J.H. Goldstein & P.H. McGhee (Eds.), *The psychology of humor: Theoretical perspectives and empirical issues* (pp. 81–100). San Diego: Academic Press.

Tager-Flusberg, H. (1981). On the nature of linguistic functioning in early infantile autism. *Journal of Autism and Developmental Disorders, 11,* 45–56.

Thurber, C., & Tager-Flusberg, H. (1993). Pauses in narratives produced by autistic, mentally retarded, and normal children as an index of cognitive demand. *Journal of Autism and Developmental Disorders, 23*(2), 309–322.

Turkstra, L. (2001). Partner effects in adolescent conversations. *Journal of Communication Disorders, 34,* 151–162.

Turkstra, L., Ciccia, A., & Seaton, C. (2003). Interactive behaviors in adolescent conversation dyads. *Language, Speech, and Hearing Services in Schools, 34,* 117–127.

Vallance, D.D., & Wintre, M.G. (1997). Discourse processes underlying social competence in children with language learning disabilities. *Developmental Psychopathology, 9,* 95–108.

Volden, J. (2004). Conversational repair in speakers with autism spectrum disorder. *International Journal of Language and Communication Disorders, 39,* 171–189.

Volden, J., & Johnston, J. (1999). Cognitive scripts in autistic children and adolescents. *Journal of Autism and Developmental Disorders, 29,* 203–211.

Volden, J., Magill-Evans, J., Goulden, K., & Clarke, M. (2006). Varying language register according to listener needs in speakers with autism spectrum disorders. *Journal of Autism and Developmental Disorders* [ePub ahead of print]. DOI 10.1007/s10803-006-0256-1.

Volkmar, F., Klin, A., Schultz, R., Bronen, R., Maranas, W., Sparrow, S., et al. (1996). Grand rounds: Asperger syndrome. *Journal of the American Academy of Child and Adolescent Psychiatry, 35,* 118–123.

Volkmar, F., Klin, A., Schultz, R., Rubin, E., & Bronen, R. (2000). Clinical case conference: Asperger's disorder. *American Journal of Psychiatry, 157,* 262–267.

Volkmar, F.R., Klin, A., Siegel, B., Szatmari, P., Lord, C., Campbell, M., et al. (1994). Field trial for autistic disorder I *DSM-IV. American Journal of Psychiatry, 151,* 1361–1367.

Volkmar, F.R., Lord, C., Bailey, A., Schultz, R.T., & Klin, A. (2004). Autism and pervasive developmental disorders. *Journal of Child Psychology and Psychiatry, 45,* 135–170.

Walker, D.R., Thompson, A., Zwaigenbaum, L., Goldberg, J., Bryson, S.E., Mahoney, W.J., et al. (2004). Specifying PDD-NOS: A comparison of PDD-NOS, Asperger syndrome, and autism. *Journal of the American Academy of Child and Adolescent Psychiatry, 43,* 172–180.

Wang, A.T., Lee, S.S., Sigman, M., & Dapretto, M. (2006). Neural basis of irony comprehension in children with autism: The role of prosody and context. *Brain, 129,* 932–943.

White, S.W., Keonig, K., & Scahill, L. (2006). Social skills development in children with autism spectrum disorders: A review of the intervention research. *Journal of Autism and Developmental Disorders* [ePub before print]. DOI 10.1007/s10803-006-0320-x.

Wiig, E., & Secord, W. (1985). *Test of Language Competence–Extended edition technical manual.* San Antonio, TX: Psychological Corporation.

World Health Organization. (1994). *International Classification of Diseases, tenth revision (ICD-10).* Geneva: Author.

7

Autism Spectrum Disorders in the First 3 Years of Life

Rebecca Landa

Autism spectrum disorders (ASDs), including autism, pervasive developmental disorder-not otherwise specified (PDD-NOS), and Asperger syndrome, are a class of neurodevelopmental disorders characterized by social and communication impairments, often accompanied by patterns of restricted interests and stereotyped behaviors (American Psychiatric Association [APA], 1994). Development must be disrupted by the third birthday to qualify for an ASD diagnosis. ASDs are usually diagnosed between 3 and 6 years of age (Mandell, Novak, & Zubritsky, 2005; Rice, 2007). Although there are no diagnostic criteria for ASDs for children younger than 36 months, detection of ASDs before this age is possible (Charman et al., 2005; Landa, Holman, & Garrett-Mayer, 2007; Lord, 1995; Stone et al., 1999).

ASDs are usually diagnosed considerably later than the age at which parents first recognize disrupted development in their children (i.e., an average of 2 years, as reviewed by Gray & Tonge, 2001) or the age of first evaluation by a qualified professional (i.e., an average delay of 13 months) (Wiggins, Baio, & Rice, 2006). A major emphasis has been placed on diagnosing ASDs earlier in life. In response to the call for earlier detection, evidence-based information about the early signs of ASDs has become widely available to the public (Centers for Disease Control and Prevention, n.d.). In addition, an ASD toolkit (American Acad-

emy of Pediatrics, 2007) is available to pediatricians and other health care providers, summarizing the literature on early signs of ASDs, as well as providing information about ASD screeners and referral information. This chapter reviews the current information available about the early signs of ASDs.

WHY DETECT AUTISM SPECTRUM DISORDERS EARLY IN LIFE?

The impetus for earlier detection of ASDs stems from several factors. First, the retrospective literature converges with the prospective literature on young children with ASDs, indicating that developmental disruption occurs prior to the third birthday, sometimes in the first year of life. Second, studies focusing on neurobiological mechanisms of ASDs (Bailey et al., 1998; Bauman & Kemper, 2005; Chugani, 2002; Courchesne, Carper, & Aksoomoff, 2003; Nelson et al., 2006; Rodier, Ingram, Risdale, Nelson, & Romano, 1996) have provided compelling evidence that the neurobiological underpinnings of atypical brain development in ASDs begins very early in life, possibly even during fetal life, but behavioral manifestation of such impairment may not be detected until later. Third, the neuroscience literature has revealed that experience affects brain development and that the impact of experience is greater for some aspects of brain development and functioning (i.e., experience-dependent neuroplasticity) (Sanders, Weber-Fox, & Neville, in press; Stevens & Neville, 2006). This phenomenon, in combination with evidence that children with ASDs benefit from early intervention (Kasari, Freeman, & Paparella, 2006; Landa & Holman, 2005; Rogers & Lewis, 1989; Smith, Groen, & Wynn, 2000), is the major motivation for detecting and beginning treatment for ASDs as early in life as possible.

EARLY CHARACTERISTICS OF AUTISM SPECTRUM DISORDERS

Two research approaches have been employed in an effort to characterize the features of ASDs in the first 3 years of life. One approach has been to utilize retrospective material such as parent recall and analysis of home videos made before the ASD diagnosis. Both types of retrospective studies indicate that signs of developmental disruption occur as early as the first year of life, although for some children this may occur later (Baghdadli, Picot, Pascal, Pry, & Aussilloux, 2003; De Giacomo & Fombonne, 1998; Gray & Tonge, 2001). The mean age at which parents report concerns to a professional is 18–24 months (De Giacomo & Fombonne, 1998; Rogers & DiLalla, 1990; Young, Brewer, & Pattison, 2003). The retrospective literature suggests that multiple developmental systems may be disrupted early in the lives of children with ASDs, affecting one or more of the following domains: perceptual/sensory; motor; social; and communication (reviewed by Charman et al., 2000; Palomo, Belinchon, & Ozonoff, 2006; Young, Brewer, & Pattison, 2003).

Another approach to understanding the early features of ASDs has involved prospective examination of children at risk for ASD diagnoses. Studies involving these approaches have involved children identified through screenings and clinical referrals, as well as children who are at high genetic risk for ASDs (i.e., having an older sibling with an ASD, as ASDs and milder variants are heritable) (Bailey et al., 1995; Folstein et al., 1999; Landa & Garrett-Mayer, 2006).

The prospective literature involving infant siblings of children with autism (AU sibs) is beginning to show that, as a group, 6-month-old AU sibs may show subtle differences compared with age-matched low-risk controls, but the implications of these differences for later diagnostic outcome or level of functioning are not yet known. In this chapter, evidence from the retrospective and prospective literatures is used to characterize what is currently known about the early emergence of ASDs from infancy.

Perceptual and Sensory

The literature on this aspect of development is quite small and comes from retrospective studies. It indicates an early tendency for infants to engage in unusual visual inspection of objects before the first birthday (Baranek, 1999), to have dysregulated sleep and disruptions in other regulatory functions (Dahlgren & Gillberg, 1989), and to exhibit unusual sensory responses (Dahlgren & Gillberg, 1989).

Motor

Evidence for early disruption in the motor system is emerging in infants at high risk for ASDs. For example, Iverson and Wozniak (2007) found that infant AU sibs, who had not yet reached the age at which a diagnostic classification can be established, showed delays in acquisition of motor milestones, had less stable posture, and displayed attenuation in limb movements at the time of babble onset compared with low-risk controls. In addition, data from our lab showed a variety of subtle motor differences at 6 months of age in AU sibs diagnosed with ASDs or milder language and social impairments at 36 months of age compared with low-risk controls and unimpaired AU sibs (Flanagan & Landa, 2007). These differences included problems with motor coordination, low muscle tone, passivity, and atypical patterns of motor behavior. Some of the AU sibs also showed motor delays (Flanagan & Landa, 2007), as was reported by Iverson and Wozniak (2007). These motor features are not expected to be specific to children later diagnosed with ASDs, but their presence represents a risk for later impairment (Flanagan & Landa, 2007). Atypical motor behaviors including posturing, repetitive motor behaviors (i.e., with and without objects), and excessive mouthing have also been reported in numerous retrospective studies of children with ASDs. Infants later diagnosed with ASDs showed decreased flexibility, variety, and appropriateness of play with objects or in gesture production (Colgan et al., 2006) compared with infants later diagnosed with intellectual disability (ID) based on retrospective videotape analysis. These symptoms could be related to disrupted motor functions.

Social

Deficits in social orienting, joint attention, imitation, and affective engagement are considered central to ASDs, resulting in impaired interpersonal synchrony in the first 2 years of life (Baranek, 1999; Charman et al., 2000; Dawson et al., 2004; Iverson & Wozniak, 2007; Landa et al., 2007; Maestro et al., 2001; Maestro et al., 2002; Sullivan et al., 2007). Impairment in social orienting and joint attention (e.g., pointing, showing objects, looking at others, orienting to name) appear to be an important early marker of autism. Joint attention impairment correctly identified 10 of 11 12-month-olds later diagnosed as having ASDs (videotape analysis; Osterling & Dawson, 1994). In a prospective study, infrequent or absent response to others' joint attention cues predicted outcomes

of ASDs in 14-month-olds having an older sibling with autism (Sullivan et al., 2007). Similarly, in a longitudinal study of 2-year-olds referred due to concerns about ASDs, the failure to direct others' attention at age 2 correctly predicted diagnostic classification (i.e., having an ASD versus not having an ASD) when these children were seen for a follow-up evaluation at 3 years of age (Lord, 1995). Imitation, socioemotional reciprocity, and affective expressions have also been reported as diminished or atypical in toddlers with ASD according to findings from retrospective studies (Baranek, 1999) and prospective studies (Landa et al.,2007; Stone et al., 1999). Imitation difficulties have distinguished children with ASDs from those with non–ASD developmental delay as early as age 2 (Charman et al., 1997; Stone, Ousley, & Littleford, 1997). Expression of affect also differentiates young children with ASDs or at risk for ASDs from other groups, and is characterized by an overall attenuation in affective expression, the presence of ambiguous affective expression, and increased levels of negative affect (Adrien et al, 1991; Cassel et al., 2007; Landa et al., 2007; Yirmiya et al., 2006).

Communication

Communication impairments begin in infancy in AU sibs (Iverson & Wozniak, 2007), with disruption in babbling (Iverson & Wozniak, 2007), gesture (Colgan et al., 2006; Landa et al., 2007), language (Landa & Garrett-Mayer, 2006; Landa et al., 2007; Mitchell et al., 2006; Yirmiya et al., 2006; Zwaigenbaum et al., 2005), and social communication development (Goldberg et al., 2005; Landa et al., 2007) measurable by 12–17 months of age (Landa & Garrett-Mayer, 2006; Landa et al., 2007; Mitchell et al., 2006).

Communicative behaviors that distinguish ASDs from language disorders, developmental delays, and/or typical development in children over the age of

2 years include the initiation of social communication, the rate of communication, gestural communication, repair strategies, gaze shifts, language comprehension, and symbolic play (Wetherby, Prizant, & Hutchinson, 1998). Nonverbal social-communicative behaviors and delayed onset of speech were diagnostic characteristics of ASDs between 2 and 3 years of age (Stone et al., 1999). Higher language scores and comprehension of a few words in context at 2 years of age indicated a better outcome prognosis at 5 years of age for children with ASDs (Lord, Rutter, DiLavore, & Risi, 1999).

A restricted range of communicative forms is characteristic of young children with ASDs as indicated by undue reliance on the manipulation of others' hands, and decreased pointing and showing (McEvoy, Rogers, & Pennington, 1993; Mundy, Sigman, & Kasari, 1994; Stone et al., 1997). For the first time, this has been documented prospectively in children with ASDs (Landa et al., 2007). A reduced variety of nonverbal (i.e., gestures) and vocal (i.e., consonants in syllables) communicative forms distinguished 14-month-olds diagnosed at that age with ASDs from children with typical development (Landa et al., 2007).

Integration of communication form with gaze and affect is also impaired in the first 3 years of life in children with ASDs. Gestures tend to be isolated acts, less often integrated with vocalization than in children with typical prelinguistic development (Wetherby & Prizant, 1989). Initiation of social communicative acts (e.g., showing, initiating joint attention), which requires integrated attention to social and nonsocial aspects of context, is impaired relative to requesting (i.e., a nonsocial use of communication) in 2- and 3-year-old children with ASDs (Baron-Cohen, 1989; Loveland & Landry, 1986; McEvoy, Rogers, & Pennington, 1993; Mundy, Sigman, & Kasari, 1990; Sigman, Mundy, Sherman, & Ungerer, 1986; Stone et al., 1997; Wetherby et al., 1998)

Patterns of Onset and Progression of Autism Spectrum Disorders

The literature and the observation of infant AU sibs within Kennedy Krieger's autism research program have afforded insights into the patterns of onset and progression of ASDs throughout the first 3 years of life. Our prospective longitudinal research program enrolled infants at low risk for ASDs (i.e., no family history of ASD) and infant siblings of children with idiopathic autism (i.e., AU sibs). AU sibs are at increased genetic risk for ASDs and a range of milder but conceptually similar impairments known as the broader autism phenotype (BAP) (Bailey et al., 1995; Landa & Garrett-Mayer, 2006). Children entered the study at 6 or 14 months of age and were assessed at 6-month intervals until they were 36 months of age. In some infants, signs of atypical development were clearly present by 6 months of age. These signs varied from child to child, including such symptoms as gaze aversion, infrequent vocalization, delays in babbling, a decreased variety of vocalizations, attenuated affect displays, difficulty disengaging attention, immature patterns of motor coordination, hypotonicity, an overall passivity toward people and objects, reduced levels of social orientation and reciprocity within social exchanges, decreased social endurance (i.e., brief attention within an engagement), atypical movement patterns, and a decreased frequency of integration of gaze + vocalization + smiling (Bhat, Rusyniak, & Landa, 2007; Flanagan & Landa, 2007). Another sign of developmental disruption in infant AU sibs involves reduced integration of rhythmic limb movement with vocalization (Iverson & Wozniak, 2007). Prospective research is needed to determine whether the impairments observed at such a young age are specific to ASDs. Our data indicate that these early signs of developmental disruption are usually rather subtle and may go unnoticed, particularly by professionals who lack expertise with infant development. The developmental disruption in the 6-month-old AU sibs in our program was most observable within novel triadic (i.e., object–child–person) contexts as opposed to familiar dyadic caregiver–child routines. However, some infants displayed multiple signs of clinically significant developmental disruption that were obviously atypical. Although it is unlikely that anyone would diagnose a 6-month-old infant with an ASD, such clear signs of developmental disruption would warrant assessment by a physician and an expert in infant development (usually a clinical psychologist or speech-language pathologist). With age, there may be increasing divergence from expected developmental patterns and timing.

In some children, signs of ASDs may be sufficiently apparent by 14 months of age that a diagnosis of ASD could be made by expert clinicians at that time (Landa et al., 2007). For most of the children in our research program diagnosed at 14 months, the ASD diagnoses were stable through 36 months. There were multiple behavioral indicators of ASDs in these young children, but the nature of these indicators varied from child to child. Social and communication indicators were always present, even in children whose language milestones were met within the expected timeframe. Social orienting and social initiation were usually impaired, as was social reciprocity. These children rarely spontaneously smiled at others, infrequently attempted to communicate, even to obtain a desired object or action, and showed a reduced variety of consonants in syllables and gestures during communicative acts. Nevertheless, they sometimes responded to favorite songs and rhymes, tickle games, and Peekaboo games, although often in a less immediate and robust way. Their initiation within these routines was usually diminished. They occasionally showed affection to their parents. Thus, they did not completely lack social and communicative skills or related-

ness. Social engagement was attainable under less diverse circumstances, more difficult to establish, and more difficult to sustain than in children with typical development or children with non–ASD language delays. Furthermore, the coordination of behaviors across developmental domains (e.g., look + smile + gesture or vocalization) was particularly infrequent. In addition, it was found that young children with ASDs were more inconsistent than children without ASDs in their display of skills, and this inconsistency (i.e., instability of skill) lasted for an unusually protracted window of development (Sullivan et al., 2007). This suggests the possibility that young children with ASDs acquire skills in a different fashion and require a longer time to do so than children with typical development.

Our data indicate that ASDs have a progressive nature, beginning in infancy. This progression is particularly robust between 14 and 36 months of age, where the pace of development decelerated, plateaued, or revealed a loss of skills (Landa et al., 2007), and atypical behavioral features associated with ASDs (e.g., echolalia, odd intonational contour, stereotyped patterns of behavior) appeared or increased. In other infants later diagnosed with an ASD, development appeared to be only mildly impaired or, less often, within the typical range until sometime later in the second or third year of life, when social and communication patterns associated with ASDs began to appear. The expert clinicians did not diagnose these children with ASDs at the 14-month-old assessment. Careful examination of the frequency and diversity of their social, communicative, and play behavior at 14 months of age indicated that they did not differ from children in the non–ASD groups (Landa et al., 2007). Signs of ASDs emerged gradually in these later diagnosed children.

The developmental pattern observed in some of the participants with ASDs outcomes was similar to the pattern described in the retrospective literature as regression.

The literature indicates that 10%–50% of children with ASDs reportedly have developmental regression at the mean age 18–24 months (Hoshino et al., 1987; Tuchman & Rapin, 1997). In 20%–40% of cases, there is a reported loss of language skills (Kurita, 1985; Rutter & Lord, 1987). Retrospective work indicates that language regression in ASDs does not reduce prognosis for later language acquisition (Goldberg et al., 2003). The implications of regression for language outcome and stability of diagnoses of ASDs are unknown.

With age, the prominence of some types of impairments may overshadow others, and new characteristics may emerge (e.g., stereotyped patterns of behavior). Early patterns of motor discoordination and delays in babbling may give way to difficulties with imitation and late onset of speech. Furthermore, delays in imitation and speech may become less concerning to family members than the child's failure to orient to their social bids or initiate social interaction.

CLINICAL APPLICATIONS

The previously summarized research has important implications for clinical practice. Practical clinical considerations pertaining to early detection, diagnosis, and intervention are discussed next.

Screening

Given the prevalence of ASDs (Fombonne, 2005; Rice, 2007), evidence that signs of ASDs are usually present during the first 2 years of life, and the importance of early intervention, screening for ASDs during the first 2 years is essential (Filipek et al., 1999). Screening may be a multiphase process, particularly for children at high risk for developmental delay. The process begins with the use of a brief assessment completed by a caregiver or professional. Screening measures are usually quite brief and require

little time or training to complete. Most available screening instruments were initially designed to identify delay in general, rather than ASDs per se; however, a few ASD-specific screeners do exist. Some of the general screening tools available for children younger than 36 months of age that have strong psychometric properties include the Ages & Stages Questionnaires® (ASQ), Second Edition (Bricker & Squires, 1999), Brigance Screens (Brigance, 1985; Glascoe, 1996), Child Development Inventories (CDIs; Ireton, 1992; Ireton & Glascoe, 1995), the Infant/Toddler Checklist from the Communication and Symbolic Behavior Scales Developmental Profile (CSBS DP™; Wetherby & Prizant, 2002), and the Parents' Evaluation of Developmental Status (PEDS; (Glascoe, 2006). Some of the ASD-specific screeners include the Modified Checklist for Autism in Toddlers (M-CHAT; Robins, Fein, Barton, & Green, 2001), the Pervasive Developmental Disorders Screening Test–Stage 1 (PDDST; Siegel, 1998; Siegel & Hayer, 1999), and the Screening Tool for Autism in Two-Year-Olds (STAT; Stone & Ousley, 1997; Stone, Coonrod, & Ousley, 2000). The result of screening is not diagnosis, but an indication of whether further screening, assessment, or surveillance is appropriate. Evidence from research indicates that screening should be conducted repeatedly at least through the third birthday for children at high genetic risk for ASDs (Landa et al., 2007), and the American Academy of Pediatrics now recommends screening twice in the second year of life (first at 18 months, and again at 24 months) (Johnson, Myers, & the Council on Children with Disabilities, 2007). A brief follow-up telephone call with parents of children who fail an autism screen greatly reduces false positive rates (Kleinman et al., 2007). When the results of developmental screening are negative but concerns about the child's development linger for parents or professionals, a referral for Level 2 screening or assessment should be made.

Diagnostic Considerations

This section briefly discusses issues related to the assessment of children younger than 3 years of age. A concept that should be borne in mind is that ASDs involve the manifestation of multiple signs of developmental disruption. In the first year of life, these may not necessarily affect social behavior.

For Children Younger than 12 Months of Age

When children are younger than 12 months of age, a diagnosis of ASD is not advisable given the state of the science. The amount of variation in typical development is considerable at this age, and signs of ASDs may be quite subtle and unstable. Furthermore, there is insufficient knowledge about the specificity of behavioral characteristics to ASDs in the first year of life. There are, however, indicators that a child should be closely monitored for ASDs, and when present in sufficient number or intensity, these indicators may warrant intervention. Red flags associated with ASDs in infants may include gaze avoidance, infrequent and brief gazing at others' faces, infrequent and immature babbling, unusually high-pitched squealing, an infrequent reciprocal social smile, infrequent to no babbling, babbling not used in social engagement, passivity with objects, unusual posturing or repetitive behaviors, a lack of alternating gaze between a novel object and caregiver, and low social anticipation. Other nonspecific signs of developmental disruption that may be associated with ASDs in the first year of life have been previously reviewed (e.g., involving the motor system). In our research program, it was found that these signs are most observable in novel tasks in which an infant's cognitive system is challenged (Bhat, Rusyniak, & Landa, 2007), rather than in highly familiar, predictable contexts in which the child must pay attention to only one major stimulus (e.g., a caregiver in a Peekaboo game).

For Children Between 12 and 36 Months of Age

Considerable expertise is needed to formulate diagnostic judgments of ASDs in toddlers. Experience is needed with toddlers with typical development, those with non–ASD delays, and those with ASDs in general. Such a range of experience is necessary due to the variation in typical development at very young ages and because the quality of behavior associated with ASDs in toddlers is usually not as strikingly atypical as it is in older children. For example, there is not usually a lack of social engagement, affect sharing, communicative initiation, turn taking, or play with objects. Rather, the characteristics of ASDs in toddlers often present themselves as an order of magnitude away from typical development where social responsivity is more difficult to elicit and maintain, affect is more attenuated and less often directed to others through gaze, spontaneous imitation occurs during less socially salient contexts and is less often connected via gaze, communicative forms are less diverse, and integration of affect, gaze, and communication occurs much less frequently. These features can be missed or all too readily dismissed because the child walked at the expected age, currently plays with toys, although often in subtly atypical, less diverse, or less imaginative ways, attempts to make needs known for highly preferred items, laughs when tickled, and even responds to highly familiar social routines such as a game of Peekaboo or a favorite song. Videotapes are available for the public to view that will help hone the watchful eyes of parents and physicians to perceive ASD–related qualities of social and communication engagement so that the very early signs of ASDs may be detected (Autism Speaks, n.d.).

Evaluation

The evaluation to rule out an ASD should consist of a thorough developmental, medical, and family history interview. This will yield valuable information about the possibility of regression, plateaued or delayed development, and the presence of sensory (e.g., hearing, vision) impairments that may contribute to the behavioral patterns that gave rise to concern. Risk for some genetic or heritable disorders (e.g., fragile X, autism) will be at least preliminarily defined, as will possible sources of pain (e.g., gastrointestinal reflux) that may be related to atypical behaviors (e.g., repetitive behaviors as in Sandifer syndrome) (Gorrotxategi et al., 1995; Werlin et al., 1980). Information should be obtained about contexts in which the child is most affectively animated, socially attentive and engaged, attentive to objects, likely to initiate communication or social interaction, and so forth. In addition, information about the child's responses to such things as strangers, sounds, and different food textures should be elicited from the parents.

Developmental assessments of young children should include measures of social and communication behavior. If indicated, clinicians must adequately sample the range of behaviors associated with ASDs. Several instruments directly administered to children are available for use in this regard. Perhaps the two most commonly used are the Autism Diagnostic Observation Schedule (ADOS; Lord, Rutter, DiLavore, & Risi, 1999) and the CSBS DP™ (Wetherby & Prizant, 2002). The ADOS will soon have a module for prelinguistic children as young as 12 months of age (Lord, personal communication, July 2006). In its current form, the ADOS module 1 may be used with children as young as 18 months of age. Although this instrument does not provide developmental norms, it does provide an algorithm with cut-off scores for ASDs based on social and communication behavior ratings. These ratings are made by the clinician based on the child's behavior during a semistructured play-based assessment in which there are a variety of presses for relevant social, communication, and play behaviors. The CSBS

DP™ is a clinician-administered assessment of communication, social, and play behavior that is normed for children aged 8–24 months of age. The assessment involves a presentation of communicative temptations, probes for receptive language, and the elicitation of a play sample. Three composite scores are generated (i.e., Social Communication, Expressive Speech and Language, and Symbolic Abilities). Although there are no guidelines for ASD diagnosis associated with the CSBS DP™, the behavior sampling procedures enable clinicians to observe qualitative and quantitative aspects of social communicative behavior and to note the presence of atypical behavior. Elicitation of parents' observations and perspectives about their children's behavior during the assessment session, as well as their children's developmental status, is essential. Such information may be gained through a formal interview such as the Autism Diagnostic Interview–Revised (ADI-R; Lord, Rutter, & LeCouteur, 1994), which is best used when a child's mental age is at least 18 months (Lord, Storoschuk, Rutter, & Pickles, 1993).

Several measurement instruments that are not ASD specific are also mentioned here because they are not commonly known but may provide useful information in the assessment of very young children when there are concerns about possible ASD diagnoses. One such tool completed by parents or through an interview given by a professional is the Language Use Inventory for Young Children (O'Neill, 2002; O'Neill & Jones, 1997). This measure, normed for children aged 18–47 months of age, is a measure of pragmatic language development. It consists of three scales that collectively gather information pertaining to children's use of communicative forms to express communicative intention (e.g., speech acts), production of conversational repairs, discourse management strategies, use of deictic markers, use of cohesive devices, and use of contextually appropriate language. Thus, this instrument provides information about social communicative behavior from the parents' perspective, which is often difficult to obtain in most assessment sessions. Another useful tool is the Sensory Experiences Questionnaire (SEQ; Baranek, 1999; Baranek, David, Poe, Stone, & Watson, 2006), which is normed for children from ages 6 months to 6 years. This caregiver-completed instrument gathers information regarding frequencies of the child's unusual sensory reactions across all sensory modalities, response patterns (i.e., hyper- and hyporesponsiveness), and parents' strategies to change these unusual sensory features in their children. This information is relevant because children with ASDs often exhibit atypical sensory behavior that may not be evident or may be difficult to interpret in the course of a single assessment session. In addition, a measure of general development, such as the Mullen Scales of Early Learning (Mullen, 1995), should be given if there are concerns about ASDs.

Outcome of Autism Spectrum Disorder Assessment for Children 12–36 Months of Age

In some cases, the signs of ASDs are unmistakable, being present in classical form and consistent across contexts. Indeed, several studies have indicated that an ASD diagnosis can be made in the second year of life (Charman et al., 2000; Chawarska, Klin, Paul, & Volkmar, 2007; Landa et al., 2007), even as young as 14 months of age (Landa et al., 2007). Diagnoses of ASDs in 1-year-olds are stable in most children, but stability of an ASD diagnosis increases after 30 months of age, at least through the third birthday (Chawarska et al., 2007; Landa, Cleary, & Holman, 2005). In very young children, ASDs are often accompanied by language or cognitive delays. In other cases, no signs of ASDs are observed or can be identified in the parents' history of their children's development, even when there are delays in language or cognitive development. In such cases, children are socially oriented, showing interest in others and reciprocating their bids. They monitor the actions and attention of others, are sensitive and responsive to facial expressions of emotion in others, spontaneously imitate in playful and socially connected ways, and play in developmentally appropriate ways with toys. There are also cases in which the results of the diagnostic assessment are mixed. A child may show signs of disruption in social development, but these may not be conceptually relevant to ASDs. One example would be a child with an extreme temperament or high levels of anxiety. Alternatively, the child may show some of the signs associated with ASDs, but these may be inconsistent, contextually specific, few in number, or mild in quality. One situation that occasionally arises involves a child who exhibits repetitive interests and/or stereotypic behaviors with or without a language delay, but his or her social interaction appears to be generally within normal limits. Finally, a child may show signs indicative of ASDs in the clinical assessment, but the parents report that the child does not show these signs elsewhere. Guidelines for follow-up have been suggested by Johnson and colleagues (2007).

Clinical judgments about the presence of ASDs are made based on all available information, including standardized developmental assessments (e.g., general development, nonverbal cognitive language and communication, motor), sensory assessments (e.g., vision, hearing), ASD-specific assessment, parent report of developmental history, adaptive functioning, and current behavior. Clinicians should systematically identify the nature of observed developmental disruption and their level of confidence in the diagnosis—or lack thereof—of an ASD. (Figure 7.1 presents a checklist for doing so; see also Appendix A at the end of this chapter for a photocopiable version.) If a clinician does not have extensive experience with ASDs in general or with ASDs in toddlers, a referral to an expert is warranted to ensure that parents are given accurate information about their child's development and diagnosis.

Clinical Impressions

Child's name _____

Date of birth _____ Date of exam _____

Examiner's name _____

0	1	2	3
No delay	**Concern**	**Mild delay**	**Significant delay**
The child appears to be developing typically based on test scores and clinical judgment.	Monitor the child, but at this time there is insufficient evidence to code as impaired or delayed.	Test scores and/or clinical judgment indicate that the child is mildly delayed.	Test scores and clinical judgment indicate a definite and clinically significant delay.

Check all of the areas in which there is concern about the child's development:

☐ Speech/articulation   ☐ Feeding/GI

☐ Language   ☐ Hearing

☐ Social communication   ☐ Vision

☐ Fine motor   ☐ General developmental delay

☐ Gross motor   ☐ Nonverbal IQ/visual reception

☐ Social anxiety   ☐ Attention

☐ Social   ☐ Repetitive behaviors

☐ Temperament   ☐ Other

☐ Behavior   ☐ ASD/autism ⟨ PDD-NOS / Autism / Asperger

☐ Sensory issues

Confidence Rating for Autism Spectrum Disorder Clinical Impression

0	1	2	3	4	5	6
Confident no ASD	Possible ASD, but not likely	Suspect ASD, but can't be sure	Confident PDD-NOS	On spectrum, not sure if PDD or autism	Confident autism	Asperger syndrome

Recommendations:

☐ Referral for further evaluation   ☐ Referral for treatment

☐ Retest at age _____

☐ Monitor via telephone

☐ None

☐ **REQUEST SECOND OPINION** Specify by whom _____ Anyone

ASD indicators	ASD contra-indicators

Additional notes/observations

Clinical Impressions Copyright © 2008 Rebecca Landa. In *Autism Frontiers: Clinical Issues and Innovations,* edited by Bruce K. Shapiro & Pasquale J. Accardo (2008, Paul H. Brookes Publishing Co., Inc.). All rights reserved.

Figure 7.1. Clinical Impressions form (Copyright © 2008 Rebecca Landa, Ph.D.). (*Key:* GI = gastrointestinal; IQ = intelligence quotient; ASD = autism spectrum disorder; PDD-NOS = pervasive developmental disorder not otherwise specified.)

If the Clinician Suspects an Autism Spectrum Disorder

In children younger than 3 years of age, clinicians must take particular care in diagnostic formulations pertaining to ASDs. First, the nature of parents' concerns, understanding of ASDs, insights into their children, reasons for seeking the assessment, the presence or absence of a family history of ASDs, and related factors must be taken into consideration. If the clinician has obtained substantial evidence during the evaluation that a child is at high risk for an ASD diagnosis, a high degree of sensitivity is required in discussing this possibility with family members. After having ascertained as much information as possible about the parents' perspectives, understanding, and preparedness to hear the results of the assessment, the clinician will decide the best way to proceed. The parents' experience in the first assessment of their child with an ASD is long remembered. This experience often marks the beginning of a long journey with various types of professionals, making it a critical time for the establishment of trust. Parents depend on honest, sensitively shared, and accurate information, which may involve explaining that insights into their child's development will be an unfolding process.

A critically important factor in the discussion of the assessment results will be parents' understanding of the nature of the developmental disruption that has been identified by the clinician. A checklist such as the Review of Observations developed by Landa (Figure 7.2; see also Appendix B at the end of this chapter for a photocopiable version) may be helpful to both the clinician and the parents. Using such a checklist, the clinician and the parents can calibrate their views of the child's performance in the assessment session and identify whether the behaviors of concern are representative of the child in day-to-day life. Seeking parents' insights into their child and his or her behavior is an essential part of the discussion—and this discussion should not be rushed. As the discussion unfolds, the clinician will glean a great deal of information that will guide the manner in which a diagnosis and associated recommendations are shared. It may not be possible or advisable to give a definitive diagnosis at the conclusion of a single assessment. Follow-up meetings, which may or may not involve further assessment of the child, are often appropriate. In some cases, it may be preferable to see the child and parents for follow-up, usually within 3 months of the first evaluation, if there are concerns about an ASD diagnosis and the child is younger than 2 years of age, or within 6 months if the child is at least 2 years old. These follow-up intervals are always determined on an individual basis. Regardless of the plan for follow-up, specific recommendations for further evaluation and intervention should be made before the family leaves, giving the parents a plan of action. Evidence-based information about social communication disorders or ASDs and early intervention, as well as appropriate resources, should be shared when relevant.

Clinicians should be sensitive to the amount of information that parents can process in the first assessment, and they should provide ample time for parents to voice their reactions, express their feelings, and ask questions. Contact information should be shared for reliable resources that parents may call within the coming days and weeks if questions or additional concerns arise. Parents should also be informed that development in the early years of life is somewhat unpredictable and that follow-up is advised, either with the present clinician or with others. Making definitive prognostic statements beyond reporting what has clearly been shown in the empirical literature about predictors of outcome is unwise (reviewed in Landa, 2007).

Review of Observations

Child's name _____

Date of birth _____ Date of assessment _____ Chronological age _____

Context of assessment _____

Examiner's name _____

Caregiver's name _____

Behavior	Clinician	Caregiver
Social		
Responds to others' smile		
Initiates smile with eye contact		
Consistent eye contact throughout session		
"Checks in" with others periodically		
Three-way gaze shift (e.g., object–person–object)		
Looks where others look (note whether child requires a pointing gesture to look)		
Points things out ___to request a desired action or object ___to show an action or object		
Can switch from own play focus to that of another person's		
Spontaneously imitates others' action		
Looks at others when imitates (indicate whether this is paired with a smile)		
Gives objects to share		
Consistently and quickly responds with eye contact to name being called		
Does not respond to name, but responds when tickled, when touched, or to a familiar song or verse		
Engages in turn-taking, showing enjoyment		
Communication		
Understands gestures and words; responds to language and gestures of others		
Makes a variety of sounds to communicate, directs communication with gaze or gesture or body language		
Communicates using conventional forms (gestures, words)		
Communicates frequently		
Echoes or says things in an unusual way		
Unusual tone of voice or loudness level		
Coordinates eye contact, smile, and gesture/vocal communication		
Play		
Explores a variety of objects		
Selects several different objects and plays with them in a variety of different ways		
Shows pretend play		
Tries to engage another person in play		
Prefers certain topics or objects (e.g., numbers, letters)		
Repeatedly focuses on small parts of objects		
Repeats actions with a toy or with body (e.g., lines toys up, rolls a toy car back and forth repeatedly)		
Has difficulty with change in routine		
Reluctant to touch certain objects		
Excessive mouthing		
Unusual gait or other motor behavior; low muscle tone; poor motor coordination		

Review of Observations Copyright © 2008 Rebecca Landa. In *Autism Frontiers: Clinical Issues and Innovations,* edited by Bruce K. Shapiro & Pasquale J. Accardo (2008, Paul H. Brookes Publishing Co., Inc.). All rights reserved.

Figure 7.2.   Review of Observations form (Copyright © 2008 Rebecca Landa, Ph.D.).

▌ EARLY INTERVENTION FOR AUTISM SPECTRUM DISORDERS

For infants and toddlers who exhibit red flags associated with ASDs, intervention may be warranted. Issues related to early intervention are discussed next.

Why Early Intervention?

The neuroscience literature has shown that experience influences the ability of neurons to modulate the strength and structure of their synaptic connections (Bliss & Collingridge, 1993; Martin & Kandel, 1996). The effects of early experience are associated with changes in developmental processes (e.g., speech perception). By the first birthday, an infant's perceptual and perceptual-motor systems are changed by experience with his or her native language. The type of developmental change that occurs does not involve traditional Skinnerian learning, where language learning is the result of externally administered reinforcement (Kuhl, 2000). Rather simply through exposure to the infant's native spoken language, he or she makes the transition from discerning differences between all the phonetic units in the world's languages at birth to a more constrained speech perceptual system by the first birthday (Eimas, Miller, & Jusczyk, 1987; Kuhl et al., 1997). In this more constrained system, the infant only discriminates between speech sounds that signal different phonetic categories in his or her own language; this is an important and necessary accomplishment for receptive language development.

Timing of exposure to particular types of information appears to be important, such that the exposure may have a more potent effect on learning at certain points in development than in others (Knudsen & Brainerd, 1995: Knudsen & Knudsen, 1990). This phenomenon has led to the concept of "sensitive periods" of development, where learning of certain types is maximal at certain times. Such concepts, as illustrated in humans and animals in the neuroscience literature, have stimulated a sense of urgency for early intervention for children with ASDs.

An Eye Toward Intervention Design

There is widespread agreement that intervention should be initiated early in life for children with ASDs (National Research Council, 2001). A consensus has been reached by the research and clinical communities that intervention for ASDs must 1) take into account the whole of ASDs to help children achieve personal independence and social responsibility through addressing cognitive, communication, social, adaptive, and behavioral challenges, and taking into account each child's strengths; 2) support family participation in the planning of the intervention and provide families with the training to employ techniques for teaching their children; and 3) measure progress frequently across a range of skill areas, making necessary adjustments in the intervention to maximize learning (National Research Council, 2001). There is, however, less agreement about specific instructional approaches and where the intervention should take place for children younger than 3 years of age. There is often a tendency to implement intervention through the utilization of a single approach (e.g., floor time, verbal behavior) rather than tailoring intervention to the learning characteristics of a child by integrating instructional ingredients represented in a variety of intervention approaches. Several intervention approaches integrate a variety of intervention ingredients and embrace a continuum of adult-imposed structure. Examples of such approaches include the SCERTS® Model (Prizant, Wetherby, Rubin, Laurent, & Rydell, 2006), the Denver Model (Rogers & Lewis, 1989), the Miller Method (Miller & Miller, 1989), and the Kennedy Krieger Institute's Achievements Model (Landa & Holman, 2005). Several studies, some with randomized group assignment, have shown that children enrolled in interventions that employ a continuum of adult-imposed structure and utilize a variety of intervention ingredients are associated with children's cognitive, social, and/or communication gains (Kasari, Freeman, & Paparella, 2006; Rogers, 2005).

The "dosage" of adult-imposed structure and adult-to-child ratio will be prescribed based on factors such as the child's attention, cognitive, and self-regulatory capacities. Intervention goals and instructional strategies must be selected with the appreciation that development is an intertwined, systematic, dynamic process involving perceptual, motor, cognitive, communication, and social domains. The ASD intervention literature, together with the literature on language learning in very young children with typical and delayed development, provides insights that guide the design of very early intervention for ASDs. First, children with ASDs show the ability to learn when intervention methods are geared toward highly explicit forms of teaching, as in Discrete Trial Training (Smith, Groen, & Wynn, 2000). They also learn, perhaps with a better generalization of skills, when taught using instructional methods that provide structured learning opportunities, but also afford a wider margin of implicit learning, as in Pivotal Response Treatment and other incidental teaching approaches (Ingersoll & Schreibman, 2006; Koegel & Koegel, 2006; Whalen & Schreibman, 2003). Second, the literature on learning in young children with typical and delayed development indicates that learning and generalization occur at higher rates when stimuli graduate from simple to complex (Jones & Smith, 2005), when the stimuli (i.e., therapy materials or other forms of input such as gesture and spoken language) provide repeated exposure to multiple exemplars of the category to be learned (Baillargeon, 1993; Quinn & Eimas, 1998; Quinn, Westerlund, & Nelson, 2006; Spelke, 1990), when there is not too much novelty introduced at once (Bloom & Beckwith, 1989), when there is high proximity between

cue and reward (Diamond, 2006), and when the topic, objects, and/or actions within the engagement are of interest to the child or extend the child's ongoing action and focus of attention (Nadel, 2006; Siller & Sigman, 2002; Watson, 1998).

Although these principles may be incorporated into early intervention programs for young children with ASDs, ongoing decisions must be made regarding how simplified the intervention targets, materials, and activities are, as well as the dosage of highly structured, explicit teaching to be employed. Observation of multiple child behaviors will ultimately enable the clinician to determine the 1) developmental complexity of intervention goals, 2) degree to which antecedent stimuli must be invariant, 3) the number of consecutive repeated response opportunities a child should be given, 4) the amount of scaffolding needed, 5) the degree to which a skill should be broken into discrete components for teaching, 6) the nature and latency of reward, 7) the amount of novelty, 8) the number of factors that can differ from the original teaching context when providing opportunities for generalization, 9) the number of immediate possible response options (i.e., distracters) that are presented, and so forth. Factors such as latency of response, accuracy of response, consistency of accurate responses, attention, and the coordination of multiple behaviors (e.g., gaze + vocalization) will be key indicators to guide intervention design pertaining to goals, intervention strategies, and therapeutic materials and activities.

An organizational framework for conceptualizing dimensions of popular ASD intervention approaches has been presented by Prizant and Wetherby (2005). The framework suggests dimensions of teaching practices, learning contexts, child characteristics, and programmatic goals that can be compared across popular ASD intervention approaches. Prizant and Wetherby (2005) discussed dimensions of teaching practices, learning contexts, child characteristics, and programmatic goals associated with highly structured, prescribed, and adult-led intervention approaches such as Discrete Trial Training (Smith, Groen, & Wynn, 2000) versus those associated with a more flexible, adult-responsive, developmental model. The dimensions discussed include theoretical/research underpinnings, the degree of prescription versus flexibility, the use of directive versus facilitative interactional and teaching styles, approaches to problem behavior and emotional dysregulation, measurement of progress, parent involvement, the use of visual supports and visually mediated activities, naturalness of teaching activities or contexts, skill-based or activity-based learning opportunities, the ways in which individual differences in learning are addressed, the ways in which emotional regulatory capacities are considered, the range of developmental domains addressed, the use of augmentative communication strategies, the prioritization of spontaneous initiation of communication, and the degree to which goals are developmentally based and functional. Consideration of these dimensions may assist interventionists to critically evaluate their selection of intervention design and delivery. Intentional selection of intervention strategies to cultivate a child's learning within a carefully designed intervention program is not an *eclectic* approach, which is the term applied by some researchers to combinations of types of intervention where there is no clear evidence of fidelity.

EARLY ACHIEVEMENTS: AN EARLY INTERVENTION PROGRAM FOR AUTISM SPECTRUM DISORDERS AT KENNEDY KRIEGER INSTITUTE'S CENTER FOR AUTISM AND RELATED DISORDERS

The Early Achievements program within Kennedy Krieger Institute's Center for Autism and Related Disorders (KKI CARD) was designed to address the multifaceted nature of impairment in ASDs. The program,

based on empirical evidence regarding neuropsychological, social-emotional, communication, and learning behavior in ASDs, emphasizes intervention to address social, communication, and cognitive development, as well as challenges with flexibility (e.g., of thought, perception, behavior), generativity, planning, self-regulation, sensory impairments, and the integration of information and behavior across multiple developmental systems. The intervention process embraces the concept that development involves both quantitative and qualitative advances reflected in behavioral features, which are observed in children's responses to the environment, as well as in their initiations directed toward their environment. Thus, intervention goals address both the acquisition of skills and the quality of the state of engagement (i.e., quality and duration of engagement with objects and people). Given Landa's data on the high degree of, and protracted duration of, instability in skills in young children with ASDs (Sullivan et al., 2007), the Early Achievements program has several features to emphasize the acquisition of meaning, functional use of skills, and intentionality. Activities, materials, and social engagement experiences are designed to teach skills and establish knowledge bases to maximize flexibility, generalization, adaptive ability, and conceptual development. Children are challenged to be consciously present and attentive rather than functioning on automatic pilot. They are also challenged to develop a consciousness of self and others, and to become practiced in functioning as a social partner.

The Early Achievements program incorporates a variety of intervention strategies, including Discrete Trial Training, Pivotal Response Treatment, augmentative communication systems, sensory-social routines, environmental engineering, joint action routines, and narrative-based teaching. The program has been empirically evaluated through the author's NIH-funded treatment efficacy study (NIMH U54 MH066417-04). Participants in the study were 2-year-olds (i.e., mean age = 27 months). The elements to the intervention are 1) direct intervention delivered by therapists within a classroom setting specially designed for toddlers, 2) home-based parent training, and 3) center-based parent education. Parents learn how to infuse daily routines with teachable moments, how to read and adapt to their children's behavior, and how to engineer the home environment to optimize their children's learning opportunities and self-regulation. They learn about evidence-based intervention strategies, developmental processes in children with ASDs, local and national resources pertaining to ASDs and developmental delay, educational and therapeutic options, ways to advocate for their children, and coping strategies.

Children attend the center-based program 4 days per week for 2½ hours per day for a period of 6 months. This amounts to 10 hours of therapist-administered intervention per week. During the classroom-based learning time, the intensity of intervention is programmed to be at a high level through frequent response opportunities. In addition, parents are asked to provide and assist in establishing social and communication enhancement within daily routines and home-based interactions with their children. Families are also assisted in making connections with local public early intervention providers, as well as in establishing individualized family service plans (IFSPs) for their children. There are five children in each class, with the intervention staff consisting of a teacher and two teaching assistants. The instructional schedule is consistent every day. Each day begins with a Learning Readiness Time in which the children make the transition from their parents to the classroom. Upon entering the classroom, the children play within a contained area in which they can select toys ranging from construction-based toys (e.g., blocks, stacking toys, puzzles, shape sorters), cause–effect toys, books, and pretend play toys. All of the children then make the transition to a circle time. Following the circle time, the children

participate in one-to-one, dyad, and larger group activities on a set schedule that includes table-time structured learning tasks—some are completely steered by the therapist and others more independent work/play activities—as well as sensory-motor activities, play-center based activities, art activities, snack time, outside time, and a closing circle time activity. Between all activities, the children check their centrally-located visual (i.e., 2- and 3-dimensional) schedules to assist them in their transition, self-regulation, planning, and symbol-based development. Goals addressed and intervention strategies utilized in each activity are predefined. The fidelity of the therapists' application of the teaching strategies are monitored monthly with ongoing review to maintain high levels of fidelity.

The curriculum for the Early Achievements program is a combination of the Assessment, Evaluation, and Programming System for Infants and Children (AEPS®), Second Edition (Bricker, 2002) curriculum, along with a newly developed social cognitive and communication curriculum developed as part of this research project. Children receive assessments before entering and upon completion of the intervention, with follow-up assessment conducted 6 months after the termination of the treatment. In the treatment study, data were taken on the children's progress toward their individual goals on a daily basis, and monthly videotapes were coded to assess frequency, complexity, and diversity of communication, social, and play behaviors, as well as the presence of atypical behaviors. Children enrolled in the intervention study made substantial gains in nonverbal cognitive, language, and social development (Landa & Holman, 2005).

Fostering Interpersonal Synchrony

One of the primary goals of the Early Achievements program is for children to learn skills and develop awareness of others that will enable them to be contingent and synchronous with peers and with adults. This emphasis permeates all aspects of the intervention implementation. Interpersonal synchrony with peers and adults is accomplished through song–gesture games, simple books with associated activities, and sensory-social routines that place the children face-to-face with others in highly motivating interactions. Through these activities, therapists hone children's attention to faces, facial features, emotional expressions, and so forth. Within all of these activities, children are placed in the role of responder and initiator, enhancing flexibility and role shifting, because these experiences may contribute to the development of intersubjectivity, as related to theory of mind or perspective taking. They are taught to respond to others' joint attention cues, initiate joint attention, recognize others and their own faces and basic emotional expressions, reciprocate in simple turn-taking exchanges, and imitate others within natural interactions.

Fostering Conceptual Development

The design of the Early Achievements program was based, in part, on the fact that the formation of concepts paves the way for numerous aspects of social and linguistic development. Children form concepts that represent relations between objects and events that they encounter (Waxman & Markow, 1995). As words are mapped onto these concepts, a rich dynamic begins wherein word learning supports the development of ever-increasing abstract and flexible mental representations. Word learning also provides children with a more sophisticated vehicle for social engagement, enabling them to express their needs, ideas, and opinions with increased levels of specificity. Simply put, children are afforded the increased ability to influence the minds and behaviors of others. Thus, building a network of concepts during the early stages of learning establishes the bedrock for social and communication development. The

carefully crafted intervention system within Early Achievements provides multimodal experiences to enhance concept development with the intention of having these concepts become embodied in the child's active engagement with objects, other children, family members, and teachers. The linguistic system is also constructed with care. Different types of words are taught to facilitate development of a flexible and generative linguistic system. Thus, language goals specifically target words that allow a grammar to be built and a rich semantic network to be established. Children learn count nouns (e.g., *book*) that extend broadly to other members of the same category (i.e., as opposed to a specific book), proper nouns that refer to a specific entity, adjectives (i.e., properties of nouns that can be extended to use with other nouns within and outside of a specific category, as in "big book, little book," "big cookie, little cookie"), prepositions referring to spatial relationships, verbs referring to event concepts, and so forth.

Theme-Based Instruction

The Early Achievements program employs theme-based instruction to enhance conceptual development, attention, generalization, emergent literacy, and cultural literacy, as well as to decrease cognitive load. Themes are aligned with seasonal events in nature, celebrations, and activities. The vocabulary, play materials, books, art, and motor and sensory activities are coordinated with the theme. Children's individualized goals are addressed within these themes, where the materials, language, and activities associated with the themes are developmentally appropriate and contoured to have a high level of interest for the children in the class. These themes create the milieu and framework within which learning activities are conceptually grounded and relevant. Themes also impose a high level of coherence across diverse learning formats. Thus, children have pragmatically appropriate opportunities to utilize and generalize the vocabulary, action schema (e.g., gestures, play), social initiations, and social responses throughout the day within different contexts with different social partners and with different materials.

Because the construction of category formation, which contributes to concept formation, is probably based on interactions (Hirsch-Pasek, Golinkoff, Hennon, & Maguire, 2004) among perceptual (Jusczyk, 1997; Quinn & Eimas, 2000; Smith, 1999), conceptual (Baillargeon, 2000; Spelke, 2003), and linguistic systems (Lidz, Waxman, & Freedman, 2003), the Early Achievements program is strategic in its selection of visual, auditory, and tactile stimuli used in the teaching materials and in constructing the learning activities in which these stimuli are used. For example, *Brown Bear, Brown Bear, What Do You See?* (Martin, Jr., & Carle, 1992), a popular children's book, provides the frame within which multiple treatment goals can be addressed, including the following: specific linguistic forms (e.g., count nouns, adjectives, the experiential verb *see*, the question form *what*, pronouns); communicative intents (e.g., requesting information, telling, showing); self-other concepts and intersubjectivity (i.e., me versus other); joint attention (i.e., various animals from the story appear in unexpected places at unexpected times); affective (i.e., sharing the emotion of surprise with another when the animal is encountered unexpectedly); and working memory (i.e., children engage in hunts for a target animal). Throughout the day, different exemplars of the animals are used within different activities. Activities afford children the opportunity to practice skills in a continuum of structured tasks. For example, matching skills may be taught 1) in highly structured discrete trials where meaning is disembedded from context, 2) in semistructured contexts where meaning is embedded in context as when the child attaches a smaller but identical picture of the animal onto the page of the book next to the animal during the storytime activity, and 3) in low

structured contexts where children select and group the different animals from a bin as they set up farm yards. Across activities representing all of these levels of structure, children encounter the same intervention targets, tailored in complexity and degree of scaffolding to the child's needs and readiness levels, and capitalizing on the familiarity and redundancy afforded by the theme.

Redundancy and Novelty

The Early Achievements program acknowledges the need for the redundancy of cues, multiple exposures to familiar stimuli within familiar contexts, multiple exposures to familiar stimuli in novel contexts (e.g., new person, new toy, new location), multiple exemplars, and so forth. Such redundancy builds familiarity and automaticity. At the same time, learning requires the ability to detect novelty as well as experience with novelty. Novelty provides the opportunity to expand existing categories and concepts, to establish new functions for existing forms, and to establish new categories and concepts (Gomez, 2002). In the case of word learning, being exposed to distinct names for individual objects appears to highlight the distinctions between them and assist children in differentiating objects (Van de Walle, Carey, & Prevor, 2000). Experience with novelty also enhances generalization when there is sufficient representation of characteristics from the initial learning context (Hayne, Boniface, & Barr, 2000). Through the use of routines and themes that are systematically varied, and within which the degree of novelty is adjusted to each child's level of readiness, redundancy and novelty are balanced to promote learning and generalization within the Early Achievements program.

Continuum of Adult-Imposed Structure

Much of what is learned by children with typical development is learned implicitly. Prior to enrollment in school, children learn by watching and engaging with others, with a relatively small proportion of their knowledge being gained through formal instruction (i.e., being taught the referent for a word or specific social conventions such as "Wave bye" or "Say thank you"). Children with ASDs, however, require a different type of learning environment to maximize their developmental potential. In the Early Achievements program, the learning environment highlights cues about what is socially and conceptually salient, makes clear connections between symbols and objects or actions, and creates contexts in which social rules are more easily recognized. Within this environment, everyday facets of experience are systematically ordered, relationships between cue and reward are proximal and consistent, material to be learned is simplified, and engagement in learning opportunities is secured. These characteristics of the learning environment are achieved with different degrees of adult-imposed structure and with different degrees of disembodying from natural, meaningful contexts, depending on a child's individual needs at any given time.

Creating Contexts for Children to Learn to Learn

By adjusting the degree of adult-imposed structure, exposing children to a continuum of visually scaffolded learning opportunities, baiting the classroom with unexpected objects and events, and creating a variety of highly motivating communicative temptations, the Early Achievements program provides a continuum of explicit to implicit learning experiences for young children with ASDs. These experiences are presented within and across activities, providing as much—but no more—structure and prompting as a child needs to be successful. Each goal addressed within a highly explicit, didactic teaching format is also addressed in a less formally structured learning context, where children are given time to initiate

and problem solve as they are assisted in accomplishing a goal. In these less explicit learning contexts, there is greater variation in antecedents, longer intervals between response and reward, use of natural rewards, and an interspersing of response opportunities for different targeted skills within an activity. The goal of these less explicit teaching contexts is to foster generalization, inspire spontaneity, encourage initiation, and reduce prompt dependence and passivity in learning style. The literature indicates that a less directive approach to interacting with children with ASDs and typical development facilitates higher frequency of communicative attempts, initiations, and social-affective signaling in the ongoing interaction (Dawson & Adams, 1984; Peck, 1985; Rydell & Mirenda, 1994; Tiegerman & Primavera, 1984), as well as better language outcomes (Akhtar, Dunham, & Dunham, 1991; Carpenter, Nagell, & Tomasello, 1998; Siller & Sigman, 2002). Thus, the degree of directiveness and explicitness of the instructional approach must be consciously determined as the daily therapeutic schedule is arranged.

In addition to consciously dosing the variables associated with the previously described explicit teaching contexts, the Early Achievements program supports the development of the ability to "learn to learn" through the use of several additional strategies. One such strategy is to teach within joint action routines. These are usually derived from the storytime activities, in which the children are exposed to an adapted book. The books provide the framework for the episode structure or event representation that the children are learning. Based on the concepts in the book, simple routines relevant to the theme at hand are created. This has the effect of increasing the children's familiarity with the words, gestures, and concepts, and thereby reduces some of the cognitive load. Routines and associated communication components (e.g., words, gestures, sequences) are expanded and varied. The degree to which children are expected to perform independently is adjusted as they learn the component parts and sequences of the routine. These routines enable children to respond and initiate within a highly familiar context, where novel forms of behavior, aligned with each child's goals, are invited and rewarded. Within the storytime and associated joint action routines, children are continually assisted or encouraged to be active participants and to practice sustained attention to salient cues (Kuhl, Tsao, & Liu, 2003). This is accomplished in part through the use of a variety of visual materials (e.g., topic boards), rewritten text using simplified icons, indicators (e.g., flashlights to point to the person who should take a turn, photographs of faces on a spin board or pin wheel, placement of a child's photograph on the hand mirror into which he or she looks during a song verse about him or her while working on oral-motor skills and self-awareness), objects that afford several types of actions related to the story and which are used in different ways to enhance comprehension of words, gestures, social events, and so forth.

Strategies to Enhance Flexibility, Attention, and Social Development

The social, communication, and play routines, which are linked conceptually to the story of the week, are also used to enhance flexibility, attention, social cognitive development, and interpersonal synchrony. Children get used to assuming different roles in the scripts associated with the stories (e.g., initiator, responder), using the same communicative forms for different functions (e.g., "cookie" to request, offer, show), using different communicative forms for the same function (e.g., "go" to describe, command, request), seeing different types of exemplars of the concept being learned (e.g., real, plastic, and paper apples, first in one color, then in multiple colors such as red and green), and so forth. Throughout the day, the children are given opportunities to use

their skills across contexts and with different people. Care is taken not to over routinize the activities in which the children participate. Care is also taken to provide opportunities for the children to make choices. The result is an activated attention system that enables the children to be vigilant for new and relevant cues, to adapt their behavior based on those cues, and to continually strengthen their sense of self. Developmentally appropriate challenges are introduced to maintain high levels of awareness and purposeful behavior, such as requiring them to feel around in the sand for the shovel, push a heavy bean bag chair away from an exit, look for the location of the cookie box, and so forth. This builds awareness and intentionality that spans a variety of functions. Whenever possible, peers assist one another in searches, pointing out elements of surprise, and sharing in other problem-solving situations.

In addition, the children's ability to infer is stimulated from very early in the intervention process. This is accomplished through a variety of means, including decreasing the physical and temporal proximity between stimulus and reward, such as the child vocalizing to request a cookie and being given a cookie, a therapist pointing to a picture in a book to establish joint engagement (but then gradually teaching the child to understand gaze as a pointing gesture), a therapist touching the child to indicate that it is his or her turn and then gradually shifting this cue to a look and nod of the head toward the child as the indicator, and related types of activities.

Implications of Early Achievements as an Evidence-Based Early Intervention Program

Data show the efficacy of the Early Achievements program for intervention with 2-year-olds with ASDs. This model has been piloted in two public schools' early intervention programs, with children's pre- and post-intervention results paralleling those from the research-based implementation of the program in the controlled laboratory setting. In addition, a Professional Immersion Training program has been initiated in which professionals may come to KKI CARD for didactic training that is followed by hands-on intensive guided practice experience, which alternates practice contexts between the training classroom and the home school district in which the professional is employed. Professionals are videotaped in the practice of intervention implementation from which fidelity of implementation of intervention ingredients is assessed before, during, and after the training. Teachers and teaching assistants in the public schools have demonstrated the ability to learn the intervention techniques and to implement them successfully in the public domain. The professional training program addresses a need voiced by all community providers who participated in Stahmer, Collings, and Palinkas's (2005) study of early intervention practices for children with ASDs. Those providers have also indicated that they did not have a clear understanding of evidence-based practice (Stahmer et al., 2005).

This has considerable implication for children with ASDs, paradigms for early intervention (e.g., adult–child ratio, parent training, home-based and center-based implementation of intervention), publicly funded early intervention service delivery, and financial aspects of education. More research is needed to examine active intervention ingredients, individual characteristics of children who show greater and lesser degrees of change, issues related to intensity of intervention, issues related to the amount of teacher training needed to maximize child change, and so forth.

CONCLUSION

ASDs can now be identified in children younger than 3 years of age, even in those as young as 14 months. Social and communi-cation impairments are the key defining features of the disorder, but these may be less severely affected in the early stages of development in children with ASDs. As the early signs of ASDs become more familiar to general practitioners and to the public, ASDs will be diagnosed earlier and children with ASDs will have greater access to early intervention. Models of very early intervention currently exist, as do training programs for professionals who work with young children with ASDs. Through ongoing research and partnerships between families, researchers, and public education systems, advances in early diagnosis and the development of increasingly effective and cost-efficient early intervention programs will continue. This raises hope for a brighter future for children with ASDs and their families.

REFERENCES

Adrien, J.L., Faure, M., Perrot, A., Hameury, L., Garreau, B., Barthelemy, C., et al. (1991). Autism and family home movies: Preliminary findings. *Journal of Autism and Developmental Disorders, 21,* 43–49.

Akhtar, N., Dunham, F., & Dunham, P.J. (1991). Directive interactions and early vocabulary development: The role of joint attentional focus. *Journal of Child Language, 18,* 41–49.

American Academy of Pediatrics. (2007). *AUTISM: Caring for children with autism spectrum disorders: A resource toolkit for clinicians.* Elk Grove Village, IL: Author.

American Psychiatric Association. (1994). *Diagnostic and Statistical Manual of Mental Disorders* (4th ed.). Washington, DC: Author.

Autism Speaks. (n.d.). *ASD video glossary.* Retrieved November 5, 2007, from http://www.autismspeaks.org/video/glossary.php

Baghdadli, A., Picot, M.C., Pascal, C., Pry, R., & Aussilloux, C. (2003). Relationship between age at recognition of first disturbances and severity in young children with autism. *European Child and Adolescent Psychiatry, 12,* 122–127.

Bailey, A., Le Couteur, A., Gottesman, I., Bolton, P., Simonoff, E., Yuzda, E., et al. (1995). Autism as a strongly genetic disorder: Evidence from a British twin study. *Psychological Medicine, 25,* 63–77.

Bailey, A., Luthert, P., Dean, A., Harding, B., Janota, I., Montgomery, M., et al. (1998). A clinicopathological study of autism. *Brain, 121,* 889–905.

Baillargeon, R. (1993). The object concept revisited: New directions in the investigation of infants' physical knowledge. In C.E. Granrud (Ed.), *Carnegie symposium on cognition: Visual perception and cognition in infancy* (pp. 265–315). Mahwah, NJ: Lawrence Erlbaum Associates.

Baillargeon, R. (2000). How do infants learn about the physical world? In D. Muir & A. Slater (Eds.), *Infant development: The essential readings. Essential readings in development psychology* (pp. 195–212). Malden, MA: Blackwell Publishers, Inc.

Baranek, G.T. (1999). Autism during infancy: A retrospective video analysis of sensory-motor and social behaviors at 9–12 months of age. *Journal of Autism and Developmental Disorders, 29,* 213–224.

Baranek, G.T., David, F.J., Poe, M.D., Stone, W.L., & Watson, L.R. (2006). Sensory Experiences Questionnaire: Discriminating sensory features in young children with autism, developmental delays, and typical development. *Journal of Child Psychology and Psychiatry, 47,* 591–601.

Baron-Cohen, S. (1989). Perceptual role taking and protodeclarative pointing in autism. *British Journal of Developmental Psychology, 7,* 113–127.

Bauman, M., & Kemper, T. (2005). Neuroanatomic observations of the brain in autism: A review and future directions. *International Journal of Developmental Neuroscience, 23,* 183–187.

Bhat, A., Rusyniak, J., & Landa, R. (2007, May). *Motor and cognitive development of infants at-risk for autism and low-risk typically developing infants.* Poster presented at International Meeting for Autism Research, Seattle, WA.

Bliss, T.V.P., & Collingridge, G.L. (1993). A synaptic model of memory: Long term potentiation in the hippocampus. *Nature, 361,* 31–39.

Bloom, L., & Beckwith, R. (1989). Talking with feeling: Integrating affective and linguistic expression in early language development. In C. Izard (Ed.), *Development of emotion-cognition relation* (pp. 313–342). Mahwah, NJ: Lawrence Erlbaum Associates.

Bricker, D. (2002). *Assessment, Evaluation, and Programming System for Infants and Children* (*AEPS®,* 2nd ed.). Baltimore: Paul H. Brookes Publishing Co.

Bricker, D., & Squires, J. (1999). *Ages & Stages Questionnaires® (ASQ): A parent-completed child-monitoring system* (2nd ed.). Baltimore: Paul H. Brookes Publishing Co.

Brigance, A. (1985). *Brigance Preschool Screen.* North Billerica, MA: Curriculum Associates, Inc.

Bryson, S.E., Zwaigenbaum, L., Brian, J., Roberts, W., Szatmari, P., Rombough, V., et al. (2007). A prospective case series of high-risk infants who developed autism. *Journal of Autism and Developmental Disorders, 37,* 12–24.

Carpenter, M., Nagell, K., & Tomasello, M. (1998). Social cognition, joint attention, and communicative competence from 9 to 15 months of age. *Monographs of the Society for Research in Child Development, 63,*1–143.

Cassel, T.D., Messinger, D.S., Ibanez, L.V., Haltigan, J.D., Acosta, S.I., & Buchman, A.C. (2007). Early social and emotional communication in the infant siblings of children with autism spectrum disorders: An examination of the broad phenotype. *Journal of Autism and Developmental Disorders, 37,* 122–132.

Centers for Disease Control and Prevention. (n.d.). *Learn the signs, act early.* Retrieved July 19, 2006, from http://www.cdc.gov/ncbddd/autism/actearly

Charman, T., Baron-Cohen, S., Swettenham, J., Baird, G., Cox, A., & Drew, A. (2000). Testing joint attention, imitation, and play as infancy precursors to language and theory of mind. *Cognitive Development, 15,* 481–498.

Charman, T., Swettenham, J., Baron-Cohen, S., Cox, A., Baird, G., & Drew, A. (1997). Infants with autism: An investigation of empathy, pretend play, joint attention, and imitation. *Developmental Psychopathology, 33,* 781–789.

Charman, T., Taylor, E., Drew, A., Cockerill, H., Brown, J., & Baird, G. (2005). Outcome at 7 years of children diagnosed with autism at age 2: Predictive validity of assessments conducted at 2 and 3 years of age and pattern of symptom change over time. *Journal of Child Psychology and Psychiatry, 46,* 500–513.

Chawarska, K., Klin, A., Paul, R., & Volkmar, F. (2007). Autism spectrum disorder in the second year of life: Stability and change in syndrome expression. *Journal of Child Psychology and Psychiatry, 48,* 128–138.

Chugani, D.C. (2002). Role of altered brain serotonin mechanisms in autism. *Molecular Psychiatry, 7,* S16–S17.

Colgan, S.E., Lanter, E., McComish, C., Watson, L.R., Crais, E.R., & Baranek, G.T. (2006). Analysis of social interaction gestures in infants with autism. *Child Neuropsychology, 12,* 307–319.

Courchesne, E., Carper, R., & Akshoomoff, N. (2003). Evidence of brain overgrowth in the first year of life in autism. *Journal of the American Medical Association, 290,* 337–344.

Dahlgren, S.O., & Gillberg, C. (1989). Symptoms in the first two years of life: A preliminary population study of infantile autism. *European Archives of Psychiatry and Neurological Sciences, 238,* 169–174.

Dawson, G., & Adams, A. (1984). Imitation and social responsiveness in autistic children. *Journal of Abnormal Child Psychology, 12,* 209–226.

Dawson, G., Toth, K., Abbott, R., Osterling, J., Munson, J., Estes, A., et al. (2004). Early social attention impairments in autism: Social orienting, joint attention, and attention to distress. *Developmental Psychology, 40,* 271–283.

De Giacomo, A., & Fombonne, E. (1998). Parental recognition of developmental abnormalities in autism. *European Child and Adolescent Psychiatry, 7,* 131–136.

Diamond, A. (2006). Bootstrapping conceptual deduction using physical connection: Rethinking frontal cortex. *Trends in Cognitive Sciences, 10,* 212–218.

Eimas, P.D., Miller, J.L., & Jusczyk, P.W. (1987). On infant speech perception and the acquisition of language. In S. Harnad (Ed.), *Categorical perception* (pp. 161–195). New York: Cambridge University Press.

Filipek, P.A., Accardo, P.J., Baranek, G.T., Cook, E.H., Jr., Dawson, G., Gordon, B., et al. (1999). The screening and diagnosis of autistic spectrum disorders. *Journal of Autism and Developmental Disorders, 29,* 439–484.

Flanagan, J.E., & Landa, R. (2007, April). *Longitudinal study of motor development in infants at high and low risk for autism.* Presentation at the American Occupational Therapy Association annual conference, St Louis, MO.

Folstein, S.E., Santangelo, S.L., Gilman, S.E., Piven, J., Landa, R., Lainhart, J., et al. (1999). Predictors of cognitive test patterns in autism families. *Journal of Child Psychology and Psychiatry, 40,* 1117–1128.

Fombonne, E. (2005). Epidemiology of autistic disorder and other pervasive developmental disorders. *Journal of Clinical Psychiatry, 66,* S3–S8.

Glascoe, F.P. (1996). *Technical manual for the Brigance Screening Tests.* North Billerica, MA: Curriculum Associates, Inc.

Glascoe, F.P. (2006). *Parents' Evaluation of Developmental Status (PEDS).* Nashville: Ellsworth & Vandermeer Press.

Goldberg, W.A., Jarvis, K.L., Osann, K., Laulhere, T.M., Straub, C., Thomas, E., et al. (2005). Brief report: Early social communication behaviors in the younger siblings of children with autism. *Journal of Autism and Developmental Disorders, 35,* 657–664.

Goldberg, W.A., Osann, K., Filipek, P.A., Laulhere, T., Jarvis, K., Modahl, C., et al. (2003). Language and other regression: Assessment and timing. *Journal of Autism and Developmental Disorders, 33,* 607–616.

Gomez, R.L. (2002). Variability and detection of invariant structure. *Psychological Science, 13,* 431–436.

Gorrotxategi, P., Reguilon, M.J., Arana, J., Gaztanaga, R., Elorza, C., de la Iglesia, E., et al. (1995). Gastroesophageal reflux in association with the Sandifer syndrome. *European Journal of Pediatric Surgery, 5,* 203–205.

Gray, K.M., & Tonge, B.J. (2001). Are there early features of autism in infants and preschool children? *Journal of Pediatrics and Child Health, 37,* 221–226.

Hayne, H., Boniface, J., & Barr, R. (2000). The development of declarative memory in human infants: Age-related changes in deferred imitation. *Behavior Neuroscience, 114,* 77–83.

Hirsch-Pasek, K., Golinkoff, R.M., Hennon, E.A., & Maguire, M.J. (2004). Hybrid theories at the frontier of developmental psychology: The emergentist coalition model of word learning as a case in point. In D.G. Hall & S.R. Waxman (Eds.) *Weaving a lexicon* (pp. 173–204). Cambridge, MA: MIT Press.

Hoshino, Y., Kaneko, M., Yashima, Y., Kumashiro, H., Volkmar, F.R., & Cohen, D.J. (1987). Clinical features of autistic children with setback course in their infancy. *The Japanese Journal of Psychiatry and Neurology, 41,* 237–245.

Ingersoll, B., & Schreibman, L. (2006). Teaching reciprocal imitation skills to young children with autism using a naturalistic behavioral approach: Effects on language, pretend play, and joint attention. *Journal of Autism and Developmental Disorders, 36,* 487–505.

Ireton, H. (1992). *Child Development Inventory.* Minneapolis, MN: Behavior Science Systems.

Ireton, H., & Glascoe, F.P. (1995). Assessing children's development using parents' reports: The Child Development Inventory. *Clinical Pediatrics, 34,* 248–255.

Iverson, J., & Wozniak, R.H. (2007). Variation in vocal-motor development in infant siblings of children with autism. *Journal of Autism and Developmental Disorders, 37,* 158–170.

Johnson, C.P., Myers, S.M., & the Council on Children with Disabilities. (2007). Identification and evaluation of children with autism spectrum disorders. *Pediatrics, 120,* 1183–1215.

Jones, S.S., & Smith, L. (2005). Object name learning and object perception: A deficit in late talkers. *Journal of Child Language, 32,* 223–240.

Jusczyk, P. (1997). *The discovery of spoken language.* Cambridge, MA: MIT Press.

Kasari, C., Freeman, S., & Paparella, T. (2006). Joint attention and symbolic play in young children with autism: A randomized controlled intervention study. *Journal of Child Psychology and Psychiatry, 47,* 611–620.

Kleinman, J.M., Ventola, P.E., Pandey, J., Verbalis, A.D., Barton, M., Hodgson, S., et al. (2007). Diagnostic stability in very young children with autism spectrum disorders. *Journal of Autism and Developmental Disorders* (ePub).

Knudsen, E.I., & Brainerd, M.S. (1995). Creating a unified representation of visual and auditory space in the brain. *Annual Review of Neuroscience, 18,* 19–43.

Knudsen, E.I., & Knudsen, P.F. (1990). Sensitive and critical periods for visual calibration of sound localization by barn owls. *Journal of Neuroscience, 10,* 222–232.

Koegel, R.L., & Koegel, L.K. (2006). *Pivotal Response Treatments for autism: Communication, social, and academic development.* Baltimore: Paul H. Brookes Publishing Co.

Kuhl, P.K. (2000). A new view of language acquisition. *Proceedings of the National Academy of Sciences of the United States of America, 24,* 11850–11857.

Kuhl, P.K., Kirtani, S., Deguchi, T., Hayashi, A., Stevens, E.B., Dugger, C.D., et al. (1997). Effects of language experience on speech perception of /ra/and/la/. *Journal of the Acoustical Society of America, 102,* 3135–3136.

Kuhl, P.K., Tsao, F.-M., & Liu, H.-M. (2003). Foreign-language experience in infancy: Effects of short-term exposure and social interaction on phonetic learning. *Proceedings of the National Academy of Sciences, 100,* 9096–9101.

Kurita, H. (1985). Infantile autism with speech loss before the age of thirty months. *Journal of the American Academy of Child and Adolescent Psychiatry, 24,* 191–196.

Landa, R. (2005, October). *Early intervention for autism.* Distinguished Lecture Series, UC Davis M.I.N.D. Institute, Davis, CA.

Landa, R. (2007). Diagnosis of autism spectrum disorders in the first 3 years of life. *Nature Clinical Practice Neurology.* DOI: 10.1038/ncpneuro0731

Landa, R., Cleary, J., & Holman, K. (2005, April). *Change in autism diagnostic classification and symptoms from 14 to 24 months.* Presentation at the Society for Research in Child Development Conference, Atlanta, GA.

Landa, R., & Garrett-Mayer, E. (2006). Development in infants with autism spectrum disorders: A prospective study. *Journal of Child Psychology and Psychiatry, 47,* 629–638.

Landa, R., & Holman, K. (2005). *The effects of targeting interpersonal synchrony on social and communication development in toddlers with autism.* Poster presented at the Annual CPEA/STAART meeting, Washington, DC.

Landa, R.J., Holman, K.C., & Garrett-Mayer, E. (2007). Social and communication development in toddlers with early and later diagnosis of autism spectrum disorders. *Archives of General Psychiatry, 64,* 853–864.

Lidz, J., Waxman, S., & Freedman, J. (2003). What infants know about syntax but couldn't have learned: Experimental evidence for syntactic structure at 18 months. *Cognition, 89,* 65–73.

Lord, C. (1995). Follow-up of two-year-olds referred for possible autism. *Journal of Child Psychology and Psychiatry, 36,* 1365–1382.

Lord, C., Rutter, M., DiLavore, P.C., & Risi, S. (1999). *Autism Diagnostic Observation Schedule (ADOS).* Los Angeles: Western Psychological Services.

Lord, C., Rutter, M., & LeCouteur, A.J. (1994). Autism Diagnostic Interview–Revised: A revised version of a diagnostic interview for caregivers of individuals with possible pervasive developmental disorders. *Journal of Autism and Developmental Disorders, 24,* 659–685.

Lord, C., Storoschuk, S., Rutter, M., & Pickles, A. (1993). Using the ADI-R to diagnose autism in preschool children. *Infant Mental Health Journal, 14,* 1234–1252.

Loveland, K., & Landry, S.H. (1986). Joint attention and language in autism and developmental language delay. *Journal of Autism and Developmental Disorders, 16,* 335–349.

Maestro, S., Muratori, F., Barbieri, F., Casella, C., Cattaneo, V., Cavallaro, M.C., et al. (2001). Early behavioral development in autistic children: The first 2 years of life through home movies. *Psychopathology, 34,* 147–152.

Maestro, S., Muratori, F., Cavallero, M.C., Pei, F., Stern, D., Golse, B., et al. (2002). Attentional skills during the first 6 months of age in autism spectrum disorder. *Journal of the American Academy of Child and Adolescent Psychiatry, 41,* 1239–1245.

Mandell, D.S., Novak, M.M., & Zubritsky, C.D. (2005). Factors associated with age of diagnosis among children with autism spectrum disorders. *Pediatrics, 116,* 1480–1486.

Martin, K.C., & Kandel, E.R. (1996). Cell adhesion molecules, CREB, and the formation of new synaptic connections. *Neuron, 17,* 567–570.

Martin, Jr., B., & Carle, E. (1992). *Brown bear, Brown bear, What do you see?* New York: Henry Holt and Company.

McEachin, J.J., Smith, T., & Lovaas, O. (1993). Long-term outcome for children with autism who received early intensive behavioral treatment. *American Journal on Mental Retardation, 97,* 359–372.

McEvoy, R.E., Rogers, S.J., & Pennington, B.F. (1993). Executive function and social communication deficits in young autistic children. *Journal of Child Psychology and Psychiatry, 34,* 563–578.

Miller, A., & Eller-Miller, E., (1989). *From ritual to repertoire: A cognitive-developmental systems approach with behavior-disordered children.* New York: Wiley.

Mitchell, S., Brian, J., Zwaigenbaum, L., Roberts, W., Szatmari, P., Smith, I., et al. (2006). Early language and communication development of infants later diagnosed with autism spectrum disorder. *Journal of Developmental and Behavioral Pediatrics, 27,* S69–S78.

Mullen, E.M. (1995). *Mullen Scales of Early Learning.* Circle Pines, MN: AGS Publishing.

Mundy, P., Sigman, M., & Kasari, C. (1990). A longitudinal study of joint attention and language development in autistic children. *Journal of Autism and Developmental Disorders, 20,* 115–128.

Mundy, P., Sigman, M., & Kasari, C. (1994). Joint attention, developmental level, and symptom presentation in autism. *Development and Psychopathology, 6,* 389–401.

Nadel, J. (2006). Does imitation matter to children with autism? In S.J. Rogers & J.H.G. Williams (Eds.), *Imitation and the social mind: Autism and typical development* (pp. 118–137). New York: Guilford Press.

National Research Council, Committee on Educational Interventions for Children with Autism, Division of Behavioral and Social Sciences and Education. (2001). *Educating children with autism.* Washington, DC: National Academy Press.

Nelson, P.G., Kuddo, T., Song, E.Y., Dambrosia, J.M., Kohler, S., Satyanarayana, G., et al. (2006). Selected neurotrophins, neuropeptides, and cytokines: Developmental trajectory and concentrations in neonatal blood of children with autism or Down syndrome. *International Journal of Developmental Neuroscience, 24,* 73–80.

O'Neill, D.K. (2002). *Language use inventory for young children: An assessment of pragmatic language development.* Unpublished document, University of Waterloo, Ontario, Canada.

O'Neill, M., & Jones, R.S.P. (1997). Sensory-perceptual abnormalities in autism: A case for more research. *Journal of Autism and Developmental Disorders, 27,* 283–293.

Osterling, J., & Dawson, G. (1994). Early recognition of children with autism: A study of first birthday home videotapes. *Journal of Autism and Developmental Disorders, 24,* 247–257.

Palomo, R., Belinchon, M., & Ozonoff, S. (2006). Autism and family home movies: A comprehensive review. *Journal of Developmental and Behavioral Pediatrics, 27,* S59–S68.

Peck, C.A. (1985). Increasing opportunities for social control by children with autism and severe handicaps: Effects on student behavior and perceived classroom climate. *Journal of the Association for Persons with Severe Handicaps, 10,* 183–193.

Prizant, B.M., & Wetherby, A. (2005). Critical issues in enhancing communication abilities for persons with autism spectrum disorders. In F.R. Volkmar, R. Paul, A. Klin, & D. Cohen (Eds.), *Handbook of autism and pervasive developmental disorders: Assessment, interventions and policy* (3rd ed., pp. 925–945). New York: Wiley.

Prizant, B.M., Wetherby, A.M., Rubin, E., Laurent, A., & Rydell, P. (2006). *The SCERTS® Model: A comprehensive educational approach for children with autism spectrum disorders.* Baltimore: Paul H. Brookes Publishing Co.

Quinn, P.C., & Eimas, P.D. (1998). Evidence for a global categorical representation of humans by young infants. *Journal of Experimental Child Psychology, 69,* 151–174.

Quinn, P.C., & Eimas, P.D. (2000). The emergence of category representations during infancy: Are separate perceptual and conceptual processes required? *Journal of Cognition and Development, 1,* 55–62.

Quinn, P.C., Westerlund, A., & Nelson, C.A. (2006). Neural markers of categorization in 6-month-old infants. *Psychological Science, 17,* 59–66.

Rice, C. (2007). Prevalence of autism spectrum disorders: Autism and developmental disabilities monitoring network, 14 sites, United States, 2002. *Morbidity and Mortality Weekly Report, 56,* 12–28.

Robins, D.L., Fein, D., Barton, M.L., & Green, J.A. (2001). The modified checklist for autism in toddlers: An initial study investigating the early detection of autism and pervasive developmental disorders. *Journal of Autism and Developmental Disorders, 31,* 131–144.

Rodier, P.M., Ingram, J.L., Risdale, B., Nelson, S., & Romano, J. (1996). Embryological origin for autism: Developmental anomalies of the cranial nerve motor nuclei. *Journal of Comparative Neurology, 370,* 247–261.

Rogers, S.J. (2005). Evidence-based practices for language development in young children with autism. In T. Charman & W. Stone (Eds.), *Social and communication development in autism spectrum disorders: Early identification, diagnosis, and intervention* (pp. 143–179). New York: Guilford Press.

Rogers, S.J., & DiLalla, D. (1990). Age of symptom onset in young children with pervasive developmental disorders. *Journal of the American Academy of Child and Adolescent Psychiatry, 29,* 863–872.

Rogers, S.J., & Lewis, H. (1989). An effective day treatment model for young children with pervasive developmental disorders. *Journal of the American Academy of Child and Adolescent Psychiatry, 28,* 207–217.

Rutter, M., & Lord, C. (1987). Language disorders associated with psychiatric disturbance. In W. Yale & M. Rutter (Eds.), *Language development and disorders* (pp. 206–233). Philadelphia: Lippincott Williams & Wilkins.

Rydell, P.J., & Mirenda, P. (1994). Effects of high and low constraint utterances on the production of immediate and delayed echolalia in young children with autism. *Journal of Autism and Developmental Disorders, 24,* 719–735.

Sanders, L.D., Weber-Fox, C.M., & Neville, H.J. (in press). Varying degrees of plasticity in different subsystems within language. In J.R. Pomerantz & M. Crair (Eds.), *Topics in integrative neuroscience: From cells to cognition.* New York: Cambridge University Press.

Siegel, B. (1998). *Early screening and diagnosis in autistic spectrum disorders: The Pervasive Developmental Disorders Screening Test (PDDST).* Paper presented at the National Institute for Child Health and Development Early Screening and Diagnosis for Autism Invitational Conference, Bethesda, MD.

Siegel, B. (2004). *Pervasive Developmental Disorders Screening Test–II (PDDST-II).* San Antonio, TX: Harcourt Assessment.

Siegel, B., & Hayer, C. (1999, April). *Detection of autism in the second and third year: The Pervasive Developmental Disorders Screening Test.* Paper presented at the symposium on Early diagnosis and screening for autism at the Society for Research in Child Development, Albuquerque, NM.

Sigman, M., Mundy, P., Sherman, T., & Ungerer, J. (1986). Social interactions of autistic, mentally retarded, and normal children and their caregivers. *Journal of Child Psychology and Psychiatry, 27,* 647–655.

Siller, M., & Sigman, M. (2002). The behaviors of parents of children with autism predict the subsequent development of their children's communication. *Journal of Autism and Developmental Disorders, 32,* 77–89.

Smith, L.B. (1999). Children's noun learning: How general learning processes make specialized learning mechanisms. In B. MacWhinney (Ed.), *The emergence of language* (pp. 277–303). Mahwah, NJ: Lawrence Erlbaum Associates.

Smith, T., Groen, A.D., & Wynn, J.W. (2000). Randomized trial of intensive early intervention for children with pervasive developmental disorder. *American Journal of Mental Retardation, 105,* 269–285.

Spelke, E.S. (1990). Principles of object segregation. *Cognitive Science, 14,* 29–56.

Spelke, E.S. (2003). Core knowledge. In N. Kanwisher & J. Duncan (Eds.), *Attention and performance, functional neuroimaging of visual cognition* (pp. 1233–1243). New York: Oxford University Press.

Stahmer, A.C., Collings, N.M., & Palinkas, L.A. (2005). Early intervention practices for children with autism: Descriptions from community providers. *Focus on Autism and Other Developmental Disabilities, 20,* 66–79.

Stevens, C., & Neville, H. (2006). Neuroplasticity as a double-edged sword: Deaf enhancements and dyslexic deficits in motion processing. *Journal of Cognitive Neuroscience, 18,* 701–714.

Stone, W.L., Coonrod, E.E., & Ousley, O.Y. (2000). Brief report: Screening Tool for Autism in Two-year-olds (STAT): Development and preliminary data. *Journal of Autism and Developmental Disorders, 30,* 607–612.

Stone, W.L., Lee E.B., Ashford, L., Brissie, J., Hepburn, S.L., Coonrod, E.E., et al. (1999). Can autism be diagnosed accurately in children under 3 years? *Journal of Child Psychology and Psychiatry, 40,* 219–226.

Stone, W.L., & Ousley, O.Y. (1997). STAT manual: *Screening Tool for Autism in Two-Year-Olds.* Unpublished manuscript, Vanderbilt University.

Stone, W.L., Ousley, O.Y., & Littleford, C.D. (1997). Motor imitation in young children with autism: What's the object? *Journal of Abnormal Child Psychology, 25,* 475–485.

Sullivan, M., Finelli, J., Marvin, A., Garrett-Mayer, E., Bauman, M., & Landa, R. (2007). Response to joint attention in toddlers at risk for autism spectrum disorder: A prospective study. *Journal of Autism and Developmental Disorders, 37,* 37–48.

Tiegerman, E., & Primavera, L.H. (1984). Imitating the autistic child: Facilitating communicative gaze behavior. *Journal of Autism and Developmental Disorders, 14,* 27–38.

Tuchman, R.F., & Rapin, I. (1997). Regression in pervasive developmental disorders: Seizures and epileptiform electroencephalogram correlates. *Pediatrics, 99,* 560–566.

Turner, L.M., & Stone, W.L. (2007). Variability in outcome for children with an ASD diagnosis at age 2. *Journal of Child Psychology and Psychiatry, 48,* 793–802.

Van de Walle, G., Carey, S., & Prevor, M. (2000). Bases for object individuation in infancy: Evidence from manual search. *Journal of Cognition and Development, 1,* 249–280.

Watson, L.R. (1998). Following the child's lead: Mothers' interactions with children with autism. *Journal of Autism and Developmental Disorders, 28,* 51–59.

Waxman, S.R., & Markow, D.B. (1995). Words as invitations to form categories: Evidence from 12-to 13-month-old infants. *Cognitive Psychology, 29,* 257–302.

Werlin, S.L., D'Souza, B.J., Hogan, W.J., Dodds, W.J., & Arndorfer, R.C. (1980). Sandifer syndrome: An unappreciated clinical entity. *Developmental Medicine and Child Neurology, 22,* 374–378.

Wetherby, A., & Prizant, B.M. (1989). Assessing the communication of infants and toddlers: Integrating a socioemotional perspective. *Zero to Three, 11,* 1–12.

Wetherby, A., & Prizant, B.M. (2002). *Communication and Symbolic Behavior Scales Developmental Profile (CSBS DP™), first normed edition.* Baltimore: Paul H. Brookes Publishing Co.

Wetherby, A.M., Prizant, B.M., & Hutchinson, T.A. (1998). Communicative, social/affective, and symbolic profiles of young children with autism and pervasive developmental disorder. *American Journal of Speech-Language Pathology, 7,* 79–91.

Whalen, C., & Schreibman, L. (2003). Joint attention training for children with autism using behavior modification procedures. *Journal of Child Psychology and Psychiatry, 44,* 456–468.

Wiggins, L.D., Baio, J., & Rice, C. (2006). Examination of the time between first evaluation and first autism spectrum diagnosis in a population-based sample. *Journal of Developmental and Behavioral Pediatrics, 27,* S79–S87.

Yirmiya, N., Gamliel, I., Pilowsky, T., Feldman, R., Baron-Cohen, S., & Sigman, M. (2006). The development of siblings of children with autism at 4 and 14 months: Social engagement, communication, and cognition. *Journal of Child Psychology and Psychiatry, 47,* 511–523.

Young, R.L., Brewer, N., & Pattison, C. (2003). Parental identification of early behavioural abnormalities in children with autistic disorder. *Autism, 7,* 125–143.

Zwaigenbaum, L., Bryson, S., Rogers, T., Roberts, W., Brian, J., & Szatmari, P. (2005). Behavioral manifestations of autism in the first year of life. *International Journal of Developmental Neuroscience, 23,* 143–152.

Clinical Impressions

Clinical Impressions

Child's name _____

Date of birth _____ Date of exam _____

Examiner's name _____

0	1	2	3
No delay	**Concern**	**Mild delay**	**Significant delay**
The child appears to be developing typically based on test scores and clinical judgment.	Monitor the child, but at this time there is insufficient evidence to code as impaired or delayed.	Test scores and/or clinical judgment indicate that the child is mildly delayed.	Test scores and clinical judgment indicate a definite and clinically significant delay.

Check all of the areas in which there is concern about the child's development:

☐ Speech/articulation   ☐ Feeding/GI

☐ Language   ☐ Hearing

☐ Social communication   ☐ Vision

☐ Fine motor   ☐ General developmental delay

☐ Gross motor   ☐ Nonverbal IQ/visual reception

☐ Social anxiety   ☐ Attention

☐ Social   ☐ Repetitive behaviors

☐ Temperament   ☐ Other

☐ Behavior   ☐ ASD/autism   ⟨ PDD-NOS / Autism / Asperger

☐ Sensory issues

Confidence Rating for Autism Spectrum Disorder Clinical Impression

0	1	2	3	4	5	6
Confident no ASD	Possible ASD, but not likely	Suspect ASD, but can't be sure	Confident PDD-NOS	On spectrum, not sure if PDD or autism	Confident autism	Asperger syndrome

Recommendations:

☐ Referral for further evaluation   ☐ Referral for treatment

☐ Retest at age _____

☐ Monitor via telephone

☐ None

☐ **REQUEST SECOND OPINION** Specify by whom _____ Anyone

ASD indicators	ASD contra-indicators

Additional notes/observations

Clinical Impressions Copyright © 2008 Rebecca Landa. In *Autism Frontiers: Clinical Issues and Innovations,* edited by Bruce K. Shapiro & Pasquale J. Accardo (2008, Paul H. Brookes Publishing Co., Inc.). All rights reserved.

Review of Observations

Review of Observations

Child's name _____

Date of birth _____ Date of assessment _____ Chronological age _____

Context of assessment _____

Examiner's name _____

Caregiver's name _____

Behavior	Clinician	Caregiver
Social		
Responds to others' smile		
Initiates smile with eye contact		
Consistent eye contact throughout session		
"Checks in" with others periodically		
Three-way gaze shift (e.g., object–person–object)		
Looks where others look (note whether child requires a pointing gesture to look)		
Points things out		
___to request a desired action or object		
___to show an action or object		
Can switch from own play focus to that of another person's		
Spontaneously imitates others' action		
Looks at others when imitates (indicate whether this is paired with a smile)		
Gives objects to share		
Consistently and quickly responds with eye contact to name being called		
Does not respond to name, but responds when tickled, when touched, or to a familiar song or verse		
Engages in turn-taking, showing enjoyment		
Communication		
Understands gestures and words; responds to language and gestures of others		
Makes a variety of sounds to communicate, directs communication with gaze or gesture or body language		
Communicates using conventional forms (gestures, words)		
Communicates frequently		
Echoes or says things in an unusual way		
Unusual tone of voice or loudness level		
Coordinates eye contact, smile, and gesture/vocal communication		
Play		
Explores a variety of objects		
Selects several different objects and plays with them in a variety of different ways		
Shows pretend play		
Tries to engage another person in play		
Prefers certain topics or objects (e.g., numbers, letters)		
Repeatedly focuses on small parts of objects		
Repeats actions with a toy or with body (e.g., lines toys up, rolls a toy car back and forth repeatedly)		
Has difficulty with change in routine		
Reluctant to touch certain objects		
Excessive mouthing		
Unusual gait or other motor behavior; low muscle tone; poor motor coordination		

Review of Observations Copyright © 2008 Rebecca Landa. In *Autism Frontiers: Clinical Issues and Innovations,* edited by Bruce K. Shapiro & Pasquale J. Accardo (2008, Paul H. Brookes Publishing Co., Inc.). All rights reserved.

8

Classroom-Based Interventions for Children with Autism Spectrum Disorders

Andrew L. Egel

The majority of children with autism spectrum disorders (ASDs) spend a considerable part of their lives in school-based programs from the time they are very young until they are 21 years of age. These individuals often spend more than 6 hours per day, 5 days per week receiving instruction in a classroom setting. The most important behaviors addressed in classrooms reflect the most serious deficits characteristic of individuals with ASDs—socialization and communication. A renewed emphasis has also been placed on understanding motivation and creating strategies for increasing the motivation of children with ASDs. This chapter reviews the research in these areas and describes its importance and relevance for school-based programs.

JOINT ATTENTION AND COMMUNICATION

One area that has received more attention in recent years is joint attention. *Joint attention* refers to a child's alternating attention between an object and a communication partner. Children display joint attention skills by initiating to others to pay attention to that which they are attending and by responding to another person's cues (e.g., pointing) to attend to a particular stimulus or set of stimuli in which the partner is interested. Joint attention skills are critical because they have been shown to be highly correlated with early acquisition of receptive and expressive language, as well as other, more complex skills in typically developing children (Charman, et al., 2003; Loveland & Landry, 1986; Mundy, Sigman, & Kasari, 1990). Unfortunately, children with ASDs show deficits in joint attention before they are 1 year old (Baron-Cohen, Allen, & Gillberg, 1992; Charman, et al., 1998; Osterling & Dawson, 1994). In fact, impairments in the development of joint attention skills are considered by some as hallmarks of children with ASDs (Mundy, 1995). The deficit in joint attention skills characteristic of children with ASDs is substantially greater than has been found in children with typical development and those with global developmental delays (Leekam, Lopez, & Moore, 2000; Mundy, Sigman, & Kasari, 1994). Kasari, Sigman, Mundy, and Yirmiya (1990) further noted that, even when joint attention is shown, children with ASDs are much less likely than either children with typical development or children with developmental delays to display positive affect along with joint attention behaviors. Several authors (e.g., Jones & Carr, 2004; Kasari, Freeman, & Paparella, 2006; Martins & Harris, 2006; Mundy, 1995; Whalen & Schreibman, 2003; Whalen, Schreibman, & Ingersoll, 2006) have suggested that the deficit in joint attention behaviors should be a high priority for intervention because their absence may be related to the core problems in social and communicative behavior.

The importance of joint attention for the development of language and social behaviors has led some researchers to investigate procedures for teaching joint attention. Whalen and Schreibman (2003) taught children with ASDs to respond to joint attention bids and to initiate joint attention using a training package with components from Discrete Trial Training (DTT; Smith, 2001) and Pivotal Response Treatment (PRT; e.g., Koegel, & Koegel, 2006). Each child was taught how to respond to joint attention bids using a training package with 6 levels. Levels 1–3 taught children to shift attention from the activity in which they were engaged when new toys were presented. Children in Level 4 were taught how to make eye contact so that they could subsequently follow when the therapist pointed to (i.e., Level 5) or gazed at a new object (i.e., Level 6).

Children were also taught two different ways in which to initiate joint attention. First, they were taught to shift their gaze from a toy to the therapist (i.e., *coordinated gaze shift* training) in order to share the object with the therapist. Children were then taught to point (i.e., *protodeclarative* point training) to new pictures or toys to share them with the therapist. The results of the study showed that all children increased their responding to the therapist's joint attention gestures and improved their initiation of joint attention. Maintenance measures were obtained 3 months after the posttreatment assessments were completed. The results showed that all of the children continued to respond to joint attention bids, although initiation of joint attention was not maintained.

Martins and Harris (2006) also examined whether or not children with ASDs could be taught to respond to joint attention bids from adults. The joint attention bids consisted of the adult saying the child's name followed by the adult turning his head

and looking at a specific object. Martins and Harris' intervention had four phases, each of which required a child to respond to closer approximations of the target behavior. The adult in Phase 1 called the child's name, turned his head toward the object, pointed and touched the object, and said, "Look." Phase 4 required the child to respond when the adult called the child's name and turned his head toward the object.

The results showed that all of the participants increased their responding to joint attention bids following training, and that such responding was maintained in the absence of additional reinforcement. Increases in responding to joint attention bids did not, however, improve the participants' initiation of joint attention behaviors. The authors suggested that responding to joint attention bids and the initiation of joint attention behaviors may be functionally different and may have to be taught separately.

Kasari and her colleagues (2006) targeted joint attention skills and symbolic play in children with ASDs using an approach that combined DTT and a more naturalistic approach. Specifically, the participants each received discrete trial instruction that was teacher-directed and used prompt hierarchies and reinforcement to begin shaping the targeted skills. This was followed by training of the previously targeted behaviors in a less structured setting where trainers continued to use prompt hierarchies and reinforcement but focused their instruction based on the activity in which the child was engaged (cf., Hancock & Kaiser, 2002). The authors measured the frequency of each child's joint attention skills, including coordinated looks, pointing and showing, and the duration of joint engagement between parent and child. The results for the joint attention intervention showed that children in this group initiated substantially more joint attention skills when compared with a control group. The results also showed that children in the joint attention intervention demonstrated greater levels of responding to joint attention bids than those in the control group. Finally, the joint attention skills generalized from the training conditions to a setting in which the children played with their mothers.

Each of the previously described studies demonstrated that children with ASDs can be taught to initiate joint attention skills and respond to joint attention bids. Neither, however, made it clear that increasing joint attention skills resulted in collateral improvements in other critical skills. Jones, Carr, and Feeley (2006) conducted a study designed to address this issue. In their three-part investigation, Jones et al. taught children with ASDs to engage in joint attention behaviors (e.g., responding, initiating) using both discrete trial instruction and PRT strategies. They also measured expressive language and social-communication behaviors to see if changes in these behaviors would occur if joint attention skills were increased.

Jones et al. (2006) showed that the combined approach was effective in teaching children with ASDs to respond to joint attention bids and to initiate behaviors to establish joint attention. Furthermore, the authors showed that both expressive language and social-communicative behaviors increased, although these behaviors had not been targeted directly during the study. Methodological issues make it difficult to establish a direct link between increases in joint attention and increases in expressive language and social-communicative behaviors, however, this study provided data that suggested that such a relationship may exist.

Whalen et al. (2006) presented more direct data on the effects of joint attention training on the occurrence of nontargeted behaviors. These authors taught joint attention skills using a methodology similar to that used by Whalen and Schreibman (2003). In addition, the authors measured the occurrence of four behaviors—social initiations, positive affect, imitative play, and

spontaneous speech—that were not targeted for intervention. The results showed that all participants increased their frequency of social initiations and positive affect on measures obtained subsequent to intervention. Similar data were found for all four participants on measures of imitative play during structured assessments and language obtained following intervention. Increases in spontaneous play were not obtained when measured in a more naturalistic setting. The levels of changes for all four behaviors were not maintained at the 3-month follow-up, although the responding of most participants was still above baseline levels.

Taken together, the results from the studies reviewed highlight the importance of targeting joint attention skills as part of a school curriculum for students with ASDs, especially as part of an early intervention program. Although data on the long-term effects of early joint attention training have not been published to date, there is enough evidence of its importance that teachers should include it as part of their instruction.

INCREASING SOCIAL BEHAVIOR

A second, fundamental feature of ASDs is social deficits. Deficits in this area are well-documented in the literature (e.g., McConnell, 2002; Rogers, 2000) and have been central to virtually all diagnostic criteria (e.g., *Diagnostic and Statistical Manual of Mental Disorders, Fourth Edition, Text Revision* [*DSM-IV-TR;* American Psychiatric Association, 2000]; *International Classification of Diseases: Diagnostic Criteria for Research* [*ICD-10;* World Health Organization, 1992]; *National Society for Autistic Children Definition of the Syndrome of Autism* [Ritvo & Freeman, 1977]). The importance of these social deficits can also be seen by the tremendous amount of research that has been conducted to develop and evaluate interventions for increasing the social behavior of individuals with ASDs (e.g., Brown, Odom, & Conroy, 2001; McConnell, 2002).

Many procedures such as peer-mediated interventions have produced positive effects for children with ASDs and other disabilities in classroom settings, although generalization of skills is often an issue. Table 8.1 lists some recommendations teachers can use to promote the social behavior of children with ASDs.

Several researchers have begun to evaluate the effects of using Social Stories to teach social skills to children with ASDs. Gray and Garand (1993) described a Social Story as a brief story that helps individuals understand social situations by describing a situation and teaching the desired responses. Gray (2000) identified the four basic types of sentences that should be included in a Social Story.

1. Descriptive: An accurate, assumption-free statement of observable facts

2. Perspective: A sentence that describes the thoughts and feelings of other people

3. Affirmative: A statement that enhances the meaning of surrounding sentences and may express a commonly shared opinion

4. Directive: A statement that identifies a possible response and/or gently directs behavior

Gray noted that a Social Story should have 0–1 directive sentences for every 2–5 descriptive, perspective, or affirmative sentences. Gray suggested that such a ratio would help ensure that the story describes

Table 8.1. Brief summary of recommendations for promoting social skills in individuals with autism spectrum disorders

Teach appropriate opening comments
Teach to seek clarification or assistance
Teach to recognize conversation cues
Use Social Stories/comic strip conversations for cuing
Be precise and avoid abstractions
Highlight key points for instruction
Use visual models

a specific situation (i.e., cues that set the occasion for a particular behavior) and possible responses.

In their review of the Social Stories literature, Sansosti, Powell-Smith, and Kincaid (2004) noted that most researchers have used Social Stories to reduce challenging behaviors (e.g., Brownell, 2002; Kuttler, Myles, & Carlson, 1998; Lorimer, Simpson, Myles, & Ganz, 2002; Scattone, Wilczynski, Edwards, & Rabian, 2002). Fewer studies have addressed whether Social Stories could be used to increase appropriate social behavior. Norris and Dattilo (1999) used an A–B design to assess whether Social Stories could be used to increase the level of peer interaction in an 8-year-old girl with an ASD. The authors had her read the story prior to lunch and measured appropriate social interactions (e.g., initiating, responding to other students), inappropriate social interactions, (e.g., delayed echolalia, noises), and the absence of social interactions (e.g., no initiations or responses) during the students' lunch period. The results indicated that, although the frequency of inappropriate behaviors decreased, there was no effect on the level of appropriate peer interactions.

Thiemann and Goldstein (2001) conducted a more comprehensive investigation of Social Stories. These authors combined Social Stories, picture cue cards, and video feedback to increase a child's attempts at 1) securing attention, 2) initiating comments, 3) initiating requests, and 4) making contingent responses. Thiemann and Goldstein measured the occurrence of these behaviors when the child with an ASD was paired with two peers with typical development. The results showed that the participants increased their targeted social behavior following intervention. The extent to which the Social Stories component per se contributed to the effectiveness of the intervention remains unclear because a component analysis was not conducted.

Scattone, Tingstrom, and Wilczynski (2006) examined whether a Social Story could be used to increase the appropriate social interactions of three children with ASDs. The authors measured six social behaviors.

1. Verbal, physical, or gestural initiations to a peer
2. Comments or questions about the activity or conversation in which they were engaged
3. The extent to which the student with an ASD continued to be engaged in the same activity as the peer with typical development
4. On-topic responses to a peer's comments or questions
5. The initiation of a comment or the asking of a question related to the conversation
6. Any physical gestures used to communicate agreement or disagreement with a peer

Social Stories were developed for each individual participant and focused on social initiations and responses that would be appropriate when interacting with peers. The intervention consisted of a teacher reading a Social Story to a particular student and then asking a set of questions to assess comprehension. After the students answered all of the questions correctly, the teacher either had them read (or read to them, depending on their reading ability) the Social Story immediately before they began free time.

The effects of the intervention varied across participants. Two of the three participants increased their appropriate social interactions with peers, although the behavior of only one of those two increased substantially. The third participant's behavior did not change after the intervention was applied. These data suggest that Social Stories alone may not be sufficient to increase the social behavior of some children with ASDs.

Delano and Snell (2006) obtained more conclusive results. These authors assessed the effects of Social Stories on the duration of appropriate social engagement and the frequency of four social skills in three children with ASDs. Social Stories that provided information on the specific play activity used during a particular session were written for each participant. The stories also included examples of the four social skills selected as target behaviors. There were three parts to the Social Story intervention.

1. A Social Story was read to the participant and a peer with typical development.
2. The experimenter subsequently asked a series of questions to determine whether the child with an ASD comprehended the story, which was defined as the child's ability to correctly answer at least 75% of the questions.
3. Both the child with an ASD and the peer went into the play area to play.

Each participant increased the duration of social engagement with the peer with typical development as well as with one who was novel. Increases were also seen in the frequency of targeted social skills during play sessions following the intervention, although the participants engaged in two of the four behaviors, contingent responding and initiating comments. Data from the generalization assessments showed that the social behaviors of two participants generalized to their classrooms. The maintenance probes demonstrated that the target behaviors occurred more frequently than in the baseline; however, responding was more variable than during intervention.

Overall, the results from the Delano and Snell (2006) article are more encouraging than those reported by Scattone, et al. (2006). Delano and Snell's data suggested that teachers could use Social Stories as a main intervention to increase the social behavior of individuals with ASDs. Further study is necessary to determine whether Social Stories must be combined with other visual supports (Thiemann & Goldstein, 2001) to promote greater generalization and maintenance.

MOTIVATION

For some time, investigators have identified motivation as a substantial problem for children with ASDs (e.g., Dunlap & Koegel, 1980; Egel, 1980, 1981; Koegel & Egel, 1979; Koegel, & Koegel, 2006). *Motivation* refers to a child's responsivity to environmental stimuli. The assumption has been that increases in motivation or responsivity may lead to generalized changes in the overall responding of children with ASDs (Koegel, Koegel, & McNerney, 2001).

Several studies have evaluated the effects of different procedures designed to increase motivation. The interventions addressed the problem of motivation by manipulating the manner in which antecedent or consequent stimuli were presented. The interventions are designed so that teachers can implement them during instruction with little difficulty. Dunlap and his colleagues (Dunlap, 1984; Winterling, Dunlap, & O'Neill, 1987) improved the motivation of children with ASDs by interspersing tasks (i.e., antecedent manipulation) that had been previously acquired with tasks that were currently being acquired.

Another antecedent manipulation that has improved motivation is child choice. Providing children with ASDs with choices during instruction requires teachers or therapists to use child-preferred or child-chosen materials, activities, topics, and toys as they are teaching. Several studies have shown that child choice can improve the responsivity of children with ASDs (e.g., Koegel, Dyer, & Bell, 1987; Moes, 1998; Reinhartsen, Garfinkle, & Wolery, 2002). It is likely that providing the child with choices and using child-preferred materials increases motiva-

tion because the teaching situation becomes more reinforcing under these conditions.

There is also evidence that manipulating consequences can increase the motivation of children with ASDs. Egel (1980, 1981) evaluated the effects of varying reinforcers systematically on the responsiveness of children with ASDs. Specifically, Egel compared a constant delivery condition in which the same reinforcer was presented on each trial to a varied delivery condition in which a child received one of three reinforcers for approximately every third response. The results showed that the varied reinforcer condition produced much higher levels of correct responding and general on-task behavior for substantially longer periods of time.

All of the procedures in this chapter can be easily incorporated into teaching opportunities within a classroom. Koegel and his colleagues (e.g., Koegel, & Koegel, 2006; Koegel et al., 2001) highlighted the importance of using procedures to increase motivation when they identified motivation as one of several pivotal responses. *Pivotal responses* are behaviors that when increased lead to improvements in other untargeted behaviors. The authors suggested that motivation should be an area targeted as early as possible to maximize the possible benefits.

CONCLUSION

There are substantial opportunities in school programs to make significant, meaningful progress for children with ASDs. Teachers and staff can take advantage of these opportunities only if they are aware of the rapid progress being made toward the development of effective instructional methodologies and can identify important target behaviors such as those described previously. When changed, these target behaviors can impact the lives of children with ASDs.

REFERENCES

American Psychiatric Association. (2000). *Diagnostic and statistical manual of mental disorders* (4th ed., text rev.). Washington, DC: Author.

Baron-Cohen, S., Allen, J., & Gillberg, C. (1992). Can autism be detected at 18 months? The needle, the haystack, and the CHAT. *British Journal of Psychiatry, 161*, 839–843.

Brown, W.H., Odom, S.L., & Conroy, M.A. (2001). An intervention hierarchy for promoting young children's interactions in natural environments. *Topics in Early Childhood Special Education, 21*, 162–175.

Brownell, M.D. (2002). Musically adapted Social Stories to modify behaviors in students with autism: Four case studies. *Journal of Music Therapy, 39*, 117–144.

Charman, T., Baron-Cohen, S., Swettenham, J., Baird, G., Drew, A., & Cox, A. (2003). Predicting language outcome in infants with autism and pervasive developmental disorder. *International Journal of Language and Communication Disorders, 38*, 265–285.

Charman, T., Swettenham, J., Baron-Cohen, S., Cox, A., Baird, G., & Drew, A. (1998). An experimental investigation of social-cognitive abilities in infants with autism: Clinical implications. *Infant Mental Health Journal, 19*, 260–275.

Delano, M., & Snell, M.E. (2006). The effects of Social Stories on the social engagement of children with autism. *Journal of Positive Behavioral Interventions, 8*, 29–42.

Dunlap, G. (1984). The influence of task variation and maintenance tasks on the learning and affect of autistic children. *Journal of Experimental Child Psychology, 37*, 41–64.

Dunlap, G., & Koegel, R.L. (1980). Motivating autistic children through stimulus variation. *Journal of Applied Behavior Analysis, 13*, 619–627.

Dunlap, G., & Koegel, R.L. (1984). Motivating autistic children through stimulus variation. *Journal of Applied Behavior Analysis, 13*, 619–627.

Egel, A.L. (1980). Effects of constant vs. varied reinforcer presentation on the responding of autistic children. *Journal of Experimental Child Psychology, 30*, 455–463.

Egel, A.L. (1981). Reinforcer variation: Implications for motivating developmentally delayed children. *Journal of Applied Behavior Analysis, 14*, 343–350.

Gray, C.A. (2000). *The new Social Story book.* Arlington, TX: Future Horizons.

Gray, C.A., & Garand, J.D. (1993). Social Stories: Improving responses of students with autism with accurate social information. *Focus on Autistic Behavior, 8*, 1–10.

Hancock, T.B., & Kaiser, A. (2002). The effects of trainer-implemented Enhanced Milieu Teaching on the social communication of children with autism. *Topics in Early Childhood Special Education, 22*, 39–54.

Jones, E.A., & Carr, E.G. (2004). Joint attention in children with autism: Theory and intervention. *Focus on Autism and Other Developmental Disabilities, 19*, 13–26.

Jones, E.A., Carr, E.G., & Feeley, K.M. (2006). Multiple effects of joint attention intervention for children with autism. *Behavior Modification, 30*, 782–834.

Kasari, C., Freeman, S., & Paparella, T. (2006). Joint attention and symbolic play in young children with autism: A randomized controlled intervention study. *Journal of Child Psychology and Psychiatry, 47*, 611–620.

Kasari, C., Sigman, M., Mundy, P., & Yirmiya, N. (1990). Affective sharing in the context of joint attention interactions of normal, autistic, and mentally retarded children. *Journal of Autism and Developmental Disorders, 20*, 87–100.

Koegel, R.L., Dyer, K., & Bell, L.K. (1987). The influence of child-preferred activities on autistic children's social behavior. *Journal of Applied Behavior Analysis, 20*, 243–252.

Koegel, R.L., & Egel, A.L. (1979). Motivating autistic children. *Journal of Abnormal Psychology, 88*, 418–426.

Koegel, R.L., & Koegel, L.K. (2006). *Pivotal Response Treatments for autism: Communication, Social, and Academic Development.* Baltimore: Paul H. Brookes Publishing Co.

Koegel, R.L., Koegel, L.K., & McNerney, E.K. (2001). Pivotal areas in intervention for autism. *Journal of Clinical Child Psychology, 30*, 19–32.

Kuttler, S., Myles, B.S., & Carlson, J.K. (1998). The use of Social Stories to reduce precursors to tantrum behavior in a student with autism. *Focus on Autism and Other Developmental Disabilities, 13*, 176–182.

Leekam, S.R., Lopez, B., & Moore, C. (2000). Attention and joint attention in preschool children with autism. *Developmental Psychology, 36*, 261–273.

Lorimer, P.A., Simpson, R.L., Myles, B.S., & Ganz, J.B. (2002). The use of Social Stories as a preventative behavioral intervention in a home setting with a child with autism. *Journal of Positive Behavior Intervention, 4,* 53–60.

Loveland, K.A., & Landry, S.H. (1986). Joint attention and language in autism and developmental language delay. *Journal of Autism and Developmental Disorders, 16,* 335–349.

Martins, M.P., & Harris, S.L. (2006). Teaching children with autism to respond to joint attention initiations. *Child and Family Behavior Therapy, 28,* 51–68.

McConnell, S.R. (2002). Interventions to facilitate social interaction for young children with autism: Review of available research and recommendations for educational intervention. *Journal of Autism and Developmental Disorders, 32,* 351–372.

Moes, D.R. (1998). Integrating choice-making opportunities within teacher-assigned academic tasks to facilitate the performance of children with autism *Journal of the Association for Persons with Severe Handicaps, 23,* 319–328.

Mundy, P. (1995). Joint attention and social-emotional approach in children with autism. *Development and Psychopathology, 7,* 63–82.

Mundy, P., Sigman, M., & Kasari, C. (1990). A longitudinal study of joint attention and language development in autistic children. *Journal of Autism and Developmental Disorders, 20,* 115–128.

Mundy, P., Sigman, M., & Kasari, C. (1994). Joint attention, developmental level, and symptom presentation in young children with autism. *Development and Psychopathology, 6,* 389–401.

Norris, C., & Dattilo, J. (1999). Evaluating effects of a Social Story intervention on a young girl with autism. *Focus on Autism and Other Developmental Disabilities, 14,* 180–186.

Osterling, J., & Dawson, G. (1994). Early recognition of children with autism: A study of first birthday home videotapes. *Journal of Autism and Developmental Disorders, 24,* 247–257.

Reinhartsen, D.B., Garfinkle, A.N., & Wolery, M. (2002). Engagement with toys in two-year-old children with autism: Teacher selection versus child choice. *Research and Practice for Persons with Severe Disabilities, 27,* 175–187.

Ritvo, E.R., & Freeman, B.J. (1977). National Society for Autistic Children definition of the syndrome of autism. *Journal of Pediatric Psychology, 2,* 146–148.

Rogers, S.J. (2000). Interventions that facilitate socialization in children with autism. *Journal of Autism and Developmental Disorders, 30,* 399–409.

Sansosti, F.J., Powell-Smith, K.A., & Kincaid, D. (2004). A research synthesis of Social Story intervention for children with autism spectrum disorders. *Focus on Autism and Other Developmental Disabilities, 19,* 194–204.

Scattone, D., Tingstrom, D.H., & Wilczynski, S.M. (2006). Increasing appropriate social interactions of children with autism using Social Stories. *Focus on Autism and Other Developmental Disabilities, 21,* 211–222.

Scattone, D., Wilczynski, S.M., Edwards, R.P., & Rabian, B. (2002). Decreasing disruptive behavior of children with autism using Social Stories. *Journal of Autism and Developmental Disorders, 32,* 535–543.

Smith, T. (2001). Discrete trial training in the treatment of autism. *Focus on Autism and Other Developmental Disabilities, 16,* 86–92.

Thiemann, K., & Goldstein, H. (2001). Social Stories, written text cues, and video feedback: Effects on social communication of children with autism. *Journal of Applied Behavior Analysis, 24,* 425–446.

Whalen, C., & Schreibman, L. (2003). Joint attention training for children with autism using behavior modification procedures. *Journal of Child Psychology and Psychiatry, 44,* 456–468.

Whalen, C., Schreibman, L., & Ingersoll, B. (2006). The collateral effects of joint attention training on social initiations, positive affect, imitation, and spontaneous speech for young children with autism. *Journal of Autism and Developmental Disorders, 29,* 154–172.

Winterling, V., Dunlap, G., & O'Neill, R.E. (1987). The influence of task variation on the aberrant behaviors of autistic students. *Education and Treatment of Children, 10,* 105–119.

World Health Organization. (1992). *International Classification of Diseases: Diagnostic criteria for research, tenth revision (ICD-10).* Geneva: Author.

9

Student, Parent, and Teacher Perspectives on Barriers to and Facilitators of School Success for Students with Asperger Syndrome

Donald P. Oswald, Martha J. Coutinho,
Jesse "Woody" Johnson, Jennifer H. Larson, and Carla A. Mazefsky

Asperger syndrome (AS) is a fairly common and complex pervasive developmental disorder (PDD) characterized by marked social impairment that negatively affects functioning and participation in home, school, and community settings. In recent years, the number of children and youth identified as having AS or high functioning autism (HFA) has increased dramatically. Prevalence estimates indicate that as many as 48 (Kadesjo, Gillberg, & Nagberg, 1999) to 76 (Ehlers & Gillberg, 1993) per 10,000 children may have AS. Students with AS/HFA are at significant risk for impaired functioning and depression, as well as other forms of emotional distress (Hedley & Young, 2006) due to their complicated learning profiles, educational needs that are often masked by average or better intelligence quotient (IQ), a lack of reciprocal friendships, and frequent victimization by their peers.

Teachers and clinicians are faced with great uncertainty when it comes to effectively addressing the complex and sometimes surprising or unusual social, academic, and behavioral needs of students with AS/HFA. In many cases, parents bring diagnoses of their children from mental health professionals and pediatricians, as well as recommendations for addressing their children's social and educational needs. Too often, the bridge between educational and other systems of care is not obvious or easy, and the relationship between home and school can be tenuous. In addition, students with AS/HFA are not likely to articulate their needs in ways teachers can readily apply; thus, students may not contribute much to the search for strategies or supports that are necessary for them to succeed.

CHARACTERISTICS OF ASPERGER SYNDROME

AS is generally understood to be first and foremost a disorder of social functioning (Frith, 1991; Wing, 1981). Individuals with AS tend to seek out social engagement, but they are likely to approach social situations in an overly rigid, moralistic, and naïve manner (Macintosh & Dissanayake, 2006a; Wing, 1981). Youth with AS often present as socially stiff or awkward due in part to their difficulty inferring the thoughts or beliefs of

Support for this chapter was provided in part by a Research and Innovation grant from the Office of Special Education Programs, U.S. Department of Education (H324C040023).

others and understanding the rules and conventions of social behavior (Myles & Simpson, 1998, 2002). Social competence does not generally improve merely as a function of age (Myles & Simpson, 2002), and as a result, many adults with AS do not have significant social relationships (Gutstein & Whitney, 2002).

Individuals with AS may display a rigid and literal use of language and have problems understanding conversational rules (Landa, 2000). During attempts at social interaction, they frequently engage in one-sided monologues consisting of facts related to their intense and often unusual interests. They may also fail to pick up on nonverbal cues regarding a listener's interest in the conversation (Frith, 1991; Klin, Pauls, Schultz, & Volkmar, 2005; Volkmar, Klin, Schultz, Rubin, & Bronen, 2000). Individuals with AS may exhibit strong preferences for nonfunctional rituals and for consistent environments and schedules (Gagnon, 2001; Safran, 2001). Additional associated characteristics may include motor clumsiness (Gillberg, 1989), abnormal tone of voice modulation (Bonnet & Gao, 1996), and other differences in prosody (Bellon-Harn & Harn, 2006).

Adolescence may be a particularly challenging time for individuals with AS because of societal expectations related to work habits, social and peer demands, and advanced academic requirements (Bauer, 1999). In fact, a deterioration in general functioning often occurs in adolescents with AS, usually resulting from the increased complexity of social demands and the students' inability to establish appropriate peer relationships (Bradley, Summers, Wood, & Bryson, 2004). Social awkwardness often leads to peer rejection (Volkmar et al., 2000), and adolescents with AS often experience victimization in the form of physical aggression or extreme teasing (Tantam, 2003).

Individuals with AS may experience extreme stress because of their social impair-

ment (Barnhill & Myles, 2001; Ozonoff, Rogers, & Pennington, 1991; Williams, 2001). They often encounter conflict with others, and this social difficulty may lead to withdrawal or decreased participation in activities. Social dysfunction in individuals with AS negatively affects not only peer relationships, but also their employment opportunities and the overall quality of their lives (Safran, 2001). Individuals with AS often do not participate in the community in a manner that is meaningful to them (Newport, 2001).

Although individuals with AS are generally less globally impaired than most individuals with classic autism, strong verbal ability and generally good cognitive skills may lead peers, educators, and other service providers to overlook or misunderstand their numerous social, behavioral, communication, and learning difficulties (Griswold, Barnhill, Myles, Hagiwara, & Simpson, 2002; Safran, 2001). Average intellectual functioning or giftedness may mask significant learning differences that include a lesser capacity to grasp the meaning of information (Happé, 1991), poor comprehension of abstract concepts, a diminished ability to discriminate relevant information, and difficulty in such areas as interpreting figures of speech (e.g., idioms or metaphors) (Myles & Simpson, 1998; Myles & Southwick, 1999), applying information in real-life situations (Attwood, 1998), and comprehending sequential instructions because of their reliance on nonconventional methods to solve problems (Myles & Simpson, 1998). Behavioral problems or aggression can occur because of the impact of the social deficits when demonstrated in school or community environments that are unprepared or unwilling to provide the necessary accommodations for students with AS (Simpson & Myles, 1998).

The need for supports for students with AS is often underestimated. Not all children and youth with AS are determined to be eligible for services and accommodations under the Individuals with Disabilities Education Act (IDEA) Amendments of 1997 (PL 105-17) or through Section 504 Plans under the Rehabilitation Act of 1973 (PL 93-112). However, it is estimated that as many as 80% of students with AS receive special education services under IDEA and have specific individual education plans (IEPs).

BARRIERS AND CHALLENGES

The qualitative data included in this chapter were generated as part of a project that investigated the implementation of a team-based approach to supporting students with AS/HFA in classrooms. The initial step of the project included student, parent, and teacher assessment through interviews and surveys. We were particularly interested in learning more about the barriers and challenges that face students with AS/HFA, and we draw on data from that project to illustrate those barriers and challenges. The information acquired through this project has yielded suggestions for pediatricians, psychologists, and other service providers as they interact with school personnel, students with AS/HFA, and their families in school settings.

Difficulty with Social Interactions

Individuals with ASDs are commonly thought to prefer social isolation, and children with prototypical autism may indeed withdraw from social contact. Students with AS, however, are typically motivated to seek social interaction with others (Howard, Cohn, & Orsmond, 2006). Klin, Pauls, Schultz, and Volkmar (2005) proposed that the presence of social motivation is a defining characteristic of AS.

Nonetheless, social motivation does not mitigate the marked ineffectiveness in social interactions generally seen in children with AS. Their pervasive inability to establish and maintain age-typical relationships, particu-

larly with peers, is indicative of a profound underlying deficit that prevents successful social engagement. This deficit has been variously conceptualized as a weakness of theory of mind (Baron-Cohen, 1995; Kaland, Smith, & Mortensen, 2007); a fundamental weakness of social and pragmatic communication skills (Volkmar & Klin, 2000); a cognitive rigidity that prevents flexible accommodation of the social partner's needs (Attwood, 1998); difficulty decoding, interpreting, and expressing complex emotions (Ben Shalom et al., 2006; Lindner & Rosen, 2006); a deficit in social problem solving or social information processing (Goddard, Howlin, Dritschel, & Patel, 2007; Meyer, Mundy, Van Hecke, & Durocher, 2006); or simply a profound lack of social interaction skills (Attwood, 1998).

Whatever the source, these interaction difficulties have a direct impact on the way children with AS are perceived by their peers and the ways in which these students experience peer interactions. Some of the more common complaints about school voiced by children with AS recalled negative experiences with peers. Students perceived themselves as frequent targets of peer teasing:

"Kids said mean things like 'I hate you.'"

"One guy is mean to me, he calls me a bad name."

"[This kid] made rude comments and wouldn't be quiet."

"It bothers me when the other kids stare at me and make fun of me."

"[They] boss me around sometimes."

"[The other kids] ignore me."

"[Some of the] older kids laugh at me outside the bathroom."

Sometimes students' complaints about peers reflected personal idiosyncrasies in that they were bothered by things that other children would most likely ignore or handle without difficulty:

"Kids sometimes . . . touch me, make noises, stick out their tongue."

"Every time we are working [another student] . . . draws pictures I don't like."

The presence of these idiosyncratic preferences further compromises the ability of children with AS to engage effectively with their peers. They frequently find themselves alienated because behavior that would be enjoyed or ignored by their peers can be particularly troubling to them.

Difficulties in social functioning in school settings are also among the concerns frequently mentioned by parents of children with AS. These parents realize that their children are not functioning typically in social situations:

"[My child has difficulty] understanding social situations."

"[My child has difficulty] learning social skills."

"[My child has] trouble with concepts of socialization."

"[The] biggest challenge . . . [is] the social aspect."

"[My child has difficulty acquiring] social training . . . to help [him] fit in well with peers."

Parents are also sensitive to their children's subjective experience in school. They recognize that children with AS/HFA are frequently isolated and lonely:

"She has no friends and feels alone."

"[He] doesn't have buddies that he can go with to games or movies."

Some parents are able to identify more specific social behavior difficulties that they believe get in their children's way when interacting with others:

"[My child] always needs to be a leader and in charge."

"[My child] doesn't care how he is perceived or what other people think."

"[My child] doesn't make new friends."

"[My child] is challenged with social skills . . . would rather work alone than face rejection from peers."

Many parents recognize that their children's social difficulties constitute their main impairment and worry about the future:

"I think [my child] will always have a problem with social situations and will have to be guided as [my child] really has no social skills to deal with others."

"He has never had a friend over to our house, and we have to force [him] to go to school sporting events, where [he] sits with parents instead of peers."

Children with AS are thought to have difficulties with inferring the thoughts or beliefs of others and understanding the rules of social behavior (Myles & Simpson, 1998, 2002). Teachers' views of the social difficulties of students with AS may emphasize such specific student characteristics that are perceived to interfere with successful adult and peer interaction. Teachers are particularly conscious of differences in awareness students with AS have of social cues and the difficulties they have in deciphering the perspectives of others:

"[There is some concern] with [the student's] ability to recognize and respond to nonverbal cues."

"[There is some concern] with [the student's] ability to accept others' point[s] of view."

"[It's] difficult to tell if he's listening."

"He tries to engage the aide . . . in conversation [when] it isn't an appropriate time."

"[The child] prefers to work alone."

"[The child has] problems with peers . . . misinterpreting their actions."

"[He] often feels he is treated unfairly and will [describe] a situation very differently than others who were present."

"[He] does not understand how he sounds when he speaks . . . he can be quite bossy and [he] makes demands of others."

"[The child is] often withdrawn."

"[The child] doesn't respond well to peers."

"[The child] has trouble reading people."

"[The child] sometimes doesn't want to participate in activities with other students."

"[The child has problems] dealing with difficult people and making new friends."

There is emerging evidence that social skill instruction is a useful approach to intervention with children and youth with AS (Elder, Caterino, & Chao, 2006). Teachers are likely to emphasize the need for social skill development as a means of overcoming the interaction difficulties of their students with AS:

"[She] desperately needs social skills instruction as she has a strong desire for friendships."

"[He has] difficulty knowing the appropriate ways of working and playing with other students."

"[The child needs to develop] social skills."

Difficulty understanding and accepting social conventions has frequently been recognized as a fundamental deficit of children with AS/HFA (Green, Gilchrist, Burton, & Cox, 2000). Teachers have frequent opportunities to observe students' difficulties in this area:

"[The child] struggles with understanding the roles of adults and people in positions of authority."

"[The child] speak[s] the same way to all people—peers and adults."

"[The child] needs assistance with [social] norms."

"[The child] has difficulty with implied boundaries of social interaction."

"[The child] prefers to do things [his] own way."

Communication Differences

The *Diagnostic and Statistical Manual of Mental Disorders, Fourth Edition, Text Revision* (*DSM-IV-TR;* APA, 2000) criteria for

Asperger's Disorder explicitly require that individuals' language is not significantly delayed. Indeed, children with AS often develop speech early and also possess and use unusually large and sophisticated vocabularies. The presence of marked verbosity is a key characteristic of children with AS (Klin et al., 2005). However, the presence of pragmatic language deficits as part of the typical picture of children with AS/HFA is well-documented (Loukusa et al., 2006). Teachers are frequently quite aware of students' pragmatic language deficits:

"[He] will dominate the conversation to share his ideas and thoughts, and it is difficult to redirect him, change the subject, or get in others' comments."

"[He needs to improve his skills in] asking for clarification."

The identified barriers and challenges often include other more fundamental communication difficulties, particularly for children who are best characterized as displaying HFA. Students themselves may recognize their own difficulties with auditory comprehension:

"Directions can be confusing."

"I have a hard time understanding my teacher."

"I get lost in class discussions."

Parents often note broader language functioning deficits, but they may also identify specific communication differences that reflect pragmatic language weaknesses:

"[My child's] expressive and receptive communication skills are limited."

"[My child] has trouble with conversations back and forth with friends."

"[My child] grabs topics from far left field and brings them into the conversation."

Intense Interests and Verbosity

The *DSM-IV-TR* criteria for a diagnosis of AS also include the presence of repetitive or stereotyped behaviors or interests that are restricted (APA, 2000). This criterion is often met by virtue of the child's expression of intense interests that are narrowly focused. These interests are generally either developmentally atypical or unusual in the intensity with which the child pursues them.

Parents often note that their children are "obsessed" with a particular interest for a period of time, eventually moving on to yet another intense interest. However, it is sometimes difficult for a diagnostician to decide whether a child's strong interest should be considered a manifestation of AS. Some children's interests are obviously peculiar, but it is not uncommon for an intense interest to be developmentally appropriate yet unusual in terms of the intensity or single-mindedness with which the child pursues it:

"[My child is] very interested in building and drawing."

"[My child is] obsessed with video games."

"[My child spends a great deal of time playing] video games and shooting basketball."

Teachers may sometimes appreciate children's interests, especially when they can be channeled toward relevant academic activities. At the same time, teachers often complain that children with AS are obsessed with certain topics to the exclusion of all else and to the detriment of their educational experience:

"[The child is] narrow in his interests [and] gets deeply into whatever he is interested in."

"[The child is] is interested only in specific activities."

"[His] imagination . . . can interfere with things he should be doing . . . focusing on what is going on in class."

Cognitive Rigidity

The presence of intense interests is sometimes seen as a manifestation of a more general feature of AS often characterized as *cognitive rigidity*. This feature frequently causes significant problems for children with AS in school. Common minor changes in the classroom routine (e.g., the presence of a substitute teacher, the introduction of a new schedule, the creation of a different physical arrangement) can have profound effects on the behavior and learning of students with AS/HFA (Adreon & Stella, 2001).

Teachers frequently comment on the difficulty students with AS/HFA have tolerating transitions and accepting changes in established patterns:

"[The child] prefers to do things his way."

"[The child] struggles when a schedule change occurs."

"[The child] needs great assistance with flexibility."

"[The child] needs reminders . . . when a new activity is beginning."

Cognitive rigidity is also sometimes manifested as "black and white thinking" or a lack of tolerance for ambiguity. This frequently appears as an unusually strong commitment to rules and rule-following, as well as an inability to accept others' violations of rules. Teachers have noted such rigidity toward rules and guidelines:

"[The child shows a] lack of forgiveness for peers who 'do wrong.'"

"[The child is] very focused on rules . . . this can work to his disadvantage if he . . . 'catches' a peer who doesn't follow a rule."

Another manifestation of cognitive rigidity that is common in children with AS is perfectionism. It is not unusual for teachers to note that students are unable to move on to another task until the last one is done to their standard of perfection or that students are easily upset by an inability to get something done just right:

"[The child] recognizes her abilities and gets upset at failures."

"Everything has to be perfect."

"[The child demonstrates] anxiety—the feeling that everything has to be perfect."

"[The child experiences] frustration when [he is not the] first to do something or be somewhere."

Parents often note their children's attachment to routines; this resistance to change can have a serious impact on a child's functioning in a typical school setting:

"[My child] hates special events at school because they cause schedule changes."

"[His biggest challenge is] overcoming rigidity."

"[My child] needs a strict routine."

Attention Difficulties

Children with AS often display marked deficits in attention and other executive functions (Hill & Bird, 2006). Attention difficulties are so common in children with PDDs that current diagnostic criteria preclude diagnosing attention-deficit/hyperactivity disorder (ADHD) in children with a diagnosis of a PDD (APA, 2000), presumably because the attention difficulties are viewed as inherent in the conditions. However, clinical practice routinely ignores this restriction, and comorbid diagnoses of AS and ADHD are very common. In any case, the symptoms of ADHD are often identified by teachers as key barriers to the academic success of children with AS:

"[The child] fiddles with various objects—pencils and pens, paper clips, rubber bands."

"[The child] struggles with task completion, time management . . . and following verbal directions."

"[The child] finds it difficult to complete tasks."

"When asked to work independently . . . [the child] will often gaze and not be able to focus until prompted."

"[The child] requires prompts and reminders from his assistant to stay on task, organized, and focused."

"[The child] is sometimes distracted by things he brings into class."

"[The child] appears distracted."

"It takes a couple minutes with him to help him refocus."

"Attention span [and] on-task behaviors are a concern."

"[The child] has trouble with organization and staying on task."

"[The child] has problems waiting until the appropriate time for things."

"[The child] does not attend to any teacher-given task without constant redirection."

"[The child tries to] escape . . . when asked to do any schoolwork."

"[The child has difficulty with] work completion/organization."

"[The child has difficulty] listening in [a] group without interruption for inappropriate reasons."

Sensory Differences

The presence of hypersensitivity, particularly to auditory stimuli, is often included in clinical descriptions of children with AS/HFA, and research evidence for this feature is emerging (Blakemore et al., 2006). Students are likely to complain about being bothered by "loud talking." Parents and teachers are often well aware of children's hypersensitivity and the impact this feature has on functioning in school settings:

"[The biggest challenge in school is] noise, lights, and sitting."

"[The child demonstrates] sensitivity to loud noises."

Learning Difficulties

The learning profile of students with AS is often uneven and perplexing to educators (Griswold et al., 2002). Students with AS/HFA frequently have difficulty grasping the meaning of information (Happé, 1991), demonstrate poor comprehension of abstract concepts, show diminished ability to problem solve and discriminate relevant information, or perform poorly when instruction relies on figures of speech (e.g., idioms, metaphors) (Myles & Southwick, 1999). Teachers may face a learner who is strong in the acquisition of fact-based material but cannot use what has been learned in other situations (Attwood, 1998). Students with AS/HFA often employ nonconventional methods to solve problems, and these strategies may be at odds with step-by-step, sequential instruction (Myles & Simpson, 1998).

Students themselves will often identify specific subjects or activities that are difficult for them or that they particularly dislike, expressing limited awareness as to why they find those subjects and activities so challenging:

"Individual special projects are really hard."

"Language arts and reading assignments [are difficult]."

Parents and teachers often express general concerns about academic material, and they may identify specific aspects of academic demands that are particularly challenging:

"Much of the material is abstract and she doesn't understand it."

"He doesn't understand what he is to do . . . but explodes if I try to help him."

"[The child has difficulty with] comprehension of basic instructions and [understanding] what he is reading."

"[The child] continues to struggle with reading."

"[The child] has problems with getting thoughts on paper."

"[His biggest challenge] is participating in class discussions."

"Math is an extremely challenging subject for [the child]."

"There are times when [the child] seems more in tune with concepts."

"[The child struggles with] comprehension and *wh-* questions."

"There are times when [the child] seems more able to learn/understand concepts and other times [the child] has difficulty grasping concepts."

One of the most frequently mentioned academic-related challenges is homework. This is an area in which students and parents often agree about the existence of difficulty:

"I don't like to do homework, it takes too much time."

"[The child's biggest challenge] is homework, big projects, and tests."

"[The child's biggest challenge] is homework . . . [he] worries about it all day and then lays in bed at night worrying about the next day's homework."

Motor Coordination Deficits

The presence of deficits in fine motor coordination is a feature that has often been mentioned in descriptions of children with AS. Hans Asperger (Asperger, 1991) commented on this feature in each of his original case reports, noting that one child was "motorically very clumsy" (p. 44), and that another displayed "general stiffness and clumsiness . . . it seemed as if he could only manage to move those muscular parts to which he directed a conscious effort of will" (p. 57); a third child "was clumsy from a motor point of view" (p. 61) and "had atrocious handwriting" (p. 63), whereas a fourth "was said to have been clumsy in all practical matters from infancy" and his "movements when catching and throwing gave him an extremely comical appearance" (p. 66). The *DSM-IV-TR* (APA, 2000) notes that if there is clumsiness, it is usually minor. There is, however, emerging evidence that subtle neuromotor deficits are common in children with AS/HFA (Jansiewicz et al., 2006).

Difficulties with tasks involving motor coordination, particularly handwriting, frequently cause problems for children in school. Students frequently complain about having to do written work:

> "Handwriting is hard for me."

> "[My biggest challenge is] writing things."

Motor coordination deficits are also frequently noted by parents and teachers:

> "[The child] works slow because of handwriting problems."

> "[Child] struggles with . . . fine motor skills."

> "Writing is difficult for [child]."

> "[The child's] actual writing is beautiful, but . . . way too slow."

> "[The child has] poor fine motor skills."

Emotional Distress

It is perhaps not surprising that students who face the many challenges noted above often find themselves experiencing significant emotional distress. Children with AS are often emotionally vulnerable, anxious (Farrugia & Hudson, 2006), or depressed (Stewart, Barnard, Pearson, Hasan, & O'Brien, 2006), and they frequently experience extreme stress because of their social impairment (Williams, 2001). Parents and teachers are likely to express concern when they perceive a child to be unhappy or otherwise emotionally distressed:

> "She has high anxiety about school."

> "[The child has trouble with] self confidence and independence."

> "[The child is] often very sad and withdrawn."

Challenging Behaviors

A common co-occurring feature in children with AS is the presence of disruptive behaviors (Macintosh & Dissanayake, 2006b). The social deficits and other difficulties experienced by individuals with AS may result in stress and frustration, which may lead to challenging behavior that should be viewed as an integral part of AS and not as willful misconduct (Myles, 2002). Parents and teachers are likely to report a variety of challenging behaviors in children with AS/HFA:

> "[The child's biggest challenge is] self-control—knowing how to behave across environments."

> "[The child's biggest challenge is] controlling his impulsive behaviors."

> "When . . . frustrated, she may engage in verbal and nonverbal refusals."

> "[The child] wants to grab [other students' things]."

> "[The child] tends to get frustrated quickly with difficult tasks."

> "[The child has] screaming fits when [he] doesn't get [his] way or when something is upsetting."

> "[The child expresses] negative comments toward others."

STRENGTHS

The focus in this chapter has been on students' barriers and challenges in school, and these difficulties are extensive and varied. There are, however, many abilities and strengths that are often displayed by students with AS/HFA. Students often identify things that they enjoy or things at which they perceive they are particularly skilled as being their greatest strengths:

> "Math and spelling are easy for me."

> "[I enjoy] science, physical education, and computer work."

Parents are likely to identify a wide variety of specific things at which their children are well-skilled:

> "[My child is good at] spelling, drawing, and telling stories."

> "[My child is] very compassionate, kind, and loving."

> "[My child has good] manners [and enjoys] physical education and music."

> "[My child enjoys] sorting, singing, bike riding, and writing."

"[My child has a] great imagination and loves being scientific."

"[My child enjoys] swimming, math, and organization."

"[My child is skilled at] reading, memorizing, [and] spelling, [and demonstrates] empathy toward others and good manners."

"[My child enjoys] math, computer [work], and art."

Teachers similarly offered a variety of comments regarding their students' strengths:

"[The child] interacts best in one-on-one situations and especially with adults."

"[The child] has a fertile imagination . . . is creative and intelligent."

"[The child] does very well on objective tests . . . [the child] has a vast amount of general knowledge and is an excellent reader."

"[The child is] always polite and hardworking."

"[The child] completes all homework assignments and projects."

"[She] truly desires to learn and please her teachers."

"[The child] has great talents in the area of written expression."

"[The child is] driven to participate and remain on task."

"[The child] tries hard and truly wants to learn."

"[The child is] very intelligent . . . knows a lot of factual information."

CONCLUSION

Overall, the barriers and challenges facing students with AS/HFA as reported by the students, parents, and teachers in this study are consistent with the *DSM-IV-TR* criteria (APA, 2000), as well as the findings of many research studies (e.g., Griswold et al., 2002). The information specifically illustrates difficulties in school settings related to the characteristics of students with AS, including social interactions, communication differences, intense interests, cognitive rigidity, attention difficulties, sensory differences, learning difficulties, motor coordination, emotional distress, and challenging behaviors. These findings expand the understanding of researchers and educators as to the ways in which the characteristics of AS are manifested in school settings.

The collaborative services of related service providers (e.g., pediatricians, psychologists, speech and language pathologists, occupational and physical therapists, school counselors) can help to remove or lessen the impact of barriers faced by students with AS/HFA. Without appropriate accommodations, individuals with AS/HFA are much less likely to experience social and academic success in schools and positive personal, social, and vocational transitions to adult life. Organized by the barriers identified in this chapter, Table 9.1 offers recommendations for collaborative involvement for service providers as they interact with educators, parents, and students with AS/HFA.

The perspectives of students, parents, and teachers reveal many of the significant challenges children and youth with AS/HFA encounter as they attempt to learn, make friends, and succeed in school environments. The complex patterns of strengths and differences that form the central characteristics of students with AS/HFA make it particularly difficult for service providers and educators to readily recognize and respond in an appropriate manner. There is a tremendous need for a collaborative and helpful relationship between service providers, schools, and families that will address the barriers that are most significant for students with AS/HFA. Pediatricians, clinicians, and other service providers may share many of the available strategies with educators and families as a starting point for planning treatment and intervention for achieving more successful outcomes for students with AS.

Table 9.1. Suggestions for addressing barriers to school success

Barrier	Suggestions and facilitators
Difficulty with social interactions • Forming and maintaining friendships • Negative experiences with peers, including teasing • Problems with perspective taking	• Encourage social skills training—individual, group, and class-wide. • Encourage innovative, site-friendly approaches to involving peers with typical development. • Consider the full range of options for social skills training (e.g., Social Stories, video modeling, published social skills curricula). • Include schoolwide responses to bullying that address the bully, the victim, and the bystanders.
Communication differences • Pragmatic language deficits • Auditory comprehension difficulties • Broader language deficits	• Encourage direct instruction and opportunities for practice in social and conversational skills. • Anticipate the need for accommodations, such as additional explanations and extra time for responding in classes where content includes inferred meanings, metaphors, abstract language, and humor.
Intense interests and verbosity • Narrow and obsessive interests	• Reward work completed in low-interest areas (e.g., homework) with access to time or conversation devoted to a special interest. • Develop social and leadership skills during times when knowledge or competence about the special interest is important for the class (i.e., assign a leadership role to the student when the curricula is related to the special interest).
Cognitive rigidity • Difficulty tolerating transitions or changes in routines • Perfectionism • Overadherence to rules	• Anticipate the likelihood that even small changes may be difficult. • Support efforts to teach the student coping strategies through Social Stories or self-monitoring. • Encourage modifications that accommodate perfectionism where possible (e.g., remembering fewer spelling words, solving every other problem, grading performance rather than written demonstrations of competence). • Teach decision-making strategies for making exceptions to rules. • Build awareness among teachers and families about cognitive rigidity as an important characteristic of those with Asperger syndrome/high-functioning autism (AS/HFA) that requires accommodations.
Attention difficulties • Procrastination or low productivity on school work • The tendency to be easily distracted • Dependence on prompts or an assistant to commence and complete work when compared with peers	• Encourage the use of choices or an agreed-upon system of frequent breaks (e.g., sensory, physical activity, down time). • Encourage instruction that is direct and includes high rates of student engagement and feedback. • Use visual or other schedules to help student stay oriented around the day's activities and goals. • Pair verbal instruction or content with visual or written information. • Teach self-monitoring with liberal payoff clauses for attending and staying on task.

(continued)

Table 9.1.   *(continued)*

Barrier	Suggestions and Facilitators

Sensory Differences
- Hypersensitivity to stimuli, particularly auditory

- Anticipate the possibility that unusual sensitivities may be overlooked.
- When problem behavior is observed, encourage teachers and caregivers to assess sensitivity to auditory, visual, olfactory, and tactile stimuli across settings.
- Involve the student directly. Ask about sensitivities and preferred environments for working and interacting with others. Adapt environments as needed.

Learning difficulties
- Use of unconventional problem solving or execution
- Difficulty comprehending content that is abstract, inferred, or relies on figures of speech
- Difficulty applying fact-based or other information

- Difficulty completing homework and typical worksheets

- Where possible, allow nonconventional approaches or algorithms if they lead the child to the correct answer.
- Encourage instructors to pair abstract or highly verbal presentations of content with visual, written, or demonstrative material that explains or depicts the concepts.
- Anticipate the need for more accommodations in course work that is less reliant on formal, fact-based classification systems.
- Pursue comprehensive assessment for learning disabilities when indicated.
- Encourage teachers and parents to provide opportunities to apply information in different settings under changing conditions.
- Homework, worksheets, or special projects:
  —Limit homework to demonstration of only essential content.
  —Encourage teachers to be flexible about response demands (e.g., allow a verbal response or performance in lieu of a written demonstration of mastery).
  —Use a behavioral contract with generous payoff clauses to communicate expectations, increase motivation, and address perfectionism.
  —Suggest a home–student–school communication system (e.g., e-mail, checklist) to keep everyone informed.
  —Encourage patience and help others avoid a preoccupation with homework over other family or school activities.

Motor coordination deficits
- Poor handwriting

- An aversion to handwriting
- Clumsiness

- Support accommodations that limit handwritten demonstrations of mastery of content, and use verbal and performance-based options wherever possible.
- Encourage instruction in keyboarding skills.
- Limit or counterbalance social participation activities where clumsiness will interfere with developing and maintaining friendships.

Emotional distress
- Anxiety or other emotional distress
- Low self-esteem or expressions of sadness and loneliness

- Support individualized or small group instruction and counseling that can teach students to identify emotional states in themselves and others and to increase the repertoire of coping skills needed to respond in settings stressful for the student (e.g., activities from *Navigating the Social World* [McAfee, 2002], *My Social Stories Book* [Gray & White, 2002]), or teacher or counselor led *social autopsies* following stressful events [Myles, 2002]).
- Encourage lifestyle changes and instruction that promote leisure and hobby endeavors (e.g., karate, building models).

Barrier	Suggestions and Facilitators
Challenging behaviors	
• Behavioral excesses, "meltdowns," verbally or physically aggressive toward others	• Encourage instruction in the social skills needed to survive social environments with others using social skills curricula such as *Navigating the Social World* (McAfee, 2002) or *My Social Stories Book* (Gray & White, 2002).
• Deficits in self-control and self-regulation	• Assist educators and others in making discriminations between behaviors that are functions of anxiety and stress rather than willful misconduct.
• Low frustration threshold	• Support efforts to teach students how to self-monitor and to learn about and demonstrate alternative, adaptive behaviors when they are overwhelmed or frustrated.
	• In situations likely to be difficult, pair students with AS with others who can provide support and model appropriate alternative behaviors.

REFERENCES

Adreon, D., & Stella, J. (2001). Transition to middle and high school: Increasing the success of students with Asperger syndrome. *Intervention in School and Clinic, 36*(5), 266–271.

American Psychiatric Association. (2000). *Diagnostic and Statistical Manual of Mental Disorders* (4th ed., text rev.). Washington, DC: Author.

Asperger, H.. (1991). 'Autistic psychopathy' in childhood (U. Frith, Trans.). In U. Frith (Ed.), *Autism and Asperger syndrome* (pp. 37–920). Cambridge, United Kingdom: Cambridge University Press. (Original work published 1944)

Attwood, T. (1998). *Asperger's syndrome: A guide for parents and professionals.* Philadelphia: Jessica Kingsley Publishers.

Barnhill, G.P., & Myles, B.S. (2001). Attributional style and depression in adolescents with Asperger syndrome. *Journal of Positive Behavior Interventions, 3,* 175–183.

Baron-Cohen, S. (1995). *Mind blindness: An essay on autism and theory of mind.* Cambridge, MA: MIT Press.

Bauer, S. (1999). *Asperger Syndrome. The O.A.S.I.S.* [Online Asperger Syndrome Information and Support Web Page]. Retrieved November 21, 2007, from http://www.udel.edu/bkirgy/asperger/asthruyears.html

Bellon-Harn, M.L., & Harn, W.E. (2006). Profiles of social communicative competence in middle school children with Asperger syndrome: Two case studies. *Child Language Teaching and Therapy, 22*(1), 1–26.

Ben Shalom, D., Mostofsky, S.H., Hazlett, R.L., Goldberg, M.C., Landa, R.J., & Faran, Y. (2006). Normal physiological emotions but differences in expression of conscious feelings in children with high-functioning autism. *Journal of Autism and Developmental Disorders, 36*(3), 395–400.

Blakemore, S.J., Tavassoli, T., Calo, S., Thomas, R.M., Catmur, C., Frith, U., et al. (2006). Tactile sensitivity in Asperger syndrome. *Brain and Cognition, 61*(1), 5–13.

Bonnet, K.A., & Gao, X. (1996). Asperger syndrome in neurologic perspective. *Journal of Child Neurology, 11,* 483–489.

Bradley, E.A., Summers, J.A., Wood, H.L., & Bryson, S.E. (2004). Comparing rates of psychiatric and behavior disorders in adolescents and young adults with severe intellectual disability with and without autism. *Journal of Autism and Developmental Disorders, 34,* 151–161.

Ehlers, S., & Gillberg, C. (1993). The epidemiology of Asperger syndrome: A total population study. *Journal of Child Psychology and Psychiatry, 34,* 1327–1350.

Elder, L.M., Caterino, L.C., & Chao, J. (2006). The efficacy of social skills treatment for children with Asperger syndrome. *Education and Treatment of Children, 29*(4), 635–663.

Farrugia, S., & Hudson, J. (2006). Anxiety in adolescents with Asperger syndrome: Negative thoughts, behavioral problems, and life interference. *Focus on Autism and Other Developmental Disabilities, 21*(1), 25–35.

Frith, U. (1991). *Autism and Asperger syndrome.* New York: Cambridge University Press.

Gagnon, E. (2001). *The Power Card strategy: Using special interests to motivate children and youth with Asperger syndrome and autism.* Shawnee Mission, KS: Autism Asperger Publishing.

Gillberg, C. (1989). Asperger syndrome in 23 Swedish children. *Developmental Medicine and Child Neurology, 31,* 520–531.

Goddard, L., Howlin, P., Dritschel, B., & Patel, T. (2007). Autobiographical memory and social problem-solving in Asperger syndrome. *Journal of Autism and Developmental Disorders, 37*(2), 291–300.

Gray, C., & White, A.L. (2002). *My Social Stories Book.* Philadelphia: Jessica Kingsley Publishers.

Green, J., Gilchrist, A., Burton, D., & Cox, A. (2000). Social and psychiatric functioning in adolescents with Asperger syndrome compared with conduct disorders. *Journal of Autism and Developmental Disorders, 30,* 279–293.

Griswold, D.E., Barnhill, G.P., Myles, B.S., Hagiwara, T., & Simpson, R.L. (2002). Asperger syndrome and academic achievement. *Focus on Autism and Other Developmental Disabilities, 17,* 94–102.

Gutstein, S.E., & Whitney, T. (2002). Asperger syndrome and the development of social competence. *Focus on Autism and Other Developmental Disabilities, 17,* 161-171.

Happé, F.G.E. (1991). The autobiographical writings of three Asperger syndrome adults: Problems of interpretation and implications for theory. In U. Frith (Ed.), *Autism and Asperger syndrome* (pp. 207–242). New York: Cambridge University Press.

Hedley, D., & Young, R. (2006). Social comparison processes and depressive symptoms in children and adolescents with Asperger syndrome. *Autism, 10*(2), 139–153.

Hill, E.L., & Bird, C.M. (2006). Executive processes in Asperger syndrome: Patterns of performance in a multiple case series. *Neuropsychologia, 44*(14), 2822–2835.

Howard, B., Cohn, E., & Orsmond, G.I. (2006). Understanding and negotiating friendships: Perspectives from an adolescent with Asperger syndrome. *Autism, 10*(6), 619–627.

Individuals with Disabilities Education Act Amendments (IDEA) of 1997, PL 105-17, 20 U.S.C. §§ 1400 *et seq.*

Jansiewicz, E.M., Goldberg, M.C., Newschaffer, C.J., Denckla, M.B., Landa, R., & Mostofsky, S.H. (2006). Motor signs distinguish children with high functioning autism and Asperger's syndrome from controls. *Journal of Autism and Developmental Disorders, 36*(5), 613–621.

Kadesjo, B., Gillberg, C., & Nagberg, B. (1999). Autism and Asperger syndrome in seven-year-old children: A total population study. *Journal of Autism and Developmental Disorders, 29,* 327–332.

Kaland, N., Smith, L., & Mortensen, E.L. (2007). Response times of children and adolescents with Asperger syndrome on an 'advanced' test of theory of mind. *Journal of Autism and Developmental Disorders, 37*(2), 197–209.

Klin, A., Pauls, D. Schultz, R., & Volkmar, F. (2005). Three diagnostic approaches to Asperger disorder. *Journal of Autism and Developmental Disorders, 35,* 221–234.

Landa, R. (2000). Social language use in Asperger syndrome and HFA. In A. Klin, F.R. Volkmar, & S.S. Sparrow (Eds.), *Asperger syndrome* (pp. 125-158). New York: The Guilford Press.

Lindner, J.L., & Rosen, L.A. (2006). Decoding of emotion through facial expression, prosody and verbal content in children and adolescents with Asperger's syndrome. *Journal of Autism and Developmental Disorders, 36*(6), 769–777.

Loukusa, S., Leinonen, E., Jussila, K., Mattila, M.L., Ryder, N., Ebeling, H., et al. (2006). Answering contextually demanding questions: Pragmatic errors produced by children with Asperger syndrome or high-functioning autism. *Journal of Communication Disorders* [Electronic version, ahead of print]. Retrieved May 29, 2007 from www.sciencedirect.com

Macintosh, K., & Dissanayake, C.A. (2006a). Comparative study of the spontaneous social interactions of children with high-functioning autism and children with Asperger's disorder. *Autism, 10*(2), 199–220.

Macintosh, K., & Dissanayake, C. (2006b). Social skills and problem behaviours in school-aged children with high-functioning autism and Asperger's disorder. *Journal of Autism and Developmental Disorders, 36*(8), 1065–1076.

McAfee, J. (2002). *Navigating the social world.* Arlington, TX: Future Horizons.

Meyer, J.A., Mundy, P.C., Van Hecke, A.V., & Durocher, J.S. (2006). Social attribution processes and comorbid psychiatric symptoms in children with Asperger syndrome. *Autism, 10*(4), 383–402.

Myles, B.S. (2002). Introduction to the special issue on Asperger syndrome. *Focus on Autism and Other Developmental Disabilities, 17,* 130–131.

Myles, B.S., & Simpson, R.L. (1998). *Asperger syndrome: A guide for educators and parents.* Austin, TX: PRO-ED.

Myles, B.S., & Simpson, R.L. (2002). Asperger syndrome: An overview of characteristics. *Focus on Autism and Other Developmental Disabilities, 17,* 132–137.

Myles, B.S., & Southwick, J. (1999). *Asperger syndrome and difficult moments: Practical solutions for tantrums, rage, and meltdowns.* Shawnee Mission, KS: Autism Asperger Publishing.

Newport, J. (2001). *Your life is not a label.* Arlington, TX: Future Horizons.

Ozonoff, S., Rogers, S.J., & Pennington, R.F. (1991). Executive function deficits in high functioning autistic individuals: Relationship to theory of mind. *Journal of Child Psychology and Psychiatry, 32,* 1107–1122.

Rehabilitation Act of 1973, PL 93-112, 29 U.S.C. §§ 701 *et seq.*

Safran, S. (2001). Asperger syndrome: The emerging challenge to special education. *Exceptional Children, 67,* 151–160.

Simpson, R.L., & Myles, B.S. (1998). Aggression among children and youth who have Asperger's syndrome: A different population requiring different strategies. *Preventing School Failure, 42*(4), 149–153.

Stewart, M.E., Barnard, L., Pearson, J., Hasan, R., & O'Brien, G. (2006). Presentation of depression in autism and Asperger syndrome: A review. *Autism, 10*(1), 103–116.

Tantam, D. (2003). The challenge of adolescents and adults with Asperger syndrome. *Child and Adolescent Psychiatric Clinics of North America, 12,* 143–163.

Volkmar, F.R., & Klin, A. (2000). Diagnostic issues in Asperger syndrome. In A. Klin, F.R. Volkmar, & S.S. Sparrow (Eds.), *Asperger syndrome* (pp. 25–71). New York: Guilford Press.

Volkmar, F.R., Klin, A., Schultz, R.T., Rubin, E., & Bronen, R. (2000). Asperger's Disorder. *American Journal of Psychiatry, 157,* 262–267.

Williams, K. (2001). Understanding the student with Asperger syndrome: Guidelines for teachers. *Intervention in School and Clinic, 36*(5), 287–292.

Wing, L. (1981). Asperger's syndrome: A clinical account. *Psychological Medicine, 11,* 115–129.

10

Psychopharmacologic Approaches to Challenging Behaviors in Individuals with Autism

Scott M. Myers

Autism spectrum disorders (ASDs; e.g., the diagnoses of Autistic Disorder, Asperger's Disorder, and Pervasive Developmental Disorder Not Otherwise Specified [PDD-NOS]), like other neurodevelopmental disabilities, are generally not curable. The primary goals of chronic management include minimizing the core impairments and associated deficits, maximizing functional independence and quality of life, and alleviating family distress. Educational interventions, including behavior analytic strategies and habilitative therapies, are the primary treatments used to 1) help to alleviate the core features of impairment in social reciprocity, deficits in communication, and restricted, repetitive behavioral repertoire, 2) facilitate daily living skills, play and leisure skills, and academic achievement, and 3) address maladaptive behaviors. Medications have not been proven effective in correcting the core deficits of ASDs, and behavioral psychologists have appropriately made the point that "there is no skill in a pill." However, associated maladaptive behaviors or psychiatric comorbidities may interfere with educational progress, socialization, health or safety, and quality of life. In some cases, these symptoms may be amenable to psychopharmacologic intervention, and effective medical management may allow children with ASDs to benefit more opti-

mally from educational and behavioral interventions.

HISTORY

Psychopharmacology is the study and use of psychotropic medications to produce behavioral, emotional, or cognitive changes. Pediatric psychopharmacology is a relatively young discipline; observations of the effects of benzedrine on behavior and academic performance of hyperactive children first appeared in the literature in 1937 (Bradley, 1937), but more scientifically rigorous clinical research did not appear until the 1960s, and widespread acceptance of the use of psychotropic medications in children did not emerge until the late 1980s (Riddle, 1995). Reports of pharmacologic manipulation of the neurochemistry of children with ASDs began to appear in the literature in the late 1950s and early 1960s. Since then, a wide variety of psychotropic agents have been studied and used in clinical practice.

The isolation of reserpine from *Rauwolfia serpentina* and the synthesis of chlorpromazine by molecular modification of the antihistamine promethazine in the 1950s heralded the modern age of psychopharmacology. The spectacular effects of chlorpromazine on patients with schizophrenia led to the development of many more antipsychotics that also worked primarily through antagonism of dopaminergic receptors, although this mechanism was not clear until 1970 (Curzon, 1990). Because of their dramatic effects on behavior in schizophrenia, reserpine (Lehman, Haber, & Lesser, 1957) and many of the first generation antipsychotics (i.e., chlorpromazine, trifluoperidol, trifluoperazine, thiothixene, fluphenazine, molindone, pimozide) were studied in children with ASDs (Campbell, Fish, Shapiro, & Floyd Jr., 1970, 1971, 1972; Engelhardt, Polizos, Waizer, & Hoffman, 1973; Ernst, Magee, Gonzalez, & Locascio, 1992; Faretra, Dooher, & Dowling, 1970; Fish, Shapiro, & Campbell, 1966; Naruse et al., 1982; Waizer, Polizos, Hoffman, Engelhardt, & Margolis, 1972; Wolpert, Hagamen, & Merlis, 1967). Haloperidol, the most thoroughly studied, was shown to have efficacy in reducing challenging behaviors in double-blind, placebo-controlled trials (Anderson et al., 1989; Anderson et al., 1984; Campbell et al., 1978; Cohen et al., 1980; Naruse et al., 1982; Remington, Sloman, Konstantareas, Parker, & Gow, 2001), but dyskinesias were found to be common (Campbell et al., 1997). Clinical and research interest in this group of medications has continued, as evidenced by the recent controlled trials and widespread use of second generation (i.e., atypical) antipsychotics, which will be subsequently reviewed.

In addition to antipsychotics, many other agents have been studied in patients with ASDs, primarily because of their effects on pertinent behavioral symptoms in other populations. Examples include stimulants, tricyclic antidepressants, alpha-2 agonists, and atomoxetine for symptoms of attention-deficit/hyperactivity disorder (ADHD), and anticonvulsants and lithium for symptoms attributed to mood instability (reviewed in Myers, 2007 and Posey & McDougle, 2000).

During the late 1950s and the 1960s, when psychogenic theories of causation were popular, the hallucinogen lysergic acid diethylamide (LSD) was administered to children with ASDs with the therapeutic goal of "undermining an intractable defense system and thereby making the patient more receptive to contact and communication with others" (Mogar & Aldrich, 1969). During the same time period, observation of the psychotomimetic effects of LSD and the discovery that it modulated serotonergic neurotransmission stimulated speculation about the role of serotonin in a variety of disorders, including ASDs. The discovery of elevated whole blood serotonin in children with ASDs (Schain & Freedman, 1961) led to attempts at pharmacological reduction with agents such as methysergide (Fish, Campbell, Shapiro, & Floyd, 1969) and levodopa (Campbell et al., 1976; Ritvo et al., 1971) based on biological findings and hypothesized neurochemistry rather than psychodynamic theory. After fenfluramine, an amphetamine analogue that reduces whole blood serotonin levels, was reported by Geller, Ritvo, Freeman, and Yuwiler in 1982 to have had beneficial effects on three boys with ASDs, the drug was studied extensively for a decade, but it was not found to be particularly efficacious or well tolerated (Aman & Kern, 1989; Leventhal et al., 1993). However, multiple lines of evidence have suggested that serotonin plays a role in the pathogenesis of ASDs (Anderson, 2005; Chugani, 2005), and in the last two decades, research efforts and clinical management have focused on manipulation of serotonergic neurotransmission with potent serotonin reuptake inhibitors.

Although no new medications have been developed based on an understanding of the pathophysiology of ASDs, available psychotropic agents that modulate a variety of neurotransmitter systems have been studied in this population based on neurobiological findings or etiologic hypotheses. Examples include the opiate antagonist naltrexone in the 1980s and 1990s, synthetic oxytocin, glutamate N-methyl-D-aspartate (NMDA) receptor modulators (e.g., antagonists amantadine, memantine, and dextromethorphan, and the partial agonist D-cycloserine), and acetylcholinesterase inhibitors (e.g., donepezil, galantamine, rivastigmine) in the late 1990s and the 2000s (reviewed in Myers, 2007).

EPIDEMIOLOGY

Studies that include children indicate that approximately 50% of all individuals with ASDs are treated with psychotropic medication (Aman, Lam, & Collier-Crespin, 2003; Green et al., 2006; Langworthy-Lam, Aman, & Van Bourgondien, 2002; Witwer & Lecavalier, 2005), and it has been reported that nearly 75% of adults with ASDs take at least one psychotropic medication (Seltzer, Shattuck, Abbeduto, & Greenberg, 2004; Tsakanikos et al., 2006). There is evidence of a trend toward increasing the use of medication in patients with ASDs, with the prevalence of psychotropic use in North Carolina increasing from 30% in 1992–1993 to 46% in 2001 (Aman, Lam, & Van Bourgondien, 2005). Factors associated with increased likelihood of medication use include greater age, lower adaptive skills and social competence, higher levels of maladaptive behavior, and residency in a place other than the parental home (Aman et al., 2005; Seltzer et al., 2004; Witwer & Lecavalier, 2005). Antidepressants, stimulants, antipsychotics, alpha agonists, and anticonvulsant mood stabilizers are the most commonly prescribed classes of psychotropic medication in this population (Aman et al., 2005; Witwer & Lecavalier, 2005). Polypharmacy is common; Martin, Scahill, Klin, and Volkmar, (1999) found that 29% of a referred clinical sample of children, adolescents, and adults with ASDs and intelligence quotient (IQ) scores of >70 were taking two or more psychotropic medications simultaneously.

THE EVIDENCE BASE: REVIEW OF SELECTED RECENT LITERATURE

Randomized controlled clinical trials with adequate sample sizes, well-defined study populations, and independent replication are the gold standard of evidence-based psychopharmacology. However, problems with syndrome definition, clinical heterogeneity, psychiatric comorbidity, determination of appropriate outcome targets and measures, self-selection of participants, ethical concerns, and issues of funding and sample size present practical barriers to the design and implementation of scientifically ideal clinical trials in ASDs (Hollander et al., 2004). Most psychotropic medications have been used in children with ASDs, but there is insufficient literature to establish a single consensus evidence-based approach to psychopharmacologic management. Fortunately, more information from randomized, double-blind, placebo-controlled clinical trials has become available to guide practice. Although clinical practice is also informed by well-designed studies conducted in populations of children with overlapping target symptoms (e.g., ADHD, intellectual disability [ID] with conduct disorder, anxiety disorders, mood disorders, psychoses), this brief review is limited to studies specifically involving patients with ASDs.

Stimulants, Atomoxetine, and Alpha-2 Agonists

ADHD symptoms (e.g., inattention, distractibility, impulsivity, hyperactivity) are common in individuals with ASDs, especially children and adolescents (Lee & Ousley, 2006). Although early studies of the effects of stimulants yielded negative results (Campbell, Fish, & David et al., 1972; Campbell et al., 1976), more recent double-blind, placebo-controlled trials of methylphenidate have demonstrated improvement in these symptoms in children with ASDs (Table 10.1) (Handen, Johnson, & Lubetsky, 2000; Quintana et al., 1995; Research Units on Pediatric Psychopharmacology [RUPP] Autism Network, 2005a). These trials have shown that methylphenidate is effective in some children with ASDs, but the response rate is lower than in children with isolated

ADHD, and adverse effects are more frequent (Aman, 2004; RUPP Autism Network, 2005a). However, a large open-label methylphenidate study found no statistically significant difference between children with an ASD plus ADHD symptoms versus children with ADHD alone in the degree of improvement or the rate of adverse effects, including worsening of tics or repetitive behaviors (Santosh, Baird, Pityaratstian, Tavare, & Gringas, 2006). It has been suggested that higher functioning patients, such as those with Asperger syndrome, may be more likely to have a positive response (Stigler, Desmond, Posey, Wiegand, & McDougle, 2004). In an open-label study, Di Martino, Melis, Cianchetti, and Zuddas (2004) provided evidence that giving a single test dose of methylphenidate was useful in identifying children with ASDs who may benefit from ongoing treatment with the medication. Although the evidence of efficacy of methylphenidate in this population is substantial, it is unclear whether the results can be generalized to other stimulants.

Three open-label studies (Jou, Handen, & Hardan, 2005; Posey, Wiegand et al., 2006; Troost, Steenhuis et al., 2006) and a small double-blind, placebo-controlled pilot trial (Arnold et al., 2006) (Table 10.1) have suggested that the selective norepinephrine reuptake inhibitor atomoxetine may be effective in children and adolescents with ASDs for symptoms including hyperactivity, impulsivity, and oppositionality. Two small, double-blind, placebo-controlled trials have documented the modest benefit of clonidine in reducing symptoms, including hyperactivity, irritability, outbursts, impulsivity, and repetitive behaviors, in youth with ASDs (Table 10.1) (Fankhauser, Karumanchi, German, Yates, & Karumanchi, 1992; Jaselskis, Cook, Jr., Fletcher, & Leventhal, 1992). In an open-label study, clonidine was shown to be effective for sedation for electroencephalography in 27 children (Mehta, Patel, & Castello, 2004). Lofexidine, an alpha-2 agonist available in Europe,

has also been found to reduce hyperactivity in children with ASDs in a double-blind, placebo-controlled crossover study (Niederhofer, Staffen, & Mair, 2002). A retrospective record review showed that open-label treatment with guanfacine was beneficial in 24% of 80 children with ASDs and suggested that patients without comorbid ID were more likely to show improvement in target symptoms, including hyperactivity, inattention, insomnia, and tics (Posey, Puntney, Sasher, Kem, & McDougle, 2004). Subsequently, a prospective open-label trial that included 25 children with ASDs who had previously failed treatment with methylphenidate demonstrated that guanfacine was effective for hyperactivity and inattention in 48% of the cases (RUPP Autism Network, 2006).

Atypical Antipsychotics

Typical antipsychotic medications currently available in the United States include clozapine, risperidone, olanzapine, quetiapine, ziprasione, and aripiprazole. Evidence suggests that atypical antipsychotics are efficacious in the treatment of children and adolescents with severe disruptive behaviors associated with ID (Aman et al., 2002; Croonenberghs et al., 2005; Snyder et al., 2002) in addition to those with psychosis, bipolar disorder, Tourette syndrome, and potentially conduct disorder and severe ADHD (Cheng-Shannon, McGough, Pataki, & McCracken, 2004).

In 1998, risperidone was demonstrated to be superior to placebo in reducing maladaptive behaviors in adults with ASDs (McDougle et al., 1998). Subsequently, four randomized controlled studies, including two large multisite trials, have confirmed the short-term efficacy of risperidone for irritability and associated severe disruptive behaviors such as tantrums, aggression, and self-injurious behavior in youths with ASDs (Arnold et al., 2003; Hellings et al., 2006; McCracken et al., 2002; Nagaraj, Singhi, & Mahli, 2006; Shea et al., 2004) (Table 10.2). Two open-label studies, each with a double-

Table 10.1. Double-blind, placebo-controlled clinical trials of stimulants, atomoxetine, and alpha-2 agonists in autism spectrum disorders: 1992–2006

Agent	Reference	Age (years)	Dose	N	Duration	Outcomes/Comments
Methylphenidate	Quintana et al. (1995)	7–11	10 mg bid and 20 mg bid	10	2 weeks	Statistically significant improvement in hyperactivity and irritability compared with placebo
Methylphenidate	Handen, Johnson, & Lubetsky (2000)	5–11	0.3-0.6 mg/kg/dose bid–tid	13	2 weeks	Superior to placebo on several measures of hyperactivity and other ADHD symptoms and also ABC Irritability, Stereotypy, and Inappropriate Speech subscales; response rate 61%
Methylphenidate	Research Units on Pediatric Psychopharmacology (RUPP) Autism Network (2005a)	5–14	7.5 mg/day–50 mg/day (0.125–0.5 mg/kg/dose bid and a third dose of approximately half of the earlier doses)	72	4 weeks (+ 8 weeks open-label for responders)	Superior to placebo for ADHD symptoms; response rate 49%; discontinuation rate 18% due to adverse effects
Atomoxetine	Arnold et al. (2006)	5–15	Range 20–100 mg/day, mean 44 mg/day	16	12 weeks	Superior to placebo for hyperactivity and impulsivity; response rate 43%
Clonidine	Fankhauser et al. (1992)	5–33	Transdermal Range 0.1–0.3 mg/day	9	4 weeks	Superior to placebo for hyperactivity and anxiety; improvement in some social behaviors
Clonidine	Jaselskis, Cook, Jr., Fletcher, & Leventhal (1992)	5–13	4–10 mcg/kg/day	8	6 weeks	Superior to placebo on measures of hyperactivity, irritability, stereotypy, and oppositional behavior; only 2 patients were still taking clonidine after a year
Lofexidine	Niederhofer, Staffen, & Mair (2002)	Mean 7.3 +/− 2.3 years (lofexidine) and 9.2 +/− 3.9 years (placebo); range not provided	Range 0.8–1.2 mg/day divided tid	12	6 weeks	Statistically significant improvement in hyperactivity as well as irritability, stereotypy, and inappropriate speech relative to placebo

From Myers, S.M. (2007). The status of pharmacotherapy for autism spectrum disorders. *Expert Opinion on Pharmacotherapy, 8*(11), 1581–1584; adapted by permission.
Key: N = total number in sample; bid–tid = twice daily to three times daily; ADHD = attention-deficit/hyperactivity disorder; ABC = Aberrant Behavior Checklist (Aman, Singh, Stewart, & Field, 1985).

blind discontinuation component, have suggested long-term benefits and tolerance (RUPP Autism Network, 2005b; Troost et al., 2005). In late 2006, the Food and Drug Administration (FDA) approved risperidone for the symptomatic treatment of irritability (i.e., aggressive behavior, deliberate self-injury, temper tantrums, quickly changing moods) in children and adolescents with ASDs.

Table 10.2. Double-blind, placebo-controlled clinical trials of atypical antipsychotics in autism spectrum disorders: 1996–2006

Agent	Reference	Age (years)	Dose	N	Duration	Outcomes/Comments
Risperidone	McDougle et al. (1998)	18–43	Range 1–6 mg/day, mean 2.9 mg/day	31	12 weeks	Superior to placebo for aggression, repetitive behavior, anxiety, irritability, and depression; response rate 57% (versus 0% in placebo group)
Risperidone (RUPP trial)	Arnold et al. (2003); McCracken et al. (2002); McDougle et al. (2005) Research Units on Pediatric Psychopharmacology (RUPP) Autism Network (2005b)	5–17	Range 0.5– 3.5 mg/day, mean 1.8 mg/day	101	8 weeks	Superior to placebo for irritability and associated tantrums, aggression, and SIB; response rate 69% (versus 12% in placebo group); benefits maintained at 6 months; decreased repetitive behavior
Risperidone	Shea et al. (2004)	5–12	Mean 1.17 mg/day, or 0.04 mg/kg/ day	77	8 weeks	Decreased irritability and associated maladaptive behaviors; superior to placebo on all 5 ABC subscales
Risperidone	Hellings et al. (2006)	8–56	Children and Adolescents: range 1.0– 2.9 mg/day Adults: range 2.0–5.2 mg/day	36	22 weeks	Superior to placebo for irritability and aggression; low doses (1.0 mg for children and 2.0 mg for adults) equally effective and better tolerated than high doses (i.e., mean 2.0 mg for children and 3.6 mg for adults); 57.5% had >50% decrease in ABC Irritability score; 87.5% had >25% decrease
Risperidone	Luby et al. (2006)	2–6	Range 0.5– 1.5 mg/day, mean 1.14 mg/day or 0.05 mg/kg/ day	24	6 months	Well-tolerated; improvement relative to placebo in global autism severity scores of questionable clinical significance
Risperidone	Nagaraj, Singhi, & Mahli (2006)	2–9	1 mg/day	39	6 months	Superior to placebo on measures of global autism severity and on parent ratings of aggression, hyperactivity
Olanzapine	Hollander, Wasserman, et al. (2006)	6–14	Range 7.5– 12.5 mg/ day; mean 10 mg/day	11	8 weeks	Significant improvement in global functioning but not superior to placebo on measures of irritability, aggression, or compulsive behavior

From Myers, S.M. (2007). The status of pharmacotherapy for autism spectrum disorders. *Expert Opinion on Pharmacotherapy,* *8*(11), 1581–1584; adapted by permission.
Key: N = total number in sample; SIB = self-injurious behavior; ABC = Aberrant Behavior Checklist (Aman, Singh, Stewart, & Field, 1985).

The impact of risperidone on core symptoms of ASDs is less dramatic. The RUPP Autism Network trial revealed that treatment with risperidone improved repetitive behaviors but did not significantly affect impairments in social interaction or communication (McDougle et al., 2005). In the Canadian multisite trial, Shea et al. (2004) also found a decrease in repetitive behaviors, but the effect of risperidone on measures of social withdrawal or isolation was mixed, with statistically significant superiority to placebo on one measure but not on another. In a randomized, placebo-controlled trial in 24 preschool-age children with ASDs, risperidone was well-tolerated, but was not significantly or meaningfully superior to placebo in improving the social competence, communication, or restriction in a range of behaviors and interests during a 6-month treatment period (Luby et al., 2006). Risperidone has not been demonstrated to improve cognitive ability, but there is some evidence that it can improve working memory as measured by a divided attention task (Troost, Althaus et al., 2006). It is promising that in the RUPP Autism Network trial, behavioral improvement on risperidone for a period of 6 months was associated with clinically meaningful gains in adaptive skills, although this phase of the study did not include a control group (Williams et al., 2006).

Evidence of efficacy of other atypical antipsychotics for the treatment of ASDs is preliminary. Currently, the evidence supporting the efficacy of clozapine, olanzapine, quetiapine, ziprasidone, and aripiprazole for the types of target symptoms that have been shown to respond to risperidone is limited to open-label trials, chart reviews, and case reports (Chen, Bedair, McKay, Bowers, & Mazure, 2001; Cohen, Fitzgerald, Khan, S.R., & Khan, A., 2004; Corson, Barkenbus, Posey, Stigler, & McDougle, 2004; Findling et al., 2004; Hardan, Jou, & Handen, 2005; Horrigan, Barnhill, & Courvoisie, 1997; Kemner, Willemsen-Swinkels, de Jonge, Tuynman-Qua, & van Engeland,

2002; Malek-Ahmadi & Simonds, 1998; Malone, Cater, Sheikh, Choudhury, & Delaney, 2001; Martin, Koenig, Scahill, & Bregman, 1999; McDougle, Kem, & Posey, 2002; Potenza, Holmes, Kanes, & McDougle, 1999; Shastri, Alla, & Sabaratnam, 2006; Stavrakaki, Antochi, & Emery, 2004; Stigler, Posey, & McDougle, 2004; Valicenti-McDermott & Demb, 2006; Zuddas, Ledda, Fratta, Muglia, & Cianchetti, 1996). The one exception is a very small randomized, placebo-controlled trial in which three of six children (50%) were considered to be responders to olanzapine, whereas one of five (20%) responded to placebo, and there was a statistically significant linear trend × group interaction on the Clinical Global Impressions–Improvement (CGI-I) scale (Hollander, Wasserman, et al., 2006) (Table 10.2).

Antidepressants

The tricyclic antidepressant clomipramine, which is a potent but nonselective inhibitor of serotonin reuptake, and the selective serotonin reuptake inhibitors (SSRIs) fluoxetine and fluvoxamine have been demonstrated in double-blind trials to be superior to placebo for treatment of repetitive and other maladaptive behaviors in patients with ASDs (Buchsbaum et al., 2001; Gordon, State, Nelson, Hamburger, & Rapoport, 1993; Hollander et al., 2005; Lewis, Bodfish, Powell, & Golden, 1995; McDougle et al., 1996) (Table 10.3). McDougle and colleagues found fluvoxamine to be beneficial and well-tolerated in adults but not in children, suggesting age-dependent effects (McDougle et al., 1996; McDougle, Kresch, & Posey, 2000). However, Sugie et al. (2005) conducted a controlled crossover trial and reported moderate or marked improvement in 28% and mild improvement in another 28% of children with ASDs on fluvoxamine, although the placebo response rate was not documented in the paper.

In a large open-label retrospective study of fluoxetine, DeLong, Ritch, and Burch

Table 10.3. Double-blind, placebo-controlled clinical trials of potent serotonin reuptake inhibitors in autism spectrum disorders: 1996–2006

Agent	Reference	Age (years)	Dose	N	Duration	Outcomes/Comments
Clomipramine	Remington, Sloman, Konstantareas, Parker, & Gow (2001)	10–36	Range 100–150 mg/day; mean 128.4 mg/day	36	7 weeks	Not superior to placebo, inferior to haloperidol for irritability, hyperactivity, and global autism symptom severity; less well tolerated than haloperidol
Fluvoxamine	McDougle et al. (1996)	18–53	Range 200–300 mg/day; mean 276.7 mg/day	30	12 weeks	Superior to placebo for repetitive thoughts and behavior, aggression, general maladaptive behavior, and some aspects of social relatedness and language usage; response rate: 53% on fluvoxamine, 0% on placebo
Fluvoxamine	Unpublished but reviewed in McDougle, Kresch, & Posey (2000)	5–18	Range 25–250 mg/day; mean 107 mg/day	34	12 weeks	Response rate: 6%; adverse effects in 78% on fluvoxamine
Fluvoxamine	Sugie et al. (2005)	3–8	3 mg/kg/day	18	12 weeks	Uninterpretable; 28% much or very much improved and 28% mildly improved on fluvoxamine, but placebo response rate is not provided; however, patients with *l* serotonin transporter gene promoter region allele variants were more likely to be responders to fluvoxamine than those with *s* allele variants.
Fluoxetine	Hollander et al. (2005)	5–17	Range 2.4–20 mg/day, mean 9.9 mg/day (0.38 mg/kg/day)	39	16 weeks	Superior to placebo for repetitive behaviors by CY-BOCS compulsion scale

From Myers, S.M. (2007). The status of pharmacotherapy for autism spectrum disorders. *Expert Opinion on Pharmacotherapy,* *8*(11), 1581–1584; adapted by permission.

Key: N = total number in sample; CY-BOCS = Children's Yale-Brown Obsessive Compulsive Scale (Scahill, Riddle, & McSwiggin-Hardin, 1997).

(2002) found that 69% of 129 young children with ASDs between the ages of 2 and 8 years responded positively to fluoxetine at doses of 0.15–0.5 mg/kg/day. The most highly functioning children seemed to benefit most. Reviewers of open-label trials of various serotonin reuptake inhibitors in children and adults with ASDs note that response rates in the range of 50%–75% are reported, but publication bias and other shortcomings of uncontrolled studies must be considered when interpreting these findings (Kolevzon, Mathewson, & Hollander,

2006; Moore, Eichner, & Jones, 2004; Posey, Erickson, Stigler, & McDougle, 2006). Improvements in target symptoms (e.g., repetitive behaviors, irritability, depressive symptoms, tantrums, anxiety, aggression, difficulty with transitions, and aspects of social interaction and language) have been reported. Evidence supporting the use of other antidepressants or anxiolytics such as mirtazapine, venlafaxine, and buspirone in this population is limited to case reports and open-label trials (Buitelaar, van der Gaag, & van der Hoeven, 1998; Carminati,

Deriaz, & Bertschy, 2006; Hollander, Kaplan, Cartwright, & Reichman, 2000; Posey, Guenin, Kohn, Swiezy, & McDougle, 2001; Realmuto, August, & Garfinkel, 1989). Clomipramine is frequently associated with adverse effects and is therefore far less commonly used than SSRIs (Brasic, Barnett, Sheitman, & Tsaltas, 1997; Remington et al., 2001; Sanchez et al., 1996).

Mood Stabilizers

The literature regarding the effects of anticonvulsants on behavior in individuals with ASDs is mixed. An open retrospective review indicated that divalproex was effective in reducing aggression, impulsivity, and mood lability in children with ASDs and that the effect was sustained (Hollander, Dolgoff-Kaspar, Cartwright, Rawitt, & Novotny, 2001). In a double-blind, placebo-controlled trial, Hellings and colleagues (2005) were unable to demonstrate a significant difference between valproate and placebo for treatment of aggression and irritability. However, 10 of 16 subjects (i.e., 62%) who entered an open trial of valproate after the double-blind phase demonstrated a sustained response, and attempted tapering in 4 subjects was associated with relapse in irritability and aggression, which improved when the medication was resumed. High intra- and intersubject variability, small group size, and placebo response were problems in this study, and the authors called for a larger multisite study. Hollander, Soorya, et al. (2006) demonstrated significant improvement in repetitive behavior in a small group of children with ASDs treated with divalproex (Table 10.4). Six of the subjects went on to receive fluoxetine, and the research group published preliminary evidence that pretreatment with divalproex, in contrast to placebo, may be effective in preventing early symptoms of activation or irritability associated with fluoxetine (Anagnostou et al., 2006). In an open-label valproate trial (Hollander et al., 2001) and

several case reports (Childs & Blair, 1997; Plioplys, 1994), improvements in language and social skills were described.

Uvebrant and Bauziene (1994) reported a decrease in "autistic symptoms" in 8 of 13 patients treated with lamotrigine for intractable epilepsy, independent of efficacy in controlling the seizures. However, lamotrigine was not superior to placebo in a double-blind, placebo-controlled trial (Belsito, Law, Kirk, Landa, & Zimmerman, 2001). Similarly, levetiracetam was found to reduce mood instability, disruptive outbursts, and aggression in a small open-label trial (Rugino & Samsock, 2002), but a controlled study revealed no superiority to placebo on measures of aggression, affective instability, repetitive behavior, impulsivity and hyperactivity, or global improvement (Wasserman et al., 2006). Reports of effects of open-label use of topiramate in this population have also been mixed. Hardan, Jou, and Handen (2004) noted improvement in conduct, hyperactivity, and inattention, but others reported variable or modest effects and negative behavioral effects in some patients (Canitano, 2005; Mazzone & Ruta, 2006). Recently, oxcarbazepine has been reported to be very effective for severe disruptive behaviors in three young patients with ASDs, but it has not been studied in controlled trials (Kapetanovic, 2007).

The literature also includes several cases of patients with ASDs and comorbid atypical bipolar disorder or mania who responded well to open-label treatment with lithium (DeLong, 1994; Kerbeshian, Burd, & Fisher, 1987; Steingard & Biederman, 1987), and a controlled crossover study of 10 "severely disturbed" young children with hyperactivity showed a trend toward decreased explosiveness, aggressiveness, hyperactivity, and "psychotic speech" with lithium, with the suggestion that it deserved further study (Campbell, Fish, & Korein et al., 1972). However, controlled lithium trials in larger, well-characterized populations of patients with ASDs are lacking.

Table 10.4.   Double-blind, placebo-controlled clinical trials of mood stabilizers in autism spectrum disorders: 1996–2006

Agent	Reference	Age (years)	Dose	N	Duration	Outcomes/Comments
Divalproex sodium	Anagnostou et al. (2006); Hollander, Soorya, et al. (2006)	12 patients age 5–17 and one age 40	Range 500–1500 mg/day; mean 823 mg/day	13	8 weeks	Superior to placebo for reduction of repetitive behavior (CY-BOCS); preliminary evidence of efficacy for preventing irritability associated with treatment with fluoxetine
Valproate	Hellings et al. (2005)	6–20	20 mg/kg/day, mean trough levels 75 mcg/ml at week 4 and 77.8 mcg/ml at week 8	30	8 weeks	Not superior to placebo for aggression or irritability; however, 10 of the 16 patients who then entered an open trial demonstrated a sustained response; tapering in 4 subjects was associated with relapse in irritability and aggression, which improved when the medication was resumed
Lamotrigine	Belsito, Law, Kirk, Landa, & Zimmerman (2001)	3–11	5 mg/kg/day	28	18 weeks	Not superior to placebo for core symptoms of autism or associated maladaptive behaviors
Levetiracetam	Wasserman et al. (2006)	5–17	Target 20–30 mg/kg/day; Range 500–2500 mg/day; mean 862 mg/day	20	10 weeks	No significant efficacy compared to placebo for hyperactivity, repetitive behavior, irritability, aggression, or global improvement

From Myers, S.M. (2007). The status of pharmacotherapy for autism spectrum disorders. *Expert Opinion on Pharmacotherapy,8*(11), 1581–1584; adapted by permission.
  Key: N = total number in sample; CY-BOCS = Children's Yale-Brown Obsessive Compulsive Scale (Scahill, Riddle, & McSwiggin-Hardin, 1997).

PRINCIPLES OF CLINICAL PSYCHOPHARMACOLOGIC MANAGEMENT

Although behavioral interventions are the primary approach, consideration of psychopharmacologic intervention may arise in the setting of maladaptive behaviors such as aggression, self-injurious behavior, hyperactivity, impulsivity, inattention, repetitive behaviors (e.g., perseveration, obsessions, compulsions, stereotypic movements), sleep disturbance, mood lability, irritability, anxiety, tantrums, property destruction, or other disruptive behaviors. In some cases, the diagnosis of a comorbid psychiatric disorder (e.g., depression, bipolar disorder, anxiety disorder) can be reasonably made, although

modifications of diagnostic criteria may be necessary in individuals with ASDs or other developmental disabilities (Perry, Marston, Hinder, Munden, & Roy, 2001; Syzmanski et al., 1998). Standardized questionnaires and structured interviews may be helpful in making additional psychiatric diagnoses in this population (Brereton, Tonge, & Einfeld, 2006; Leyfer et al., 2006). More commonly, clinicians treat specific target behaviors or symptom clusters in the absence of clear comorbid psychiatric diagnoses (Bostic & Rho, 2006; Hollander, Phillips, & Yeh, 2003). Principles to guide the approach to psychopharmacologic management of ASDs in clinical practice have been proposed by several authors (Myers, 2007; Steingard, Connor, & Au, 2005; Towbin, 2003).

Evaluation of Target Symptoms

Challenging behaviors in children are most often assessed by interviewing the parents or caregivers; however, input from teachers, aides, and other observers is also desirable. Verbal patients can contribute as well. Details including frequency, intensity, and duration of the behavior, as well as the degree of interference with adaptive functioning, should be elicited. Exacerbating and ameliorating factors, including one's response to behavioral interventions, should be identified. It is important to consider time trends as well; a behavior that has been decreasing in frequency and severity may not warrant immediate psychopharmacologic intervention, whereas an escalating target behavior may require more prompt action.

Baseline data collection ideally includes behavior rating scale data and/or direct observational data (e.g., number of episodes of aggression or self-injury in a given time period). Consistent use of validated, treatment-sensitive rating scales and medication side effect scales at the baseline and for periodic monitoring is desirable. A wide variety of outcome measures have been utilized in research trials and in clinical practice to measure maladaptive behavior treatment effects in this population (Aman et al., 2004). A formal functional analysis of the behavior may be very helpful. Parents, teachers, or other caregivers may inadvertently reinforce maladaptive behaviors, and in such cases, the most appropriate and effective interventions are behavioral rather than pharmacologic. Sometimes a mismatch between educational or behavioral expectations and the cognitive ability of the child causes or exacerbates disruptive behavior, and in such cases, adjustment of the expectations and demands is the most appropriate intervention. To make informed decisions about the potential role for medication, it is necessary to assess existing and available interventions and supports, including behavioral services, educational expecta-

tions and accommodations, habilitative therapies, and family psychosocial supports (e.g., respite care, formal and informal support networks).

Medical factors can also cause or exacerbate maladaptive behaviors, and recognition and treatment of medical conditions may eliminate the need for psychopharmacologic agents in some cases. For example, history and physical examination may reveal an occult source of pain or discomfort that can be treated or may suggest the possibility of obstructive sleep apnea or a seizure disorder that requires further evaluation and possibly treatment (Table 10.5). Other medical conditions such as obesity or asthma are important to note because they may have a bearing on the choice of medication (e.g., avoiding the atypical antipsychotics that are most commonly associated with weight gain in children who are obese or β-blockers that are contraindicated in asthmatics). If the patient is taking medications or dietary supplements, this may also affect the psychotropic medication choice because of potential drug–drug interactions. Any medical tests that may have a bearing on treatment choice (e.g., EEG if there is suspicion of seizures) should be completed prior to initiating psychopharmacologic intervention.

Initiation and Monitoring of Pharmacotherapy

After treatable medical causes and modifiable environmental factors have been addressed or ruled out, a therapeutic trial of medication may be considered if the behavioral symptoms are causing significant impairment in functioning. Pharmacologic intervention is considered based on the presence of certain criteria (Myers, 2007):

1. Evidence that the target symptoms are substantially interfering with the learning/academic progress, socialization, health, or safety of the patient

Table 10.5. Examples of medical conditions that may cause or exacerbate maladaptive behaviors and potential treatment options

Medical condition	Potential medical intervention
Otitis media, otitis externa	Antimicrobial therapy, analgesia
Sinusitis	Antimicrobial therapy, analgesia
Pharyngitis	Antimicrobial therapy, analgesia
Allergic rhinitis	Antihistamine therapy, antileukotriene therapy, topical steroid therapy
Dental abscess or decay	Antimicrobial therapy, extraction, or dental repair
Headache (including migraine)	Analgesia, abortive therapies, prophylactic therapies
Esophagitis, gastritis	Acid-inhibiting therapy (e.g., proton pump inhibitors, histamine [H2] antagonists)
Constipation	Laxative therapy
Occult fracture	Casting, splinting, rest, analgesia, surgical intervention
Premenstrual discomfort or dysphoria	Analgesia, oral or injectable contraceptive therapy
Obstructive sleep apnea, other sleep disordered breathing	Weight reduction, tonsillectomy and adenoidectomy, continuous positive airway pressure
Iron deficiency, zinc deficiency	Appropriate mineral supplementation
Malnutrition	Nutritional supplementation

and/or others around him or her, or quality of life

2. Suboptimal response to available behavioral interventions and environmental modifications

3. Research evidence that the target behavioral symptoms or comorbid psychiatric diagnoses are amenable to pharmacologic intervention

The specific target symptoms should be identified and agreed upon. Medication choice is based on likely efficacy for the specific target symptoms, potential adverse effects, and practical considerations (e.g., formulations available, dosing schedule, cost, requirement for laboratory or electrocardiographic [ECG] monitoring). Some potential medication choices for particular target symptoms or clusters are outlined in Table 10.6, but there is no consensus, evidence-based approach.

All medications can have side effects, and it is important to discuss those that are common or particularly severe. Available formulations and some important possible adverse effects of selected commonly used medications are reviewed in Table 10.7. Potential benefits and risks must be explained in understandable terminology and verbal or written informed consent obtained from the parent or guardian. When possible, consent or assent should be obtained from the patient. The time course of expected effects should be discussed as part of the approach to ensure reasonable expectations, and the timing of follow-up telephone contact, completion of rating scales, reassessment of behavioral data, and clinic visits should be arranged accordingly. When necessary, baseline laboratory tests should be obtained and appropriate follow-up monitoring planned.

In general, only one medication should be initiated or adjusted at a time so that the treatment effect can be accurately judged. It is usually best to begin with a low dose and gradually titrate upward to the target effect to minimize the risk of treatment-emergent adverse events. If a medication is ineffective despite an adequate titration of the dose and appropriate duration of therapy, or if its use

Table 10.6. Selected potential medication options for common target symptoms in children with autism spectrum disorders

Target symptom cluster	Selected medication considerations
Irritability, aggression, explosive outbursts, self-injury	Atypical antipsychotic (e.g., risperidone[a], aripiprazole, olanzapine, quetiapine, ziprasidone)
	Alpha-2 agonist (clonidine[a], guanfacine)
	Anticonvulsant mood stabilizer (e.g., valproate, levitiracetam, topiramate)
	Selective serotonin reuptake inhibitor (fluoxetine, fluvoxamine[a], citalopram, escitalopram, paroxetine, sertraline)
Hyperactivity, impulsivity, inattention	Stimulant (e.g., methylphenidate[a], dextroamphetamine, mixed amphetamine salts)
	Alpha-2 agonist (e.g., clonidine[a], guanfacine)
	Atomoxetine[a]
	Atypical antipsychotic (e.g., risperidone[a], aripiprazole, olanzapine, quetiapine, ziprasidone)
	NMDA antagonists (e.g., amantadine, memantine)
Repetitive behavior, behavioral rigidity, obsessive-compulsive symptoms	Selective serotonin reuptake inhibitor (e.g., fluoxetine[a], fluvoxamine[a], citalopram, escitalopram, paroxetine, sertraline)
	Atypical antipsychotic (e.g., risperidone[a], aripiprazole, olanzapine, quetiapine, ziprasidone)
	Valproate/divalproex[a]
Sleep dysfunction	Melatonin
	Alpha-2 agonist (e.g., clonidine, guanfacine)
	Antihistamine (e.g., niaprazine, diphenhydramine, hydroxyzine)
	Ramelteon
	Mirtazapine
Anxiety	Selective serotonin reuptake inhibitor (e.g., fluoxetine, fluvoxamine, citalopram, escitalopram, paroxetine, sertraline)
	Buspirone
Depressive phenotype (marked change from baseline, including symptoms such as social withdrawal, irritability, sadness or crying spells, decreased energy, anorexia, weight loss, sleep dysfunction)	Selective serotonin reuptake inhibitor (e.g., fluoxetine, fluvoxamine, citalopram, escitalopram, paroxetine, sertraline)
	Mirtazapine
Bipolar phenotype (behavioral cycling with rages, euphoria, decreased need for sleep, manic-like hyperactivity, irritability, aggression, self-injury, sexual behaviors)	Anticonvulsant mood stabilizer (e.g., carbamazepine, gabapentin, lamotrigine, oxcarbazepine, topiramate, valproate)
	Atypical antipsychotic (e.g., risperidone, aripiprazole, olanzapine, quetiapine, ziprasidone)
	Lithium

From Myers, S.M. (2007). The status of pharmacotherapy for autism spectrum disorders. *Expert Opinion on Pharmocotherapy,* *8*(11), 1591, 1592; adapted by permission.
[a]At least one published double-blind, placebo-controlled trial supporting use in patients with autism spectrum disorders.
Key: NMDA = N-methyl-D-aspartate.

is associated with significant adverse effects, the therapeutic trial should be discontinued. Gradual tapering may be warranted, depending on the particular medication. This is particularly important when discontinuing medications known to have withdrawal-emergent adverse effects such as antipsychotics and, to a lesser extent, SSRIs.

Periodic setbacks or behavioral symptom exacerbations are to be expected, and it is wise to avoid quickly changing or adding medications to treat each behavior that arises. However, in the case of partial or suboptimal response despite titration of the medication dose, the clinician and the patient's family must decide

Table 10.7. Available formulations and side effects of selected psychotropic medications

Medication class	Examples	Formulations available	Important adverse effects (selected)
Stimulants	Mixed amphetamine salts	Tablets, extended release capsules	Appetite suppression, weight loss, insomnia, dysphoria, irritability, agitation, rebound hyperactivity, exacerbation of tics, tachycardia, hypertension
	Dextroamphetamine	Tablets, extended release capsules	
	Methylphenidate	Tablets, chewable tablets, extended release tablets, extended release capsules, liquid, transdermal patch	
	d-methylphenidate	Tablets, extended release capsules	
Selective norepinephrine reuptake inhibitors	Atomoxetine	Capsules	Gastrointestinal upset, abdominal pain, symptoms, somnolence, appetite suppression, dysphoria, liver dysfunction, suicidal ideation, agitation, dry mouth
Alpha-2 agonists	Clonidine	Tablets, transdermal patch	Fatigue, somnolence, dizziness, hypotension, dry mouth, constipation, dysphoria, irritability, agitation, sleep disturbance
	Guanfacine	Tablets	
Atypical antipsychotics	Aripiprazole	Tablets, disintegrating tablets, liquid, injectable (IM)	Sedation, appetite increase, weight gain, extrapyramidal symptoms, akathisia, neuroleptic malignant syndrome, QTc prolongation, increased salivation
	Olanzapine	Tablets, disintegrating tablets, injectable (IM)	
	Quetiapine	Tablets	
	Risperidone	Tablets, disintegrating tablets, liquid, long-acting injectable (IM)	
	Ziprasidone	Capsules, injectable (IM)	
Selective serotonin reuptake inhibitors	Citalopram	Tablets, liquid	Irritability, behavioral activation (especially in younger patients), mania/hypomania, insomnia, drowsiness, suicidal ideation, gastrointestinal upset, urinary frequency, tremor, serotonin syndrome, extrapyramidal symptoms
	Escitalopram	Tablets, liquid	
	Fluoxetine	Tablets, capsules, liquid, weekly delayed release capsules	
	Fluvoxamine	Tablets	
	Paroxetine	Tablets, controlled release tablets, liquid	
	Sertraline	Tablets, liquid	
Anticonvulsant mood stabilizers	Divalproex sodium	Sprinkle capsules, tablets, extended release tablets	Weight gain, sedation, gastrointestinal upset, thrombocytopenia, liver dysfunction, pancreatitis, tremor, hyperammonemia
	Valproic acid (e.g., valproate)	Capsules, liquid	
	Lamotrigine	Tablets, chewable tablets	Gastrointestinal upset, fatigue, dry mouth, sleep disturbance, Stevens-Johnson syndrome, abdominal pain, blood dyscrasias
	Levetiracetam	Tablets, liquid	Somnolence, dizziness, agitation, anxiety, coordination problems, depression, apathy

Medication class	Examples	Formulations available	Important adverse effects (selected)
	Oxcarbazepine	Tablets, liquid	Somnolence, dizziness, gastrointestinal upset, tremor, ataxia, nystagmus, headache, Stevens-Johnson syndrome, hyponatremia
	Topiramate	Tablets, sprinkle capsules	Appetite suppression, weight loss, somnolence, cognitive dulling, speech problems, psychomotor slowing, dizziness, tremor, metabolic acidosis, kidney stones, glaucoma, oligohydrosis, hyperthermia

From Myers, S.M. (2007). The status of pharmacotherapy for autism spectrum disorders. *Expert Opinion on Pharmocotherapy,* *8*(11), 1591, 1592; adapted by permission.
Key: IM = intramuscular.

whether to substitute another agent or add a second medication to address the same target symptoms. While monotherapy is desirable, augmentation or combination strategies are sometimes found to be necessary, particularly in the setting of significant mood instability and severe aggression or self-injury. In some cases, a medication may be very effective for some target symptoms but not others, and a different medication may be added to address additional target symptoms that remain problematic. When polypharmacy is necessary, the clinician must be aware of potential interactions among certain drugs and monitor accordingly. Careful withdrawal of a medication should be considered after a period of stability (i.e., approximately 6–12 months) so that it is possible to determine whether the medication is still necessary.

CONCLUSION

The use of psychotropic agents as a component of treatment for individuals with ASDs is common, and a substantial body of literature describing controlled and open-label clinical trials now exists to guide clinical practice. Although psychotropic medications are effective for some important associated maladaptive behaviors, evidence of significant impact on the core features of

ASDs is quite limited, and educational and behavioral interventions remain the primary treatment strategies.

Although the quantity and quality of psychopharmacologic studies have increased, additional important information is needed to guide clinical practice and improve patient outcomes. There is a need for more rigorous evaluation of the safety and efficacy of psychotropic agents for maladaptive behaviors in patients with ASDs in randomized, double-blind, placebo-controlled trials with appropriate outcome measures and adequate sample size and duration. Because patients with ASDs are a heterogeneous group in terms of etiology and clinical phenotype, as well as response to various interventions, efforts to delineate clinical and biological subgroups of patients (i.e., endophenotypes) that may be responsive to particular treatments are likely to become an increasingly important focus of research.

Some important issues, such as psychopharmacologic management of sleep disturbances, have received very little attention; recommendations are typically based on case reports and open-label trials, extrapolation from the adult sleep disorders literature, and expert consensus due to the lack of controlled clinical trials in children with ASDs. Concurrent use of two or more psychotropic medications (i.e., polypharmacy) is another area in which there is a wide gap between the available empirical scientific evidence and the reality of clinical practice. Although there is substantial evidence that certain medications are effective in reducing some maladaptive behaviors often associated with ASDs, the effectiveness of psychopharmacologic treatments for core language, social, and cognitive deficits remains to be determined.

Researchers are beginning to investigate the value of combining behavioral and medical interventions. For example, the RUPP Autism Network has conducted a study comparing the effectiveness of the combination of risperidone and behavior therapy to medication alone, with the results expected to be published soon (Vitiello, 2006). Future research may be able to determine whether short-term pharmacologic treatment can allow behavioral interventions to be successful more rapidly, reduce the overall cost of intensive behavioral intervention, or improve effectiveness by increasing parent or caregiver compliance because of more prompt and robust response. It is possible that behavioral interventions will be shown to reduce the required medication dose and thereby reduce adverse effects.

Although independently replicated randomized controlled clinical trials with adequate sample sizes and well-defined study populations are the gold standard of evidence-based medicine, long-term open-label extensions of these trials are also important, especially for establishing safety and lasting efficacy. Another type of study design that is likely to play an important role is the large practical clinical trial, which relies on participation of nonacademic clinicians in traditional clinical settings and employs more broad inclusion criteria to capture "real-world" patients. This type of trial has been extremely successful in pediatric oncology, and an infrastructure for similar research in child and adolescent psychiatry is being developed (March et al., 2004; March et al., 2005; Vitiello, 2006). Practical clinical trials have the potential to help to establish the duration of treatment effect, detect adverse

effects, evaluate polypharmacy, and close the gap between research and clinical practice by studying patients under more naturalistic circumstances.

The emergence of pharmacogenomics is likely to have a significant impact on clinical psychopharmacology, and future research may reveal specific applications for ASD management. Genotyping is already commercially available for some hepatic cytochrome P450 enzyme genes (e.g., CYP2D6, CYP2C19), and this may have some utility in safely and effectively treating patients with risperidone, typical antipsychotics, venlafaxine, tricyclic antidepressants, and possibly citalopram, escitalopram, sertraline, aripiprazole, and atomoxetine (De Leon, Armstrong, & Cozza, 2006).

REFERENCES

Aman, M.G. (2004). Management of hyperactivity and other acting-out problems in patients with autism spectrum disorder. *Seminars in Pediatric Neurology, 11,* 225–228.

Aman, M.G., De Smedt, G., Derivan, A., Lyons, B., Findling, R.L., & the Risperidone Disruptive Behavior Study Group. (2002). Double-blind, placebo-controlled study of risperidone for the treatment of disruptive behaviors in children with subaverage intelligence. *American Journal of Psychiatry, 159,* 1337–1346.

Aman, M.G., & Kern, R.A. (1989). Review of fenfluramine in the treatment of the developmental disabilities. *Journal of the American Academy of Child and Adolescent Psychiatry, 28,* 549–565.

Aman, M.G., Lam, K.S., & Collier-Crespin, A. (2003). Prevalence and patterns of use of psychoactive medicines among individuals with autism in the Autism Society of Ohio. *Journal of Autism and Developmental Disorders, 33,* 527–534.

Aman, M.G., Lam, K.S., & Van Bourgondien, M.E. (2005). Medication patterns in patients with autism: Temporal, regional, and demographic influences. *Journal of Child and Adolescent Psychopharmacology, 15,* 116–126.

Aman, M.G., Novotny, S., Samango-Sprouse, C., Lecavalier, L., Leonard, E., Gadow, K.D., et al. (2004). Outcome measures for clinical drug trials in autism. *CNS Spectrums, 9,* 36–47.

Aman, M.G., Singh, N.N., Stewart, A.W., & Field, C.J. (1985). The Aberrant Behavior Checklist: A behavior rating scale for the assessment of treatment effects. *American Journal of Mental Deficiency, 89*(5), 485–491.

Anagnostou, E., Esposito, K., Soorya, L., Chaplin, W., Wasserman, S., & Hollander, E. (2006). Divalproex versus placebo for the prevention of irritability associated with fluoxetine treatment in autism spectrum disorder. *Journal of Clinical Psychopharmacology, 26*, 444–446.

Anderson, G.M. (2005). Serotonin in autism. In M.L. Bauman & T.L. Kemper (Eds.), *The neurobiology of autism* (2nd ed., pp. 303–318). Baltimore: The Johns Hopkins University Press.

Anderson, L.T., Campbell, M., Adams, P., Small, A.M., Perry, R., & Shell, J. (1989). The effects of haloperidol on discrimination learning and behavioral symptoms in autistic children. *Journal of Autism and Developmental Disorders, 19*, 227–239.

Anderson, L.T., Campbell, M., Grega, D.M., Perry, R., Small, A.M., & Green, W.H. (1984). Haloperidol in the treatment of infantile autism: Effects on learning and behavioral symptoms. *American Journal of Psychiatry, 141*, 1195–1202.

Arnold, L.E., Aman, M.G., Cook, A.M., Witwer, A.N., Hall, K.L., Thompson, S., et al. (2006). Atomoxetine for hyperactivity in autism spectrum disorders: Placebo-controlled crossover pilot trial. *Journal of the American Academy of Child and Adolescent Psychiatry, 45*, 1196–1205.

Arnold, L.E., Vitiello, B., McDougle, C., Scahill, L., Shah, B., Gonzalez, N.M., et al. (2003). Parent-defined target symptoms respond to risperidone in RUPP autism study: Customer approach to clinical trials. *Journal of the American Academy of Child and Adolescent Psychiatry, 42*, 1443–1450.

Belsito, K.M., Law, P.A., Kirk, K.S., Landa, R.J., & Zimmerman, A.W. (2001). Lamotrigine therapy for autistic disorder: A randomized, double-blind, placebo-controlled trial. *Journal of Autism and Developmental Disorders, 31*, 175–181.

Bostic, J.Q., & Rho, Y. (2006). Target-symptom psychopharmacology: Between the forest and the trees. *Child and Adolescent Psychiatric Clinics of North America, 15*, 289–302.

Bradley, C. (1937). The behavior of children receiving benzedrine. *American Journal of Psychiatry, 94*, 577–585.

Brasic, J.R., Barnett, J.Y., Sheitman, B.B., & Tsaltas, M.O. (1997). Adverse effects of clomipramine. *Journal of the American Academy of Child and Adolescent Psychiatry, 36*, 1165–1166.

Brereton, A.V., Tonge, B.J., & Einfeld, S.L. (2006). Psychopathology in children and adolescents with autism compared to young people with intellectual disability. *Journal of Autism and Developmental Disorders, 36*, 863–870.

Buchsbaum, M.S., Hollander, E., Haznedar, M.M., Tang, C., Spiegel-Cohen, J., & Wei, T.C., et al. (2001). Effect of fluoxetine on regional cerebral metabolism in autistic spectrum disorders: A pilot study. *International Journal of Neuropsychopharmacology, 4*, 119–125.

Buitelaar, J.K., van der Gaag, R.J., & van der Hoeven, J. (1998). Buspirone in the management of anxiety and irritability in children with pervasive developmental disorders: Results of an open-label study. *Journal of Clinical Psychiatry, 59*, 56–59.

Campbell, M., Anderson, L.T., Meier, M., Cohen, I.L., Small, A.M., & Samit, C. et al. (1978). A comparison of haloperidol and behavior therapy and their interaction in autistic children. *Journal of the American Academy of Child Psychiatry, 17*, 640–655.

Campbell, M., Armenteros, J.L., Malone, R.P., Adams, P.B., Eisenberg, Z.W., & Overall, J.E. (1997). Neuroleptic-related dyskinesias in autistic children: A prospective, longitudinal study. *Journal of the American Academy of Child and Adolescent Psychiatry, 36*, 835–843.

Campbell, M., Fish, B., David, R., Shapiro, T., Collins, P., & Koh, C. (1972). Response to triiodothyronine and dextroamphetamine: A study of preschool schizophrenic children. *Journal of Autism and Childhood Schizophrenia, 2*, 343–358.

Campbell, M., Fish, B., Korein, J., Shapiro, T., Collins, P., & Koh, C. (1972). Lithium and chlorpromazine: A controlled crossover study of hyperactive severely disturbed young children. *Journal of Autism and Childhood Schizophrenia, 2*, 234–263.

Campbell, M., Fish, B., Shapiro, T., & Floyd, A., Jr. (1970). Thiothixene in young disturbed children: A pilot study. *Archives of General Psychiatry, 23*, 70–72.

Campbell, M., Fish, B. Shapiro, T., & Floyd, A., Jr. (1971). Study of molindone in disturbed preschool children. *Current Therapeutic Research, Clinical, and Experimental, 13*, 28–33.

Campbell, M., Fish, B., Shapiro, T., & Floyd, A., Jr. (1972). Acute responses of schizophrenic children to a sedative and a "stimulating" neuroleptic: A pharmacologic yardstick. *Current Therapeutic Research, Clinical, and Experimental, 14*, 759–766.

Campbell, M., Small, A.M., Collins, P.J., Friedman, E., David, R., & Genieser, N. (1976). Levodopa and levoamphetamine: A crossover study in young schizophrenic children. *Current Therapeutic Research, Clinical, and Experimental, 19*, 70–86.

Canitano, R. (2005). Clinical experience with topiramate to counteract neuroleptic induced weight gain in 10 individuals with autistic spectrum disorders. *Brain Development, 27*, 228–232.

Carminati, G.G., Deriaz, N., & Bertschy, G. (2006). Low-dose venlafaxine in three adolescents and young adults with autistic disorder improves self-injurious behavior and attention deficit/hyperactivity disorders (ADHD)-like symptoms. *Progress in Neuropsychopharmacology and Biological Psychiatry, 30*, 312–315.

Chen, N.C., Bedair, H.S., McKay, B., Bowers, M.B.J., & Mazure, C. (2001). Clozapine in the treatment of aggression in an adolescent with autistic disorder. *Journal of Clinical Psychiatry, 62*, 479–480.

Cheng-Shannon, J., McGough, J.J., Pataki, C., & McCracken, J.T. (2004). Second-generation antipsychotic medications in children and adolescents. *Journal of Child and Adolescent Psychopharmacology, 14*, 372–394.

Childs, J.A., & Blair, J.L. (1997). Valproic acid treatment of epilepsy in autistic twins. *Journal of Neuroscience Nursing, 29*, 244–248.

Chugani, D.C. (2005). Positron emission tomography studies of autism. In M.L. Bauman & T.L. Kemper (Eds.), *The neurobiology of autism* (2nd ed., pp. 164–176). Baltimore: The Johns Hopkins University Press.

Cohen, I.L., Campbell, M., Posner, D., Small, A.M., Triebel, D., & Anderson, L.T. (1980). Behavioral effects of haloperidol in young autistic children: An objective analysis using a within-subjects reversal design. *Journal of the American Academy of Child Psychiatry, 19*, 665–677.

Cohen, S.A., Fitzgerald, B.J., Khan, S.R., & Khan, A. (2004). The effect of a switch to ziprasidone in an adult population with autistic disorder: Chart review of naturalistic, open-label treatment. *Journal of Clinical Psychiatry, 65*, 110–113.

Corson, A.H., Barkenbus, J.E., Posey, D.J., Stigler, K.A., & McDougle, C.J. (2004). A retrospective analysis of quetiapine in the treatment of pervasive developmental disorders. *Journal of Clinical Psychiatry, 65*, 1531–1536.

Croonenberghs, J., Fegert, J.M., Findling, R.L., De Smedt, G., Van Dongen, S., & the Risperidone Disruptive Behavior Study Group. (2005). Risperidone in children with disruptive behavior disorders and subaverage intelligence: A 1-year, open-label study of 504 patients. *Journal of the American Academy of Child and Adolescent Psychiatry, 44*, 64–72.

Curzon, G. (1990). How reserpine and chlorpromazine act: The impact of key discoveries on the history of psychopharmacology. *Trends in Pharmacological Sciences, 11*, 61–63.

De Leon, J., Armstrong, S.C., & Cozza, K. (2006). Clinical guidelines for psychiatrists for the use of pharmacogenetic testing for CYP450 2D6 and CYP450 2C19. *Psychosomatics, 47*, 75–85.

DeLong, G.R., Ritch, C.R., & Burch, S. (2002). Fluoxetine response in children with autistic spectrum disorders: Correlation with familial major affective disorder and intellectual achievement. *Developmental Medicine and Child Neurology, 44*, 652–659.

DeLong, R. (1994). Children with autistic spectrum disorder and a family history of affective disorder. *Developmental Medicine and Child Neurology, 36*, 674–687.

Di Martino, A., Melis, G., Cianchetti, C., & Zuddas, A. (2004). Methylphenidate for pervasive developmental disorders: Safety and efficacy of acute single dose test and ongoing therapy. An open-pilot study. *Journal of Child and Adolescent Psychopharmacology, 14*, 207–218.

Engelhardt, D.M., Polizos, P., Waizer, J., & Hoffman, S.P. (1973). A double-blind comparison of fluphenazine and haloperidol in outpatient schizophrenic children. *Journal of Autism and Childhood Schizophrenia, 3*, 128–137.

Ernst, M., Magee, H.J., Gonzalez, N.M., & Locascio, J.J. (1992). Pimozide in autistic children. *Psychopharmacology Bulletin, 28*, 187–191.

Fankhauser, M.P., Karumanchi, V.C., German, M.L., Yates, A., & Karumanchi, S.D. (1992). A double-blind, placebo-controlled study of the efficacy of transdermal clonidine in autism. *Journal of Clinical Psychiatry, 53*, 77–82.

Faretra, G., Dooher, L., & Dowling, J. (1970). Comparison of haloperidol and fluphenazine in disturbed children. *American Journal of Psychiatry, 126*, 1670–1673.

Findling, R.L., McNamara, N.K., Gracious, B.L., O'Riordan, M.A., Reed, M.D., Demeter, C., et al. (2004). Quetiapine in nine youths with autistic disorder. *Journal of Child and Adolescent Psychopharmacology, 14*, 287–294.

Fish, B., Campbell, M., Shapiro, T., & Floyd, A. (1969). Schizophrenic children treated with methysergide (Sansert). *Diseases of the Nervous System, 30*, 534–540.

Fish, B., Shapiro, T., & Campbell, M. (1966). Long-term prognosis and the response of schizophrenic children to drug therapy: A controlled study of trifluoperazine. *American Journal of Psychiatry, 123*, 32–39.

Geller, E., Ritvo, E.R., Freeman, B.J., & Yuwiler, A. (1982). Preliminary observations on the effect of fenfluramine on blood serotonin and symptoms in three autistic boys. *New England Journal of Medicine, 307*, 165–169.

Gordon, C.T., State, R.C., Nelson, J.E., Hamburger, S.D., & Rapoport, J.L. (1993). A double-blind comparison of clomipramine, desipramine, and placebo in the treatment of autistic disorder. *Archives of General Psychiatry, 50*, 441–447.

Green, V.A., Pituch, K.A., Itchon, J., Choi, A., O'Reilly, M., & Sigafoos, J. (2006). Internet survey of treatments used by parents of children with autism. *Research in Developmental Disabilities, 27*, 70–84.

Handen, B.L., Johnson, C.R., & Lubetsky, M. (2000). Efficacy of methylphenidate among children with autism and symptoms of attention-deficit hyperactivity disorder. *Journal of Autism and Developmental Disorders, 30*, 245–255.

Hardan, A.Y., Jou, R.J., & Handen, B.L. (2004). A retrospective assessment of topiramate in children and adolescents with pervasive developmental disorders. *Journal of Child and Adolescent Psychopharmacology, 14*, 426–432.

Hardan, A.Y., Jou, R.J., & Handen, B.L. (2005). Retrospective study of quetiapine in children and adolescents with pervasive developmental disorders. *Journal of Autism and Developmental Disorders, 35*, 387–391.

Hellings, J.A., Weckbaugh, M., Nickel, E.J., Cain, S.E., Zarcone, J.R., Reese, R.M., et al. (2005). A double-blind, placebo-controlled study of valproate for aggression in youth with pervasive developmental disorders. *Journal of Child and Adolescent Psychopharmacology, 15*, 682–692.

Hellings, J.A., Zarcone, J.R., Reese, M.R., Valdovinos, M.G., Marquis, J.G., Fleming, K.K., et al. (2006). A crossover study of risperidone in children, adolescents, and adults with mental retardation. *Journal of Autism and Developmental Disorders, 36*, 401–411.

Hollander, E., Dolgoff-Kaspar, R., Cartwright, C., Rawitt, R., & Novotny, S. (2001). An open trial of divalproex sodium in autism spectrum disorders. *Journal of Clinical Psychiatry, 62*, 530–534.

Hollander, E., Kaplan, A., Cartwright, C., & Reichman, D. (2000). Venlafaxine in children, adolescents, and young adults with autism spectrum disorders: An open retrospective clinical report. *Journal of Child Neurology, 15*, 132–135.

Hollander, E., Phillips, A., Chaplin, W., Zagursky, K., Novotny, S., Wasserman, S., et al. (2005). A placebo controlled crossover trial of liquid fluoxetine on repetitive behaviors in childhood and adolescent autism. *Neuropsychopharmacology, 30*, 582–589.

Hollander, E., Phillips, A., King, B.H., Guthrie, D., Aman, M.G., Law, P., et al. (2004). Impact of recent findings on study design of future autism clinical trials. *CNS Spectrums, 9*, 49–56.

Hollander, E., Phillips, A.T., & Yeh, C.C. (2003). Targeted treatments for symptom domains in child and adolescent autism. *Lancet, 362*, 732–734.

Hollander, E., Soorya, L., Wasserman, S., Esposito, K., Chaplin, W., & Anagnostou, E. (2006). Divalproex sodium vs. placebo in the treatment of repetitive behaviours in autism spectrum disorder. *International Journal of Neuropsychopharmacology, 9*, 209–213.

Hollander, E., Wasserman, S., Swanson, E.N., Chaplin, W., Schapiro, M.L., & Zagursky, K., et al. (2006). A double-blind placebo-controlled pilot study of olanzapine in childhood/adolescent pervasive developmental disorder. *Journal of Child and Adolescent Psychopharmacology, 16*, 541–548.

Horrigan, J.P., Barnhill, L.J., & Courvoisie, H.E. (1997). Olanzapine in PDD. *Journal of the Amer-*

ican Academy of Child and Adolescent Psychiatry,
36, 1166–1167.

Jaselskis, C.A., Cook, E.H., Jr., Fletcher, K.E., & Leventhal, B.L. (1992). Clonidine treatment of hyperactive and impulsive children with autistic disorder. *Journal of Clinical Psychopharmacology, 12*, 322–327.

Jou, R.J., Handen, B.L., & Hardan, A.Y. (2005). Retrospective assessment of atomoxetine in children and adolescents with pervasive developmental disorders. *Journal of Child and Adolescent Psychopharmacology, 15*, 325–330.

Kapetanovic, S. (2007). Oxcarbazepine in youths with autistic disorder and significant disruptive behaviors. *American Journal of Psychiatry, 164*, 832–833.

Kemner, C., Willemsen-Swinkels, S.H., de Jonge, M., Tuynman-Qua, H., & van Engeland, H. (2002). Open-label study of olanzapine in children with pervasive developmental disorder. *Journal of Clinical Psychopharmacology, 22*, 455–460.

Kerbeshian, J., Burd, L., & Fisher, W. (1987). Lithium carbonate in the treatment of two patients with infantile autism and atypical bipolar symptomatology. *Journal of Clinical Psychopharmacology, 7*, 401–405.

Kolevzon, A., Mathewson, K.A., & Hollander, E. (2006). Selective serotonin reuptake inhibitors in autism: A review of efficacy and tolerability. *Journal of Clinical Psychiatry, 67*, 407–414.

Langworthy-Lam, K.S., Aman, M.G., & Van Bourgondien, M.E. (2002). Prevalence and patterns of use of psychoactive medicines in individuals with autism in the Autism Society of North Carolina. *Journal of Child and Adolescent Psychopharmacology, 12*, 311–321.

Lee, D.O., & Ousley, O.Y. (2006). Attention-deficit/hyperactivity disorder symptoms in a clinic sample of children and adolescents with pervasive developmental disorders. *Journal of Child and Adolescent Psychopharmacology, 16*, 737–746.

Lehman, E., Haber, J., & Lesser, S.R. (1957). The use of reserpine in autistic children. *Journal of Nervous and Mental Disorders, 125*, 351–356.

Leventhal, B.L., Cook, E.H., Morford, M., Ravitz, A.J., Heller, W., & Freeman, D.X. (1993). Clinical and neurochemical effects of fenfluramine in children with autism. *Journal of Neuropsychiatry and Clinical Neurosciences, 5*, 307–315.

Lewis, M.H., Bodfish, J.W., Powell, S.B., & Golden, R.N. (1995). Clomipramine treatment for stereotyped and related repetitive movement disorders associated with mental retardation. *American Journal of Mental Retardation, 100*, 299–312.

Leyfer, O.T., Folstein, S.E., Bacalman, S., Davis, N.O., Dinh, E., & Morgan, J., et al. (2006). Comorbid psychiatric disorders in children with autism: Interview development and rates of disorders. *Journal of Autism and Developmental Disorders, 36*, 849–861.

Luby, J., Mrakotsky, C., Stalets, M.M., Belden, A., Heffelfinger, A., Williams, M., et al. (2006). Risperidone in preschool children with autistic spectrum disorders: An investigation of safety and efficacy. *Journal of Child and Adolescent Psychopharmacology, 16*, 575–587.

Malek-Ahmadi, P., & Simonds, J.F. (1998). Olanzapine for autistic disorder with hyperactivity. *Journal of the American Academy of Child and Adolescent Psychiatry, 37*, 902.

Malone, R.P., Cater, J., Sheikh, R.M., Choudhury, M.S., & Delaney, M.A. (2001). Olanzapine versus haloperidol in children with autistic disorder: An open pilot study. *Journal of the American Academy of Child and Adolescent Psychiatry, 40*, 887–894.

March, J.S., Silva, S.G., Compton, S., Anthony, G., DeVeaugh-Geiss, J., & Califf, R., et al. (2004). The Child and Adolescent Psychiatry Trials Network (CAPTN). *Journal of the American Academy of Child and Adolescent Psychiatry, 43*, 515–518.

March, J.S., Silva, S., Compton, S., Shapiro, M., Califf, R., & Krishnan, R. (2005). The case for practical clinical trials in psychiatry. *American Journal of Psychiatry, 162*, 836–846.

Martin, A., Koenig, K., Scahill, L., & Bregman, J. (1999). Open-label quetiapine in the treatment of children and adolescents with autistic disorder. *Journal of Child and Adolescent Psychopharmacology, 9*, 99–107.

Martin, A., Scahill, L., Klin, A., & Volkmar, F.R. (1999). Higher-functioning pervasive developmental disorders: Rates and patterns of psychotropic drug use. *Journal of the American Academy of Child and Adolescent Psychiatry, 38*, 923–931.

Mazzone, L., & Ruta, L. (2006). Topiramate in children with autistic spectrum disorders. *Brain Development, 28*, 668.

McCracken, J.T., McGough, J., Shah, B., Cronin, P., Hong, D., Aman, M.G., et al. (2002). Risperidone in children with autism and serious behavioral problems. *The New England Journal of Medicine, 347*, 314–321.

McDougle, C.J., Holmes, J.P., Carlson, D.C., Pelton, G.H., Cohen, D.J., & Price, L.H. (1998). A double-blind, placebo-controlled study of risperidone in adults with autistic disorder and other pervasive developmental disorders. *Archives of General Psychiatry, 55*, 633–641.

McDougle, C.J., Kem, D.L., & Posey, D.J. (2002). Case series: Use of ziprasidone for maladaptive symptoms in youths with autism. *Journal of the American Academy of Child and Adolescent Psychiatry, 41*, 921–927.

McDougle, C.J., Kresch, L.E., & Posey, D.J. (2000). Repetitive thoughts and behavior in pervasive developmental disorders: Treatment with serotonin reuptake inhibitors. *Journal of Autism and Developmental Disorders, 30*, 427–435.

McDougle, C.J., Naylor, S.T., Cohen, D.J., Volkmar, F.R., Heninger, G.R., & Price, L.H. (1996). A double-blind, placebo-controlled study of fluvoxamine in adults with autistic disorder. *Archives of General Psychiatry, 53*, 1001–1008.

McDougle, C.J., Scahill, L., Aman, M.G., McCracken, J.T., Tierney, E., Davies, M., et al. (2005). Risperidone for the core symptom domains of autism: Results from the study by the Autism Network of the Research Units on Pediatric Psychopharmacology. *American Journal of Psychiatry, 162*, 1142–1148.

Mehta, U.C., Patel, I., & Castello, F.V. (2004). EEG sedation for children with autism. *Journal of Developmental and Behavioral Pediatrics, 25*, 102–104.

Mogar, R.E., & Aldrich, R.W. (1969). The use of psychedelic agents with autistic schizophrenic children. *Psychedelic Review, 10*, 5–13.

Moore, M.L., Eichner, S.F., & Jones, J.R. (2004). Treating functional impairment of autism with selective serotonin-reuptake inhibitors. *Annals of Pharmacotherapy, 38*, 1515–1519.

Myers, S.M. (2007). The status of pharmacotherapy for autism spectrum disorders. *Expert Opinion on Pharmacotherapy, 8*, 1579–1603.

Myers, S.M., & Challman, T.D. (2008). Psychopharmacology: An approach to management in autism and intellectual disabilities. In P.J. Accardo (Ed.), *Capute and Accardo's neurodevelopmental disabilities in infancy and childhood: Vol. I. Neurodevelopmental diagnosis and treatment* (3rd ed., pp 577–614). Baltimore: Paul H. Brookes Publishing Co.

Nagaraj, R., Singhi, P., & Mahli, P. (2006). Risperidone in children with autism: Randomized, placebo-controlled, double-blind study. *Journal of Child Neurology, 21*, 450–455.

Naruse, H., Nagahata, M., Nakane, Y., Shirahashi, K., Takesada, M., & Yamazaki, K. (1982). A multi-center double-blind trial of pimozide (Orap), haloperidol and placebo in children with behavioral disorders, using crossover design. *Acta Paedopsychiatrica, 48*, 173–184.

Niederhofer, H., Staffen, W., & Mair, A. (2002). Lofexidine in hyperactive and impulsive children with autistic disorder. *Journal of the American Academy of Child and Adolescent Psychiatry, 41*, 1396–1397.

Perry, D.W., Marston, G.M., Hinder, S.A., Munden, A.C., & Roy, A. (2001). The phenomenology of depressive illness in people with a learning disability and autism. *Autism, 5*, 265–275.

Plioplys, A.V. (1994). Autism: Electroencephalogram abnormalities and clinical improvement with valproic acid. *Archives of Pediatrics and Adolescent Medicine, 148*, 220–222.

Posey, D.J., Erickson, C.A., Stigler, K.A., & McDougle, C.J. (2006). The use of selective serotonin reuptake inhibitors in autism and related disorders. *Journal of Child and Adolescent Psychopharmacology, 16*, 181–186.

Posey, D.J., Guenin, K.D., Kohn, A.E., Swiezy, N.B., & McDougle, C.J. (2001). A naturalistic open-label study of mirtazapine in autistic and other pervasive developmental disorders. *Journal of Child and Adolescent Psychopharmacology, 11*, 267–277.

Posey, D.J., & McDougle, C.J. (2000). The pharmacotherapy of target symptoms associated with autistic disorder and other pervasive developmental disorders. *Harvard Review of Psychiatry, 8*, 45–63.

Posey, D.J., Puntney, J.I., Sasher, T.M., Kem, D.L., & McDougle, C.J. (2004). Guanfacine treatment of hyperactivity and inattention in pervasive developmental disorders: A retrospective analysis of 80 cases. *Journal of Child and Adolescent Psychopharmacology, 14*, 233–241.

Posey, D.J., Wiegand, R.E., Wilkerson, J. Maynard, M., Stigler, K.A., & McDougle, C.J. (2006). Open-label atomoxetine for attention-deficit/hyperactivity disorder symptoms associated with high-functioning pervasive developmental disorders. *Journal of Child and Adolescent Psychopharmacology, 16*, 599–610.

Potenza, M.N., Holmes, J.P., Kanes, S.J., & McDougle, C.J. (1999). Olanzapine treatment of children, adolescents, and adults with pervasive developmental disorders: An open-label pilot study. *Journal of Clinical Psychopharmacology, 19*, 37–44.

Quintana, H., Birmaher, B., Stedge, D., Lennon, S., Freed, J., Bridge, J., et al. (1995). Use of methylphenidate in the treatment of children with autistic disorder. *Journal of Autism and Developmental Disorders, 25*, 283–294.

Realmuto, G.M., August, G.J., & Garfinkel, B.D. (1989). Clinical effect of buspirone in autistic children. *Journal of Clinical Psychopharmacology, 9*, 122–125.

Remington, G., Sloman, L., Konstantareas, M., Parker, K., & Gow, R. (2001). Clomipramine versus haloperidol in the treatment of autistic disorder: A double-blind, placebo-controlled, crossover study. *Journal of Clinical Psychopharmacology, 21*, 440–444.

Research Units on Pediatric Psychopharmacology (RUPP) Autism Network. (2005a). Randomized, controlled, crossover trial of methylphenidate in pervasive developmental disorders with hyperactivity. *Archives of General Psychiatry, 62*, 1266–1274.

Research Units on Pediatric Psychopharmacology (RUPP) Autism Network. (2005b). Risperidone treatment of autistic disorder: Longer-term benefits and blinded discontinuation after 6 months. *American Journal of Psychiatry, 162*, 1361–1369.

Research Units on Pediatric Psychopharmacology (RUPP) Autism Network. (2006). A prospective open trial of guanfacine in children with pervasive developmental disorders. *Journal of Child and Adolescent Psychopharmacology, 16*, 589–598.

Riddle, M.A. (1995). Pediatric psychopharmacology I: Preface. *Child and Adolescent Psychiatric Clinics of North America, 4*, xii–xv.

Ritvo, E.R., Yuwiler, A., Geller, E., Kales, A., Rashkis, S., & Schicor, A., et al. (1971). Effects of L-dopa in autism. *Journal of Autism and Childhood Schizophrenia, 1*, 190–205.

Rugino, T.A., & Samsock, T.C. (2002). Levetiracetam in autistic children: An open-label study. *Journal of Developmental and Behavioral Pediatrics, 23*, 225–230.

Sanchez, L.E., Campbell, M., Small, A.M., Cueva, J.E., Armenteros, J.L., & Adams, P.B. (1996). A pilot study of clomipramine in young autistic children. *Journal of the American Academy of Child and Adolescent Psychiatry, 35*, 537–544.

Santosh, P.J., Baird, G., Pityaratstian, N., Tavare, E., & Gringas, P. (2006). Impact of comorbid autism spectrum disorders on stimulant response in children with attention deficit hyperactivity disorder: A retrospective and prospective effectiveness study. *Child Care, Health, & Development, 32*, 575–583.

Scahill, L., Riddle, M., & McSwiggin-Hardin, M. (1997). Children's Yale-Brown Obsessive Compulsive Scale: Reliability and validity. *Journal of the American Academy of Child and Adolescent Psychiatry, 36*, 844–852.

Schain, R.J., & Freedman, D.X. (1961). Studies on 5-hydroxyindole metabolism in autistic and other mentally retarded children. *Journal of Pediatrics, 58*, 315–320.

Seltzer, M.M., Shattuck, P., Abbeduto, L., & Greenberg, J.S. (2004). Trajectory of development in adolescents and adults with autism. *Mental Retardation and Developmental Disabilities Research Reviews, 10*, 234–247.

Shastri, M., Alla, L., & Sabaratnam, M. (2006). Aripiprazole use in individuals with intellectual disability and psychotic or behavioural disorders: a case series. *Journal of Psychopharmacology, 20*, 863–867.

Shea, S., Turgay, A., Carroll, A., Schulz, M., Orlik, H., Smith, I., et al. (2004). Risperidone in the treatment of disruptive behavioral symptoms in children with autistic and other pervasive developmental disorders. *Pediatrics, 114*, e634–e641.

Snyder, R., Turgay, A., Aman, M., Binder, C., Fisman, S., Carroll, A., et al. (2002). Effects of risperidone on conduct and disruptive behavior disorders in children with subaverage IQs. *Journal of the American Academy of Child and Adolescent Psychiatry, 41*, 1026–1036.

Stavrakaki, C., Antochi, R., & Emery, P.C. (2004). Olanzapine in the treatment of pervasive developmental disorders: A case series analysis. *Journal of Psychiatry and Neuroscience, 29*, 57–60.

Steingard, R., & Biederman, J. (1987). Lithium responsive manic-like symptoms in two individuals with autism and mental retardation. *Journal of the American Academy of Child and Adolescent Psychiatry, 26*, 932–935.

Steingard, R.J., Connor, D.F., & Au, T. (2005). Approaches to psychopharmacology. In M.L.

Bauman & T.L. Kemper (Eds.), *The neurobiology of autism* (2nd ed., pp. 77–102). Baltimore: The Johns Hopkins University Press.

Stigler, K.A., Desmond, L.A., Posey, D.J., Wiegand, R.E., & McDougle, C.J. (2004). A naturalistic retrospective analysis of psychostimulants in pervasive developmental disorders. *Journal of Child and Adolescent Psychopharmacology, 14,* 49–56.

Stigler, K.A., Posey, D.J., & McDougle, C.J. (2004). Aripiprazole for maladaptive behavior in pervasive developmental disorders. *Journal of Child and Adolescent Psychopharmacology, 14,* 455–463.

Sugie, Y., Sugie, H., Fukuda, T., Ito, M., Sasada, Y., Nakabayashi, M., et al. (2005). Clinical efficacy of fluvoxamine and functional polymorphism in a serotonin transporter gene on childhood autism. *Journal of Autism and Developmental Disorders, 35,* 377–385.

Syzmanski, L.S., King, B., Goldberg, B., Reid, A.H., Tonge, B.J., & Cain, N. (1998). Diagnosis of mental disorders in people with mental retardation. In S. Reiss & M.G. Aman (Eds.), *Psychotropic medications and developmental disabilities: The international consensus handbook* (pp. 3–17). Columbus: The Ohio State University Nisonger Center.

Towbin, K.E. (2003). Strategies for pharmacologic treatment of high functioning autism and Asperger syndrome. *Child and Adolescent Psychiatric Clinics of North America, 12,* 23–45.

Troost, P.J., Althaus, M., Lahuis, B.E., Buitelaar, J.K., Minderaa, R.B., & Hoekstra, P.J. (2006). Neuropsychological effects of risperidone in children with pervasive developmental disorders: A blinded discontinuation study. *Journal of Child and Adolescent Psychopharmacology, 16,* 561–573.

Troost, P.W., Lahuis, B.E., Steenius, M.P., Ketelaars, C.E., Buitelaar, J.K., & van Engeland, H. (2005). Long-term effects of risperidone in children with autism spectrum disorders: A placebo discontinuation study. *Journal of the American Academy of Child and Adolescent Psychiatry, 44,* 1137–1144.

Troost, P.W., Steenhuis, M.P., Tuynman-Qua, H.G., Kalverdijk, L.J., Buitelaar, J.K., Minderaa, R.B., et al. (2006). Atomoxetine for attention-deficit/hyperactivity disorder symptoms in children with pervasive developmental disorders: A pilot study. *Journal of*

Child and Adolescent Psychopharmacology, 16, 611–619.

Tsakanikos, E., Costello, H., Holt, G., Bouras, N., Sturmey, P., & Newton, T. (2006). Psychopathology in adults with autism and intellectual disability. *Journal of Autism and Developmental Disorders, 36,* 1123–1129.

Uvebrant, P., & Bauziene, R. (1994). Intractable epilepsy in children: The efficacy of lamotrigine treatment, including non-seizure-related benefits. *Neuropediatrics, 25,* 284–289.

Valicenti-McDermott, M.R., & Demb, H. (2006). Clinical effects and adverse reactions of off-label use of aripiprazole in children and adolescents with developmental disabilities. *Journal of Child and Adolescent Psychopharmacology, 16,* 549–560.

Vitiello, B. (2006). An update on publicly funded multisite trials in pediatric psychopharmacology. *Child and Adolescent Psychiatric Clinics of North America, 15,* 1–12.

Waizer, J., Polizos, P., Hoffman, S.P., Engelhardt, D.M., & Margolis, R.A. (1972). A single-blind evaluation of thiothixene with outpatient schizophrenic children. *Journal of Autism and Childhood Schizophrenia, 2,* 378–386.

Wasserman, S., Iyengar, R., Chaplin, W.F., Watner, D., Waldoks, S.E., & Anagnostou, E., et al. (2006). Levetiracetam versus placebo in childhood and adolescent autism: A double-blind placebo-controlled study. *International Clinical Psychopharmacology, 21,* 363–367.

Williams, S.K., Scahill, L., Vitiello, B., Aman, M.G., Arnold L.E., & McDougle, C.J., et al. (2006). Risperidone and adaptive behavior in children with autism. *Journal of the American Academy of Child and Adolescent Psychiatry, 45,* 431–439.

Witwer, A., & Lecavalier, L. (2005). Treatment incidence and patterns in children and adolescents with autism spectrum disorders. *Journal of Child and Adolescent Psychopharmacology, 15,* 671–681.

Wolpert, A., Hagamen, M.B., & Merlis, S. (1967). A comparative study of thiothixene and trifluoperazine in childhood schizophrenia. *Current Therapeutic Research, Clinical & Experimental, 9,* 482–485.

Zuddas, A., Ledda, M.G., Fratta, A., Muglia, P., & Cianchetti, C. (1996). Clinical effects of clozapine on autistic disorder. *American Journal of Psychiatry, 153,* 738.

11

Complementary and Alternative Medicine in Autism

Promises Kept?

Thomas D. Challman

Despite H.L. Mencken's admonition that "there is always a well-known solution to every human problem—neat, plausible, and wrong" (Mencken, 1920, p.158), people faced with a medical problem that defies easy treatment often resort to unproven remedies in an effort to ameliorate their condition. Few topics in health care generate as many strong feelings as the issue of complementary and alternative medicine (CAM). An aberrant sociocultural phenomenon, the CAM movement has popularized nonstandard therapies as alternatives to scientific medicine for a variety of disorders. CAM use is common among children with developmental disabilities, including autism spectrum disorders (ASDs).

Caregivers of children with ASDs face the daunting challenge of sorting through a myriad of potential treatments promoted by various individuals and groups. It is understandable that parents will consider using almost any intervention that they feel provides hope of therapeutic benefit for their children. It is often quite difficult, however, for families to distinguish among therapies with an acceptable evidence base, those that are potentially plausible but untested, and those that arise from purely pseudoscientific notions. This problem has been made even more acute by advancements in information technology and the ease with which questionable theories and practices can spread via the Internet. Groups that advocate unsubstantiated etiologic theories, and in turn promote remedies based on theories of questionable validity, are grossly out of step with the process of rational scientific inquiry. Health care practitioners have a responsibility to protect children from interventions that are ineffective or potentially harmful and should adopt a stance that demands the critical analysis of therapeutic claims.

DEFINITIONS AND CONCEPTUALIZATION OF COMPLEMENTARY AND ALTERNATIVE MEDICINE

Some writers have justifiably argued that the concept of *alternative* medicine is inherently nonsensical—there is only medicine that works and medicine that does not (Angell & Kassirer, 1998). Over the past 20 years, a number of disparate therapeutic practices have come to be viewed under the conceptual umbrella of complementary and alternative medicine. A variety of definitions of what should be considered CAM have been proposed, including "interventions not taught widely in medical schools or generally available at U.S. hospitals" (Eisenberg et al., 1993, p. 246); "diagnosis, treatment and/or prevention which complements mainstream medicine by contributing to a common whole, by satisfying a demand not met by orthodoxy or by diversifying conceptual frameworks of medicine" (Ernst et al., 1995, p. 506); and "a broad domain of healing resources that encompasses all health systems, modalities, and practices and their accompanying theories and beliefs, other than those intrinsic to the politically dominant health systems of a particular society or culture in a given historical period" (Zollman & Vickers, 1999, p. 693). *Complementary medicine* (or *integrative medicine*) has commonly been used to refer to nonstandard practices used in concert with accepted medical interventions, whereas alternative medicine describes interventions used in place of conventional medicine. CAM practices are often touted as contributing to overall "wellness" as opposed to taking a disease-oriented approach to care, although it is certainly common for claims to be made that a particular CAM practice possesses therapeutic efficacy for a specific disorder. The National Center for Complementary and Alternative Medicine (NCCAM), which defines CAM as diagnostic or therapeutic practices "not presently considered an integral part of conventional medicine" (National Center for Complementary and Alternative Medicine, 2000, p. 10), organizes CAM practices into five domains: mind–body medicine, manipulative and body-based practices, energy medicine, biologically based practices, and a fifth domain comprised of alternative medical "systems" that may utilize therapies found in the other four domains (Table 11.1). The NCCAM created this classification in an effort to provide some organization to a concept that has shifting borders and imprecise terminology.

The boundary between alternative medical therapies and accepted medicine is purported to be dynamic. Some alternative therapies aspire eventually to be viewed as conventional or mainstream, if they are able to accumulate sufficient evidence of effectiveness. It is also clear, however, that certain practices presented as CAM overlap substantially with spirituality and cultural beliefs.

Table 11.1.   The National Center for Complementary and Alternative Medicine's classification of complementary and alternative practices, with examples

Whole Medical Systems
  Homeopathy
  Naturopathy
  Traditional Chinese medicine
  Ayurvedic medicine

Mind–Body Medicine
  Meditation
  Biofeedback
  Prayer
  Hypnosis
  Yoga

Manipulative and Body-Based Practices
  Chiropractic
  Massage
  Reflexology

Energy Medicine
  Therapeutic touch
  Qi gong
  Reiki
  Magnet therapy
  Acupuncture

Biologically Based Practices
  Herbs
  Diets
  Vitamins and other supplements

From Challman, T.D., Voigt, R.G., & Myers, S.M. (2008). Nonstandard therapies. In P.J. Accardo (Ed.), *Caputo and Accardo's neurodevelopmental disabilities in infancy and childhood: Vol. 1. Neurodevelopmental diagnoses and treatment* (3rd ed., p. 722). Baltimore: Paul H. Brookes Publishing Co.; reprinted by permission.
  Sources: Challman, Voigt, and Myers (2008) and National Center for Complementary and Alternative Medicine (2007; http://nccam.nih.gov/health/whatiscam).

A representation of this view of CAM is presented in Figure 11.1. It is also important to recognize that a particular intervention might be considered either CAM or conventional depending on the context in which it is being used. For instance, vitamin B_{12} is an accepted treatment for pernicious anemia, but it is considered CAM when promoted for the treatment of a developmental disorder. Certain practices (e.g., therapeutic touch) should be viewed as nonstandard in all situations if there is no acceptable evidence base that indicates therapeutic efficacy for any condition (or even any plausibility that such efficacy could exist).

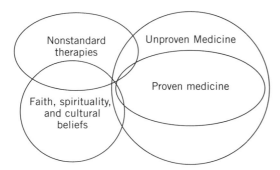

Figure 11.1. One view of the relationship between nonstandard therapies, medicine, and spirituality. (From Challman, T.D., Voigt, R.G., & Myers, S.M. [2008]. Nonstandard therapies. In P.J. Accardo [Ed.], *Capute and Accardo's neurodevelopmental disabilities in infancy and childhood: Vol. 1. Neurodevelopmental diagnoses and treatment* [3rd ed., p. 722]. Baltimore: Paul H. Brookes Publishing Co.; reprinted by permission.)

The boundary that separates medicine (defined here per *Stedman's Medical Dictionary*, 2000, p. 1077) from the other activities in Figure 11.1 may be perceived as arbitrary. Supporters of a *holistic* approach to medical care often espouse a highly inclusive view of what human activities should be considered a part of medicine (Kaptchuk & Eisenberg, 1998). However, it is reasonable to put some limits on what should be considered within the purview of the health care practitioner. For instance, a person's choice of religious orientation or marital status, although potentially associated with various health outcomes, should not be viewed as a target of potential manipulation by the health care system. Once a particular practice is promoted as treatment for a specific disorder, however, it is appropriate to fully engage the machinery of scientific investigation to look for evidence for or against the claim.

Therapies not presently accepted as part of conventional medicine but in which testable claims are made can fall into one of several categories: those that are potentially plausible based on current knowledge but are insufficiently tested; those that have very weak (or nonexistent) plausibility; and those that should be more properly viewed as part of religion, spirituality, or cultural practice and are unlikely to be rejected by believers

in the face of negative evidence. Limited research resources dictate that effort should primarily be directed to the investigation of therapies in the first category. This schema also highlights a specific practical consideration—and the approach taken in providing advice to families about specific nonstandard practices may need to vary depending upon the category in which the particular practice is judged to reside.

PREVALENCE AND COST OF NONSTANDARD PRACTICES

Most definitions of CAM have the potential to be interpreted rather broadly; this has contributed to the variability in estimates of the prevalence of CAM use. Proponents would argue that surveys indicate the widespread use of these practices among adults in the United States, although increasingly inclusive interpretations of what should be considered CAM have led to the inflation of these estimates. The first national survey to determine patterns of use of nonstandard therapies in American adults was published in 1993. It showed that roughly one third of the respondents used at least one unconventional therapy during the previous year, although only 10% actually saw a practitioner who provided these therapies (Eisenberg et al., 1993). When spiritual practices such as prayer are included in the definition of CAM, estimates of the use of CAM are uniformly high. In the 1999 National Health Interview Survey (NHIS), 28.9% of U.S. adults reported using at least one CAM therapy in the previous year, with the most commonly used therapies consisting of spiritual healing or prayer, herbal medicine, and chiropractic (Ni, Simile, & Hardy, 2002). This estimate was even higher (i.e., 62%) in the 2002 NHIS (Barnes, Powell-Griner, McFann, & Nahin, 2004). Most adults who utilize CAM practices do not eschew conventional medicine (in other words, they embrace a complementary approach), but they do report a philosophical orientation congruent with the world-view that such practices promote (Astin, 1998; Eisenberg et al., 2001).

CAM use among children is also common. There have been a variety of estimates in the frequency of nonstandard therapy use in various pediatric populations, ranging from 11%–53% (Fong & Fong, 2002; Madsen et al., 2003; Ottolini et al., 2001; Sawni-Sikand, Schubiner, & Thomas, 2002; Sibinga, Ottolini, Duggan, & Wilson, 2004; Simpson & Roman, 2001; Spigelblatt, Laine-Ammara, Pless, & Guyver, 1994; Wilson & Klein, 2002). A number of potential biases, including ascertainment bias and variations in CAM definition, may affect the validity of these estimates. Lower estimates of CAM use among children and young adults in the United States (1.8%–2%) have been derived from population-based data (Davis & Darden, 2003; Yussman, Ryan, Auinger, & Weitzman, 2004). Consistently identified factors that predict pediatric CAM use include higher levels of parental education and parental CAM use.

Children with chronic medical conditions utilize CAM at higher rates than the general population (Feldman et al., 2004; Friedman et al., 1997; Johnston, Bilbao, & Graham-Brown, 2003; Junker, Oberwittler, Jackson, & Berger, 2004; Kelly, 2004; Markowitz et al., 2004; Orhan et al., 2003). Similar high rates of CAM use have been reported among various populations of children with developmental disabilities, including attention-deficit/hyperactivity disorder (ADHD), cerebral palsy, Down syndrome, and spina bifida (Bussing, Zima, Gary, & Garvan, 2002; Gross-Tsur, Lahad, & Shalev, 2003; Hurvitz, Leonard, Ayyangar, & Nelson, 2003; Miller, Brehaut, Raina, McGrail, & Armstrong, 2004; Prussing, Sobo, Walker, Dennis, & Kurtin, 2004; Sanders et al., 2003; Sinha & Efron, 2005). CAM use is also widespread among children with ASDs. In one highly selected population, 95% of parents of children with ASDs indicated that they had used at least one CAM therapy (Harrington, Rosen,

Garnecho, & Patrick, 2006). A recent case-control study showed that 52% of parents had used a nonstandard therapy for their children with ASDs, the most commonly utilized being biological therapies (Wong & Smith, 2006). Children with ASDs may be exposed to CAM therapies even prior to formal diagnosis. In a study of recently diagnosed children with ASDs, a history of CAM use was found in approximately 30%, with a substantial minority of these children using therapies that could be potentially harmful (Levy, Mandell, Merhar, Ittenbach, & Pinto-Martin, 2003).

Complementary and alternative medicine is a multibillion dollar per year business. In 1997, annual out-of-pocket expenditures for CAM services in the U.S. population were estimated to be $27 billion (Eisenberg et al., 1998). CAM therapies have been embraced by some health insurance plans, primarily as a marketing tool to be used in an increasingly competitive marketplace, although it has been argued that health plans that offer CAM services may actually face increased net costs (Schulman, 2004). Strong political forces—and not scientific merit—have driven a dramatic increase in federal funding directed toward CAM over the past 15 years. In October 1991, the U.S. Congress created the Office of Alternative Medicine (OAM) within the National Institutes of Health (NIH), with an initial annual budget of $2 million. In 1999, the NCCAM was created, its primary mission being to investigate CAM practices by utilizing rigorous scientific methodology. The NCCAM appropriation for fiscal year 2006 was more than $122 million. Despite this substantial funding, there has been extremely slow progress toward the goal of proving or disproving the clinical value of specific CAM therapies. Although CAM use in children with developmental disabilities is widespread, the NIH has funded few studies in this population to evaluate the safety or efficacy of these therapies.

WHAT DOES THE EVIDENCE SHOW?

For a number of reasons, including barriers in study design and execution, published research into CAM practices has been plagued by poor methodological quality. Despite their widespread use, there have only been a limited number of controlled trials of CAM therapies in children with developmental disabilities (Challman, Voigt, & Myers, 2008). Although the paucity of well-designed studies makes the provision of evidence-based recommendations difficult, there are currently no therapies that fall under the NCCAM conceptualization of CAM that have a clear and convincing role in the treatment of ASDs.

No controlled studies of mind–body therapies, energy medicine (including therapeutic touch, acupuncture, Reiki, and qi gong), homeopathy, or chiropractic are identified in a search of Medline (1950–2007) and the Cochrane Central Register of Controlled Trials. A single randomized controlled trial of massage in children with ASDs showed short-term improvements in certain aspects of behavior (Escalona, Field, Singer-Strunck, Cullen, & Hartshorn, 2001); the clinical value of this therapy remains uncertain. There have been several trials of auditory integration therapy in children with ASDs, results of which have been mixed (Sinha, Silove, Wheeler, & Williams, 2004), and the use of this therapy in children with ASDs is not recommended (American Academy of Pediatrics [AAP], Committee on Children with Disabilities, 1998). Similarly, although sensory integration therapy is frequently used by occupational therapists in the treatment of children with ASDs, there remains a substantial lack of empirical evidence suggesting a clinical benefit for these techniques (Schaaf & Miller, 2005).

Many different biological interventions (e.g., herbs, diets, vitamins) have been used over the years to try to treat developmental disorders. These interventions comprise the largest group of CAM therapies that have been used in children with ASDs (Green et al., 2006). Although there is obviously a long history in medicine of effective agents being derived from botanical and other natural sources, most of the biologically based CAM treatments suffer from the same lack of experimental evidence of effectiveness that is a common feature of the other previously discussed CAM methods. Some of these therapies manifest the highly unfavorable juxtaposition of the absence of proven benefits and the presence of potentially serious risks. In light of the significant placebo and other expectancy effects observed in clinical trials of ASD therapies, the results of any uncontrolled, open-label studies should be interpreted with great caution.

Various vitamins and minerals, probiotics, antifungals, and immunological agents have been widely used in children with ASDs, and current evidence has recently been reviewed (Levy & Hyman, 2005). A number of trials of vitamin B_6 and magnesium treatment have been published, although most have had significant methodological shortcomings. The best available data do not support a benefit of vitamin B_6 and magnesium treatment (Findling et al., 1997; Tolbert, Haigler, Waits, & Dennis, 1993), and their combined use in the treatment of ASDs currently is not supported (Nye & Brice, 2006). Open-label trials have suggested that melatonin may be effective in shortening sleep latency in children with ASDs (Giannotti, Cortesi, Cerquiglini, & Bernabei, 2006; Paavonen, Nieminen-von Wendt, Vanhala, Aronen, & von Wendt, 2003), although controlled trials are not available. The use of intravenous or oral immunoglobulin, omega-3 fatty acids, or dimethylglycine is not supported by the current literature, and at present, there are no supplements that are accepted as safe and effective in the treatment of ASDs (AAP, Committee on Children with Disabilities, 2001b).

Concern over the possibility of a toxic environmental trigger in the etiology of ASDs, a contention that currently lacks empiric support, has led to the use of chelation therapy, in which various drugs are used to remove heavy metals from the body, in children with ASDs. There have been no published clinical trials regarding the effectiveness of chelation therapy in individuals with ASDs. There are potentially serious risks of toxicity related to chelation (Brown, Willis, Omalu, & Leiker, 2006), and its use should be actively avoided in the absence of a clear indication (e.g., lead poisoning). Despite the low *a priori* likelihood that chelation therapy should have any beneficial effect in children with ASDs, an NIH-funded trial is underway.

The dietary intervention that has gained the most popularity in children with ASDs has been the gluten- and casein-free (GF-CF) diet. This diet is based on the unproven and improbable hypothesis that peptides from gluten and casein exert a central nervous system (CNS) effect that leads to the behavioral features seen in ASDs. There have been several trials of this diet in children with ASDs (Christison & Ivany, 2006). The one (single-blind) controlled trial of this diet has certain methodological limitations, including the fact that parents were not blinded to group assignment (Knivsberg, Reichelt, Hoien, & Nodland, 2002). The GF-CF diet is currently not a validated therapy in ASDs, although an NIH-funded study is in progress.

PLACEBO AND OTHER EXPECTANCY EFFECTS: THE EXAMPLE OF SECRETIN

In 1998, a small case series was published that reported improvement in certain language and social features in three children with ASDs who had undergone gastrointestinal endoscopy (Horvath et al., 1998). Attention quickly focused on the hormone secretin, which had been used during the

procedures. Rapid spread of these observations soon followed on the Internet and in the mainstream media, creating a sudden and explosive interest in the use of secretin as a therapeutic agent for the treatment of ASDs. Thousands of children with ASDs were subsequently treated with secretin prior to any attempts to demonstrate the safety and efficacy of this agent. The medical research community was then compelled to try to establish an evidence base after the use of secretin was already widespread. Numerous randomized controlled trials have failed to show that secretin is any more effective than placebo in improving language or behavioral functioning in children with ASDs (Sturmey, 2005).

A number of these trials did, however, reveal interesting information relating to placebo effects in this population. In one of the first published controlled trials of secretin in children with ASDs (Sandler et al., 1999), improvement in certain behavioral and communication features was reported by parent and teacher observation in 30% of patients in both the secretin and placebo groups. Even more interestingly, a high percentage of parents (i.e., 69%) continued to express an interest in secretin as a therapy for their children even after they were informed of the negative results of the study. Clearly, something more than a rational, objective pursuit of effective treatments was occurring among these parents. Belief in the potential power of a therapy, combined with high expectations fueled by media hype, appears to have the ability to override contrary scientific evidence—even overwhelming evidence—in the minds of some parents looking for a treatment for a particular condition.

There has been a recent revival of interest in placebo effects, with a shift toward viewing these effects as a topic of scientific inquiry in their own right as opposed to merely being confounding factors that must be controlled for in clinical trials. A number of factors associated with treatment response have been subsumed under the umbrella of placebo effects, including patient and clinician attributes, expectancy effects, participation effects, conditioning phenomena, and biological effects (Sandler, 2005). Although the reality of an inherent placebo effect has been challenged based on analyses of studies comparing placebo with no treatment (Hrobjartsson & Gotzsche, 2004a, 2004b), it is apparent that a number of diverse psychological and other factors can contribute to the appearance of treatment efficacy when none truly exists. Clinical trials in conditions in which outcome measures are often subjective (e.g., depression, pain) have consistently revealed notable positive responses among participants receiving placebo. In fact, a systematic review suggested only small differences between antidepressants and active placebos that mimic certain side effects of the active drug in the treatment of depression (Moncrieff, Wessely, & Hardy, 2004).

Clinical trials of various medications in ASDs have revealed the presence of similarly robust placebo effects (Hollander et al., 2004). An additional layer of complexity in the assessment of placebo effects is introduced in trials in children with developmental disabilities, as often the outcomes being studied are being measured indirectly (i.e., through caregiver report of behavior change). The various placebo effects therefore have the potential to operate on parental behavior or perception in addition to any effect on the patient. Several other points relevant to placebo effects are important to highlight. An open-label trial of any therapy in children with ASDs is likely to overestimate the true efficacy of the intervention, and the results should be viewed with caution. The randomized, blinded, controlled trial remains the best tool for determining whether a therapy has specific beneficial effects.

CAM therapies, which have rarely been subject to any rigorous scientific scrutiny,

are likely to acquire the appearance of effectiveness as a result of various placebo and expectancy effects. Although the value of placebos in the research setting is widely accepted, it is much less clear whether placebos have any therapeutic role in modern clinical medicine. Some proponents of nonstandard therapies suggest that it does not matter if a treatment is biologically inert; what matters is that benefits are observed (Mastrangelo & Lore, 2005). However, it is difficult to conceive that true family- and patient-centered care can be based on such a fundamental deception. An argument has been made that an acceptable role for placebos in the treatment of children with developmental disorders might be possible (Sandler, 2005), although the scientific merits and ethical implications of this idea will require further analysis and debate.

HOW TO RECOGNIZE PSEUDOSCIENTIFIC THINKING: A PRIMER

Caregivers of children with ASDs, and sometimes health care providers or other professionals, can be ill-equipped to recognize the difference between a potentially valid therapy and one that is pseudoscientific. A false dichotomy is admittedly created by the suggestion that therapies are either scientific or pseudoscientific. This distinction is better viewed as a continuum, and it has as much to do with the approach proponents of the therapy take vis-à-vis building an evidence base as it does with the details of the therapy itself. One must also recognize that a lack of critical thinking that leads to the reflexive rejection of a new idea can be as detrimental as blind acceptance. Principles of skepticism and critical thinking can—and should—be taught to families to provide them with practical tools that will help them navigate the maze of etiologic theories and therapies they will encounter on the Internet and in the media. These principles can be as helpful for the analysis of mainstream medical practices as they are in the evaluation of CAM therapies.

There are a number of characteristic features that can serve as warning signs regarding the questionable validity of a particular therapy. Families should exercise caution if they encounter a nonstandard therapy based on an overly simple theory, advertised as curative, or reported to have no potential side effects (Nickel, 1996). The following questions can also be extremely helpful in allowing families and health care providers to recognize a treatment claim that may be pseudoscientific (Lilienfeld, Lynn, & Lohr, 2003):

1. Is the treatment claim testable? Do proponents attempt to explain away contradictory evidence and try to preserve an original theory by using layers of additional hypotheses without efforts to consider alternative and simpler explanations? A claim that is not potentially falsifiable falls outside the realm of science.

2. Has the treatment changed over time in response to new evidence? Therapies that remain static for decades or centuries—a characteristic often viewed as desirable by CAM proponents—have not undergone the self-correction that is an essential component of the scientific process.

3. Have studies of the treatment been published in the peer-reviewed medical literature? What is the quality of these studies? For the benefits of a therapy to be believable, purported evidence must be available for scrutiny by members of the scientific community.

4. Do proponents of the treatment selectively seek evidence that confirms the effectiveness of the therapy and ignore contradictory data? Science is a double-edged sword. Physicians, patients, and patients' families must be as willing to reject treatments and theo-ries in the face of appropriate evidence as they are to accept them.

5. Do proponents suggest that it is all right to assume the treatment is effective until proven otherwise? As shown by the example of secretin, widespread use of a therapy prior to the development of any acceptable evidence of effectiveness is a sadly recurring event in the history of ASD treatment.

6. Does the treatment show a disconnection with knowledge in other scientific disciplines? Is the treatment based on new forces or principles that are inconsistent with a current understanding of the natural world? Therapies that are based on such unverified forces (e.g., energy healing) have extremely low *prima facie* plausibility.

7. Is the treatment promoted primarily through the use of anecdotes and testimonials as opposed to a body of evidence from controlled trials? The high rate of placebo response in trials of ASD therapies shows that broad extrapolations should not be made from the observation of a single child's response to a treatment. Therapies that are supported only by anecdote should be viewed with great caution.

8. Is the treatment described in scientific-sounding jargon that upon closer analysis is very imprecise or meaningless? Such language is commonly used to hide the absence of a true scientific basis for the therapy.

9. Are claims made that the treatment is effective for a wide range of conditions? A single intervention can rarely, if ever, effectively treat diverse conditions with disparate pathophysiologies.

10. Are claims made that the treatment can only be viewed as part of a larger package of interventions and practices? This is often a ploy designed to obstruct the scientific analysis of a claim or to explain away evidence of ineffectiveness.

Pseudoscience at Academic Medical Centers

Energy therapy, also referred to as therapeutic touch, may be the most implausible of all CAM therapies. It involves a practitioner performing smoothing movements above the body with the intent to manually manipulate a purported biofield around the human body. Practitioners of this therapy believe that this balances a nonphysical "life energy" and restores the body to a state of good health, although the existence of such biofields that can be manually detected and manipulated has never been proven (Rosa, Rosa, Sarner, & Barrett, 1998). In June 2003, the Kennedy Krieger Institute in Baltimore announced that researchers were embarking on investigations to scientifically study the efficacy of energy therapy. One study involved functional brain imaging before and after the use of energy therapy in children ages 8–12 with ADHD; another study investigated behavior in children with ASDs before and after energy therapy sessions. Although a strong case can be made that the extreme implausibility of energy therapy makes its scientific investigation unwarranted, these studies had the potential to contribute to an evidence base that either supports or refutes the value of this therapy.

Certain elements that exemplify pseudoscientific thinking, however, can be gleaned from the available information regarding these studies. In the initial press release (Kennedy Krieger Institute, June 10, 2003), presumably prior to completion of the studies, a Kennedy Krieger administrator stated, "The positive results of these studies will only allow Kennedy Krieger to broaden our interdisciplinary treatments of children. Incorporating this type of therapy to our regimen can only improve our quality of patient care." This is an example of the pseudoscientific stance of expecting confirmation of a belief while ignoring the possibility of refutation and assuming some value for a therapy in the absence of supportive evidence. Additional indications of pseudoscientific thinking in the supporters of these studies (i.e., overreliance on anecdotes, uncritical acceptance of unproven physical forces and the value of such forces to heal the body) were evident in a subsequent article describing these investigations (McGrath, 2003).

Perhaps not surprisingly, results of these studies have yet to be published. In CAM research, initial hoopla regarding the scientific analysis of a treatment may not be followed by the wide dissemination of study results if those results conflict with the investigators' beliefs about the value of the therapy. The recent substantial rise in federal funding to study nonstandard therapies has been accompanied by an increase in the number of academic medical centers with research programs in CAM (NCCAM, 2004). As shown by the previous example, even reputable academic medical centers should remain on guard against the threat of being tainted by pseudoscience.

COUNSELING FAMILIES REGARDING NONSTANDARD PRACTICES

The critical analysis of treatment claims and the ability to recognize pseudoscience are skills that can help caregivers of children with ASDs develop an optimal package of interventions for their children. The education of families in critical thinking principles and the scientific method should surely be a fundamental element of family-centered care. To effectively provide this education, health care providers must be informed about the various CAM therapies that are currently popular, as well as any evidence base that exists and the potential risks that might be associated with particular treatments. The American Academy of Pediatrics makes the following recommendations to pediatricians who discuss CAM with families (AAP, Committee on Children with Disabilities, 2001a):

1. Seek information and be prepared to share it with families.

2. Evaluate the scientific merits of specific therapies.

3. Identify risks or potential harmful effects.

4. Provide families with information on a range of treatment options.

5. Educate families so they can effectively evaluate all treatment approaches.

6. Avoid dismissal of CAM in ways that communicate a lack of sensitivity or concern for the family's perspective.

7. Recognize when one is feeling threatened and guard against becoming defensive.

8. If a CAM approach is pursued, offer to monitor the patient's response.

9. Actively listen to the family and the child with a chronic illness.

Because of the diversity of practices included under the CAM umbrella, a provider may need to make adjustments in the counseling approach depending upon the specific therapy being considered and the context in which it may be employed. Therapies that have sufficient evidence to be considered safe and effective should be actively recommended; however, at the present time no CAM approaches for children with ASDs fall into this category. Therapies that are potentially plausible but insufficiently tested cannot be endorsed, but should undergo more rigorous scientific testing to prove or disprove their worth. Practices that are more appropriately viewed as part of a religious belief or cultural tradition important to the family that are unlikely to be rejected despite any amount of negative evidence probably should be tolerated, assuming that potential risks to the child are low.

The fact that a treatment is generally safe is not by itself sufficient justification to support its use. Both direct and indirect risks are recognized for many nonstandard therapies (AAP, Committee on Children with Disabilities, 2001a), and even a low risk of harm is unacceptable if a treatment is worthless. Direct risks can include toxic effects of biological agents or manipulative techniques, interference with appropriate nutrition, and the interruption or postponement of valid therapies. Financial burdens, time demands, and the risk of parental guilt related to imperfect treatment compliance are additional indirect hazards. Alternative medicine practitioners may also foster attitudes against medical practices, such as vaccination, that are known to be effective (Busse, Kulkarni, Campbell, & Injeyan, 2002). Health care providers should be well aware that the endorsement of nonstandard therapies known to be potentially harmful or the development of supervisory relationships with CAM providers could have liability implications (Cohen & Kemper, 2005; Studdert et al., 1998).

REFERENCES

American Academy of Pediatrics, Committee on Children with Disabilities. (1998). Auditory integration training and facilitated communication for autism. *Pediatrics, 102*(2, Pt. 1), 431–433.

American Academy of Pediatrics, Committee on Children with Disabilities. (2001a). Counseling families who choose complementary and alternative medicine for their child with chronic illness or disability. *Pediatrics, 107*(3), 598–601.

American Academy of Pediatrics, Committee on Children with Disabilities. (2001b). Technical report: The pediatrician's role in the diagnosis and management of autistic spectrum disorder in children. *Pediatrics,* 107, 1221–1226.

Angell, M., & Kassirer, J.P. (1998). Alternative medicine: The risks of untested and unregulated remedies. *New England Journal of Medicine, 339*(12), 839–841.

Astin, J.A. (1998). Why patients use alternative medicine: Results of a national study. *Journal of the American Medical Association, 279*(19), 1548–1553.

Barnes, P.M., Powell-Griner, E., McFann, K., & Nahin, R.L. (2004). Complementary and alternative medicine use among adults: United States, 2002. *Advance Data, 343,* 1–19.

Brown, M.J., Willis, T., Omalu, B., & Leiker, R. (2006). Deaths resulting from hypocalcemia after administration of edetate disodium: 2003–2005. *Pediatrics, 118*(2), e534–e536.

Busse, J.W., Kulkarni, A.V., Campbell, J.B., & Injeyan, H.S. (2002). Attitudes toward vaccination: A survey of Canadian chiropractic students. *Canadian Medical Association Journal, 166*(12), 1531–1534.

Bussing, R., Zima, B.T., Gary, F.A., & Garvan, C.W. (2002). Use of complementary and alternative medicine for symptoms of attention-deficit hyperactivity disorder. *Psychiatric Services, 53*(9), 1096–1102.

Challman, T.D., Voigt, R.G., & Myers, S.M. (2008). Nonstandard therapies. In P.J. Accardo (Ed.), *Caputo and Accardo's neurodevelopmental disabilities in infancy and childhood: Vol. I. Neurodevelopmental diagnoses and treatment* (3rd ed., pp. 721–741). Baltimore: Paul H. Brookes Publishing Co.

Christison, G.W., & Ivany, K. (2006). Elimination diets in autism spectrum disorders: Any wheat amidst the chaff? *Journal of Developmental and Behavioral Pediatrics, 27*(2, Suppl.), S162–S171.

Cohen, M.H., & Kemper, K.J. (2005). Complementary therapies in pediatrics: A legal perspective. *Pediatrics, 115*(3), 774–780.

Davis, M.P., & Darden, P.M. (2003). Use of complementary and alternative medicine by children in the United States. *Archives of Pediatrics and Adolescent Medicine, 157*(4), 393–396.

Eisenberg, D.M., Davis, R.B., Ettner, S.L., Appel, S., Wilkey, S., Van Rompay, M., et al. (1998). Trends in alternative medicine use in the United States, 1990–1997: Results of a follow-up national survey. *Journal of the American Medical Association, 280*(18), 1569–1575.

Eisenberg, D.M., Kessler, R.C., Foster, C., Norlock, F.E., Calkins, D.R., Delbanco, T.L. (1993). Unconventional medicine in the United States: Prevalence, costs, and patterns of use. *New England Journal of Medicine, 328*(4), 246–252.

Eisenberg, D.M., Kessler, R.C., Van Rompay, M.I., Kaptchuk, T.J., Wilkey, S.A., Appel, S., et al. (2001). Perceptions about complementary

therapies relative to conventional therapies among adults who use both: Results from a national survey. *Annals of Internal Medicine, 135*(5), 344–351.

Ernst, E., Resch, K.L., Mills, S., Hill, R., Mitchell, A., Willoughby, M., et al. (1995). Complementary medicine: A definition. *British Journal of General Practice, 45,* 506.

Escalona, A., Field, T., Singer-Strunck, R., Cullen, C., & Hartshorn, K. (2001). Brief report: Improvements in the behavior of children with autism following massage therapy. *Journal of Autism and Developmental Disorders, 31*(5), 513–516.

Feldman, D.E., Duffy, C., De Civita, M., Malleson, P., Philibert, L., Gibbon, M., et al. (2004). Factors associated with the use of complementary and alternative medicine in juvenile idiopathic arthritis. *Arthritis and Rheumatism, 51*(4), 527–532.

Findling, R.L., Maxwell, K., Scotese-Wojtila, L., Huang, J., Yamashita, T., & Wiznitzer, M. (1997). High-dose pyridoxine and magnesium administration in children with autistic disorder: An absence of salutary effects in a double-blind, placebo-controlled study. *Journal of Autism and Developmental Disorders, 27*(4), 467–478.

Fong, D.P., & Fong, L.K. (2002). Usage of complementary medicine among children. *Australian Family Physician, 31*(4), 388–391.

Friedman, T., Slayton, W.B., Allen, L.S., Pollock, B.H., Dumont-Driscoll, M., Mehta, P., et al. (1997). Use of alternative therapies for children with cancer. *Pediatrics, 100*(6), E1.

Giannotti, F., Cortesi, F., Cerquiglini, A., & Bernabei, P. (2006). An open-label study of controlled-release melatonin in treatment of sleep disorders in children with autism. *Journal of Autism and Developmental Disorders, 36*(6), 741–752.

Green, V.A., Pituch, K.A., Itchon, J., Choi, A., O'Reilly, M., & Sigafoos, J. (2006). Internet survey of treatments used by parents of children with autism. *Research in Developmental Disabilities, 27*(1), 70–84.

Gross-Tsur, V., Lahad, A., & Shalev, R.S. (2003). Use of complementary medicine in children with attention-deficit/hyperactivity disorder and epilepsy. *Pediatric Neurology, 29*(1), 53–55.

Harrington, J.W., Rosen, L., Garnecho, A., & Patrick, P.A. (2006). Parental perceptions and use of complementary and alternative medicine practices for children with autistic spectrum disorders in private practice. *Journal of Developmental and Behavioral Pediatrics, 27*(2, Suppl.), S156–S161.

Hollander, E., Phillips, A., King, B.H., Guthrie, D., Aman, M.G., Law, P., et al. (2004). Impact of recent findings on study design of future autism clinical trials. *CNS Spectrums, 9*(1), 49–56.

Horvath, K., Stefanatos, G., Sokolski, K.N., Wachtel, R., Nabors, L., & Tildon, J.T. (1998). Improved social and language skills after secretin administration in patients with autistic spectrum disorders. *Journal of the Association for Academic Minority Physicians, 9*(1), 9–15.

Hrobjartsson, A., & Gotzsche, P.C. (2004a). Is the placebo powerless? Update of a systematic review with 52 new randomized trials comparing placebo with no treatment. *Journal of Internal Medicine, 256*(2), 91–100.

Hrobjartsson, A., & Gotzsche, P.C. (2004b). Placebo interventions for all clinical conditions. Update of Cochrane Database systematic review. 2003;(1):CD003974; PMID: 12535498. *Cochrane Database of Systematic Reviews, 3,* 003974.

Hurvitz, E.A., Leonard, C., Ayyangar, R., & Nelson, V.S. (2003). Complementary and alternative medicine use in families of children with cerebral palsy. *Developmental Medicine and Child Neurology, 45*(6), 364–370.

Johnston, G.A., Bilbao, R.M., & Graham-Brown, R.A. (2003). The use of complementary medicine in children with atopic dermatitis in secondary care in Leicester. *British Journal of Dermatology, 149*(3), 566–571.

Junker, J., Oberwittler, C., Jackson, D., & Berger, K. (2004). Utilization and perceived effectiveness of complementary and alternative medicine in patients with dystonia. *Movement Disorders, 19*(2), 158–161.

Kaptchuk, T.J., & Eisenberg, D.M. (1998). The persuasive appeal of alternative medicine. [review] [84 refs]. *Annals of Internal Medicine, 129*(12), 1061–1065.

Kelly, K.M. (2004). Complementary and alternative medical therapies for children with cancer. *European Journal of Cancer, 40*(14), 2041–2046.

Kennedy Krieger Institute. (2003, June 10). *Researchers at Kennedy Krieger studying efficacy of energy therapy* (press release).

Knivsberg, A.M., Reichelt, K.L., Hoien, T., & Nodland, M. (2002). A randomised, controlled study of dietary intervention in autistic syndromes. *Nutritional Neuroscience, 5*(4), 251–261.

Levy, S.E., & Hyman, S.L. (2005). Novel treatments for autistic spectrum disorders. *Mental Retardation and Developmental Disabilities Research Reviews, 11*(2), 131–142.

Levy, S.E., Mandell, D.S., Merhar, S., Ittenbach, R.F., & Pinto-Martin, J.A. (2003). Use of complementary and alternative medicine among children recently diagnosed with autistic spectrum disorder. *Journal of Developmental and Behavioral Pediatrics, 24*(6), 418–423.

Lilienfeld, S.O., Lynn, S.J., & Lohr, J.M. (Eds.). (2003). *Science and pseudoscience in clinical psychology.* New York: Guilford Press.

Madsen, H., Andersen, S., Nielsen, R.G., Dolmer, B.S., Host, A., & Damkier, A. (2003). Use of complementary/alternative medicine among paediatric patients. *European Journal of Pediatrics, 162*(5), 334–341.

Markowitz, J.E., Mamula, P., delRosario, J.F., Baldassano, R.N., Lewis, J.D., Jawad, A.F., et al. (2004). Patterns of complementary and alternative medicine use in a population of pediatric patients with inflammatory bowel disease. *Inflammatory Bowel Diseases, 10*(5), 599–605.

Mastrangelo, D., & Lore, C. (2005). The growth of a lie and the end of "conventional" medicine. *Medical Science Monitor, 11*(12), SR27–SR31.

McGrath, C. (2003). Hands that heal: Researchers at Kennedy Krieger investigate whether energy therapy can benefit children with developmental disabilities. *Touch Magazine, 5*(3), 5.

Mencken, H.L. (1920). *Prejudices: Second series.* New York: Knopf.

Miller, A.R., Brehaut, J.C., Raina, P., McGrail, K.M., & Armstrong, R.W. (2004). Use of medical services by methylphenidate-treated children in the general population. *Ambulatory Pediatrics, 4*(2), 174–180.

Moncrieff, J., Wessely, S., & Hardy, R. (2004). Active placebos versus antidepressants for depression. Update of Cochrane Database systematic review. 2001;(2):CD003012; PMID: 11406060. *Cochrane Database of Systematic Reviews, 1,* 003012.

National Center for Complementary and Alternative Medicine. (2000). *Expanding horizons of healthcare: Five year strategic plan 2001–2005.* Washington, DC: U.S. Department of Health and Human Services.

National Center for Complementary and Alternative Medicine. (2004). *NCCAM's research centers program.* Retrieved May 30, 2005, from http://nccam.nih.gov/training/centers/index.htm

National Center for Complementary and Alternative Medicine. (2007). *What is CAM?* Retrieved November 27, 2007, from http://nccam.nih.gov/health/whatiscam

Ni, H., Simile, C., & Hardy, A.M. (2002). Utilization of complementary and alternative medicine by United States adults: Results from the 1999 national health interview survey. *Medical Care, 40*(4), 353–358.

Nickel, R. (1996). Controversial therapies for young children with developmental disabilities. *Infants and Young Children, 8,* 29–40.

Nye, C., & Brice, A. (2006). Combined vitamin B6-magnesium treatment in autism spectrum disorder. *Cochrane Database of Systematic Reviews, 4,* CD003497.

Orhan, F., Sekerel, B.E., Kocabas, C.N., Sackesen, C., Adalioglu, G., & Tuncer, A. (2003). Complementary and alternative medicine in children with asthma. *Annals of Allergy, Asthma, and Immunology, 90*(6), 611–615.

Ottolini, M.C., Hamburger, E.K., Loprieato, J.O., Coleman, R.H., Sachs, H.C., Madden, R., et al. (2001). Complementary and alternative medicine use among children in the Washington, DC area. *Ambulatory Pediatrics, 1*(2), 122–125.

Paavonen, E.J., Nieminen-von Wendt, T., Vanhala, R., Aronen, E.T., & von Wendt, L. (2003). Effectiveness of melatonin in the treatment of sleep disturbances in children with Asperger disorder. *Journal of Child and Adolescent Psychopharmacology, 13*(1), 83–95.

Prussing, E., Sobo, E.J., Walker, E., Dennis, K., & Kurtin, P.S. (2004). Communicating with pediatricians about complementary/alternative medicine: Perspectives from parents of children with Down syndrome. *Ambulatory Pediatrics, 4*(6), 488–494.

Rosa, L., Rosa, E., Sarner, L., & Barrett, S. (1998). A close look at therapeutic touch. *Journal of the American Medical Association, 279*(13), 1005–1010.

Sanders, H., Davis, M.F., Duncan, B., Meaney, F.J., Haynes, J., & Barton, L.L. (2003). Use of complementary and alternative medical therapies among children with special health care needs in southern Arizona. *Pediatrics, 111*(3), 584–587.

Sandler, A. (2005). Placebo effects in developmental disabilities: Implications for research and practice. *Mental Retardation and Developmental Disabilities Research Reviews, 11*(2), 164–170.

Sandler, A.D., Sutton, K.A., DeWeese, J., Girardi, M.A., Sheppard, V., & Bodfish, J.W. (1999). Lack of benefit of a single dose of synthetic human secretin in the treatment of autism and pervasive developmental disorder. *New England Journal of Medicine, 341*(24), 1801–1806.

Sawni-Sikand, A., Schubiner, H., & Thomas, R.L. (2002). Use of complementary/alternative therapies among children in primary care pediatrics. *Ambulatory Pediatrics, 2*(2), 99–103.

Schaaf, R.C., & Miller, L.J. (2005). Occupational therapy using a sensory integrative approach for children with developmental disabilities. *Mental Retardation and Developmental Disabilities Research Reviews, 11*(2), 143–148.

Schulman, K.A. (2004). Commentary: The unknown benefit of complementary and alternative medicine. *Journal of Alternative and Complementary Medicine, 10*(6), 911.

Sibinga, E.M., Ottolini, M.C., Duggan, A.K., & Wilson, M.H. (2004). Parent-pediatrician communication about complementary and alternative medicine use for children. *Clinical Pediatrics, 43*(4), 367–373.

Simpson, N., & Roman, K. (2001). Complementary medicine use in children: Extent and reasons. A population-based study. *British Journal of General Practice, 51*(472), 914–916.

Sinha, D., & Efron, D. (2005). Complementary and alternative medicine use in children with attention deficit hyperactivity disorder. *Journal of Paediatrics and Child Health, 41*(1–2), 23–26.

Sinha, Y., Silove, N., Wheeler, D., & Williams, K. (2004). Auditory integration training and other sound therapies for autism spectrum disorders. *Cochrane Database of Systematic Reviews,* (1), CD003681.

Spigelblatt, L., Laine-Ammara, G., Pless, I.B., & Guyver, A. (1994). The use of alternative medicine by children. *Pediatrics, 94*(6, Pt. 1), 811–814.

Stedman's Medical Dictionary (27th ed.). (2000). Philadelphia: Lippincott Williams & Wilkins.

Studdert, D.M., Eisenberg, D.M., Miller, F.H., Curto, D.A., Kaptchuk, T.J., & Brennan, T.A. (1998). Medical malpractice implications of alternative medicine. *Journal of the American Medical Association, 280*(18), 1610–1615.

Sturmey, P. (2005). Secretin is an ineffective treatment for pervasive developmental disabilities: A review of 15 double-blind randomized controlled trials. *Research in Developmental Disabilities, 26*(1), 87–97.

Tolbert, L., Haigler, T., Waits, M.M., & Dennis, T. (1993). Brief report: Lack of response in an autistic population to a low dose clinical trial of pyridoxine plus magnesium. *Journal of Autism and Developmental Disorders, 23*(1), 193–199.

Wilson, K.M., & Klein, J.D. (2002). Adolescents' use of complementary and alternative medicine. *Ambulatory Pediatrics, 2*(2), 104–110.

Wong, H.H., & Smith, R.G. (2006). Patterns of complementary and alternative medical therapy use in children diagnosed with autism spectrum disorders. *Journal of Autism and Developmental Disorders, 36*(7), 901–909.

Yussman, S.M., Ryan, S.A., Auinger, P., & Weitzman, M. (2004). Visits to complementary and alternative medicine providers by children and adolescents in the United States. *Ambulatory Pediatrics, 4*(5), 429–435.

Zollman, C., & Vickers, A. (1999). What is complementary medicine? *British Medical Journal, 319*(7211), 693–696.

12

Can Autism Resolve?

Juhi Pandey, Leandra Wilson, Alyssa Verbalis, and Deborah Fein

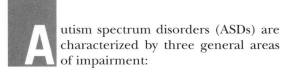utism spectrum disorders (ASDs) are characterized by three general areas of impairment:

1. Delayed or impaired social skills
2. Impairments in functional communication
3. Repetitive, stereotyped patterns of behavior and restricted interests and activities (American Psychiatric Association [APA], 2000; Rogers, 2001)

Within the domain of socialization, behaviors of interest include a lack of peer relationships; impairments in nonverbal behaviors to communicate and regulate social interaction, such as the use of eye contact and facial expression; impaired shared attention with others, manifested by a lack of pointing, showing, and following a point; and a lack of social and emotional reciprocity. Qualitative impairments within the communication domain include delayed and stereotyped language, poor conversational skills, and a lack of make-believe or pretend play. Restricted, repetitive, and stereotyped patterns of behavior include motor mannerisms, preoccupations with parts of objects, inflexible adherence to nonfunctional routines, and resistance to change (APA, 2000; Rogers, 2001). Diagnoses of pervasive developmental disorder-not otherwise specified (PDD-NOS) are provided to children who demonstrate impairments in the social domain and in either the communication or

stereotyped and repetitive behavior domains (APA, 2000). In contrast, children diagnosed with Asperger syndrome do not have a language delay but do have impairments within the domains of socialization and restrictive and repetitive behaviors (APA, 2000). Currently, many researchers and clinicians use the term *autism spectrum disorders (ASDs)* to refer to all of these disorders.

Diagnoses of ASDs are generally associated with a high likelihood of permanent disability, although increasing attention has been drawn to cases with excellent outcomes, even including those with a loss of diagnosis. This chapter reviews some of the literature concerning how ASDs can be screened for and diagnosed at an early age, the typical outcomes for children with early diagnoses of ASDs, and the transition of an early diagnosis of ASD to a later diagnosis of attention-deficit/hyperactivity disorder (ADHD). Speculations will be presented regarding possible underlying mechanisms by which early intervention facilitates movement off the autism spectrum.

SCREENING FOR AUTISM SPECTRUM DISORDERS

To identify symptoms of ASDs at earlier ages, autism screening instruments have been developed. Currently, no biological markers for ASDs have been identified (Volkmar, Lord, Bailey, Schultz, & Klin, 2004), necessitating the creation of screeners focusing on specific behaviors to help identify children at risk for ASDs. Level 1 screeners identify children at risk for any type of atypical development (Filipek et al., 1999). Level 2 screening, however, involves more in-depth investigation of children previously identified as being at risk for possible developmental disorders. The American Academy of Pediatrics has endorsed ongoing developmental surveillance of all children at specific ages and ASD-specific screening at 18 months of age (American Academy of Pediatrics, 2006). While autism screeners identify symptoms of ASDs in young children, a comprehensive evaluation is required to make a diagnosis of an ASD.

These diagnostic assessments consist of several components (Lord, Storoschuk, Rutter, & Pickles, 1993), including the child's developmental history, direct observation of the child, and parental descriptions of the child's daily social interactive behaviors (Rogers, 2001; Volkmar et al., 1994). Several different diagnostic measures have been found to be reliable in categorizing those symptoms consistent with ASDs (Volkmar et al., 2004). Autism diagnostic measures include the Autism Diagnostic Interview–Revised (ADI-R), a semistructured clinician-administered interview for parents or caregivers designed to assess day-to-day behaviors and developmental history in children for whom ASDs are possible diagnoses (Rutter, LeCouteur, & Lord, 2003). The Autism Diagnostic Observation Schedule–Generic (ADOS-G) is a semistructured assessment of communication, social interaction and relatedness, play, and imagination (Lord, Rutter, DiLavore, & Risi, 1999). The assessment consists of planned social interactions to encourage social initiations and responses and provides opportunities for spontaneous social communication. The child is also given opportunities to engage in make-believe and imaginative play activities. Schopler, Reichler, DeVellis, and Daly

(1980) developed the Childhood Autism Rating Scale (CARS), which is tailored to young children and can be completed based on observations of interactions with the children or interviews with their parents. The CARS is a 15-item scale intended to measure the presence and severity of pervasive developmental disorders and includes items involving social impairments and communication, as well as emotional responses and sensory sensitivities.

In addition to diagnostic measures, the diagnoses of expert clinicians experienced with ASDs have been shown to be consistently accurate in differentiating toddlers with ASDs from children with other developmental delays (Charman & Baird, 2002; Filipek et al., 1999; Rogers, 2001). As a result, it is important that Level 2 evaluations (i.e., assessments aimed at the diagnosis of ASDs and other developmental disorders) be conducted by professionals who have specific expertise with the evaluation and treatment of ASDs. Whereas less experienced professionals rely on various screening instruments, checklists, and diagnostic manuals, such as the *Diagnostic and Statistical Manual of Mental Disorders, Fourth Edition, Text Revision* (*DSM-IV-TR;* APA, 2000) and the *International Classification of Diseases, tenth revision* (*ICD-10;* World Health Organization, 1994), expert clinicians mainly rely on their clinical judgment when evaluating children on the autism spectrum (Filipek et al., 1999).

Screening in Younger Children

It should be noted that procedures and criteria designed for older children are not always valid in the youngest age group. In the youngest children, researchers have found support for the presence of symptoms in the social and communication domains (Baron-Cohen, Cox, Baird, Swettenham, & Nightingale, 1996; Cox et al., 1999; Gillberg et al., 1990; Osterling & Dawson, 1994; Robins, Fein, Barton, & Green, 2001; Stone et al., 1999). Symptoms seen in 2-year-olds with ASDs include a lack of eye contact, decreased pointing and joint attention behaviors, a decreased number of communicative acts, delayed speech, a decreased amount of imitation, and a lack of symbolic play.

Repetitive and stereotyped behaviors, when demonstrated with social and communicative impairments, were highly indicative of a diagnosis on the autism spectrum (Charman & Baird, 2002). Whereas repetitive and stereotyped behaviors confirmed the ASD diagnosis, the social and communication impairments represented necessary deficits for this age group, as supported by the differential diagnosis of ASD versus developmental language delay (DLD). Repetitive behaviors did not reliably differentiate children with these nonspectrum diagnoses from children on the autism spectrum. Communication and social impairments, however, were critical to the diagnoses of ASDs and reliably differentiated children with ASDs from children with other delays and from children with typical development.

Filipek et al. (1999) and Rogers (2001) discussed the importance of the fact that 2-year-old children on the autism spectrum present with more negative symptoms (i.e., decreased social and communicative behaviors) rather than positive symptoms (i.e., higher rates of unusual behaviors). Examples of negative symptoms included a lack of speech, a decreased interest in peer interactions, decreased social or emotional reciprocity, lack of eye contact, decreased or absent orientation to one's name, and reduced imitation. This presentation of mostly negative symptoms differentiated 2-year-old children with ASDs from older children with ASDs because older children not only exhibited these negative symptoms, but they also displayed positive symptoms such as stereotyped use of language, adherence to routines, and preoccupations or circumscribed interests.

THE BENFITS OF EARLY DIAGNOSIS

Early identification studies support the importance and possibility of early diagnosis, even in children as young as 2 years (Baird et al., 2000; Baron-Cohen et al., 1996). In general, these early identification studies focused on children 2 years of age or younger, demonstrating that deficits within the domains of socialization and communication were most predictive of later ASDs. Specific examples of deficits for this age group include the lack of eye contact, pointing, and pretend play (Baird, et al., 2000).

Increasing examination of ASDs in preschool-age children has allowed clinicians to follow them over time, presenting opportunities for consequent examination of the stability of their early diagnoses. Empirical evidence suggests that an early diagnosis of Autistic Disorder (i.e., occurring at approximately 3–4 years of age) is generally stable over time (Charman et al., 2005; Cox et al., 1999; Gillberg, 1990; Lord, 1995; Moore & Goodson, 2003; Sigman & Ruskin, 1999; Stone et al., 1999). However, diagnosis of an ASD (e.g., PDD-NOS) is less stable, perhaps because the less stringent diagnosis of an ASD includes less severely affected children.

Lord (1995) found evidence of diagnostic stability, as 88% of her sample of 16 children who received a diagnosis of autism (i.e., Autistic Disorder) at 2 years of age also received an independent diagnosis of autism at 3 years of age. Similarly, Stone et al. (1999) reported that 95% of a sample of 37 children diagnosed with an ASD at 2 years of age retained an ASD diagnosis 1 year later. In a group of children evaluated at 30 months and reevaluated at 54 months for whom clinical judgment was used to assign diagnosis, diagnostic stability was found to be 79%, with 93% of the sample remaining on the spectrum and 7% of the sample no longer meeting criteria for an ASD at reevaluation (Eaves & Ho, 2004). Reliability was greater for children with autism than for those with PDD-NOS. Moore and Goodson (2003) reported an impressive 100% diagnostic stability for their sample of children diagnosed with an ASD between 29 and 40 months and then reassessed 1 year later. Consistent with earlier findings, Charman et al. (2005) followed a sample of 26 children diagnosed with ASDs at 2 years of age and found that 25 of these children (i.e., 96%) continued to meet diagnostic criteria for ASDs at 7 years of age.

EVIDENCE OF CHANGES IN OR THE LOSS OF A DIAGNOSIS

Although ample evidence supports the notion that an ASD diagnosis based on clinical judgment is highly stable over time, other research indicates that a minority of children diagnosed with ASDs at young ages may eventually lose their diagnoses.

Studies examining outcome for children with ASDs published in the 1960s and 1970s suggested generally poor outcomes for children with ASDs. Initial studies (Lockyer & Rutter, 1969, 1970; Rutter, Greenfeld, & Lockyer, 1967) examined the cognitive, social, behavioral, psychological, and educational/vocational outcomes of 63 children diagnosed with "infantile psychosis" (which is now generally accepted as ASD). At 5 to 15 years after initial diagnosis, with the mean age at follow-up being 15 years, 7 months, 14% were said to have achieved a "good" adjustment (i.e., leading a typical or nearly typical social life and functioning satisfactorily at school or work), 25% were described as having a "fair adjustment" (i.e., making social and educational progress despite significant abnormalities in behavior or relationships), and 13% were noted to have made a "poor" adjustment (i.e., diagnosed as severely handicapped, unable to lead an independent life, but with some amount of social adjustment and potential for continued progress). The majority of children (i.e., 48%) were said to be "very poorly" adjusted, as defined by being unable

to lead an independent life. All children with infantile psychosis were initially described as socially "autistic," although at follow-up, 14% of the sample reportedly evidenced sufficient social skills such that this description was no longer appropriate.

Lotter (1974a, 1974b) followed 32 children with ASDs from initial diagnosis at 8–10 years of age to follow-up approximately 8 years later. Children with ASDs were found to have outcomes similar to those found by Rutter, Greenfeld, and Lockyer (1967). Specifically, 14% of children with ASDs had a "good" outcome at follow-up, 24% had a "fair" outcome, and 62% had a "poor" or "very poor" outcome. Lotter (1974a, 1974b) also found higher intelligence quotient (IQ) and language levels to be related to better outcome. Findings of DeMyer and colleagues (1973) were consistent with these studies. These authors followed 126 children with ASDs from initial evaluation (i.e., mean age = 5.5 years) to follow-up at 12 years, noting that 60%–75% of participants had a poor outcome and a small minority (1%–2%) were said to have a "normal" recovery. Higher levels of functioning at initial evaluation were associated with a greater likelihood of improvements in speech and social skills. Initial levels of functioning in work and educational settings were found to be the best predictors of later functioning in these respective areas.

In keeping with previous research, Gillberg and Steffenburg (1987) found early levels of speech and IQ to be associated with outcome in a follow-up study of individuals 16–23 years old who had originally been diagnosed with infantile autism or other childhood psychoses. Furthermore, the majority (i.e., 44%) of young adults originally diagnosed with infantile autism had "poor" or "very poor" outcomes, 35% had "restricted but acceptable" outcomes, and a minority (17%) had "fair" or "good" outcomes. In sum, these early follow-up studies helped to establish several important findings.

1. Children who demonstrate higher levels of functioning initially evidence greater improvement over time.

2. Early cognitive levels and early development of speech are important predictors of outcome.

3. The likelihood of positive outcome is generally low in children with ASDs.

Intervention and Positive Outcome

While relatively few studies have examined "recovery" from ASDs, more empirical attention has been devoted to exploring relationships between intervention and positive outcome as defined by a decrease in autistic symptomatology. In some studies, although intervention was significant in facilitating positive outcomes, prognosis was also found to be related to other variables, including initial levels of language and imitation skills and the amount of intervention provided (Bono, Daley, & Sigman, 2004). It has been suggested that certain pivotal areas or skills (e.g., spontaneous initiations of social behavior) are associated with positive responses to treatment and that children can be taught such pivotal skills, thereby increasing the likelihood of favorable treatment outcomes (Koegel, Koegel, & McNerney, 2001; Koegel, Koegel, Shoshan, & McNerney, 1999). Self-initiated social communication prior to receiving intervention, in particular, was found to be associated with positive treatment outcomes.

The Significance of Cognitive Ability

In children with ASDs, cognitive ability has also been found to have a significant impact on outcome (Fein, et al., 1999; Gabriels, Hill, Pierce, Rogers, & Wehner, 2001). Furthermore, cognitive level has also been found to be the best single predictor of developmental trajectory (Fein et al., 1999). When compared with children with lower levels of nonverbal intelligence, children

with higher levels of nonverbal intelligence have been found to be more likely to demonstrate communicative skills, symbolic play, and social improvement over time (Fein et al., 1999). Children's responsiveness to bids for joint attention has also been found to be associated with improvement in language skills over time (Bono et al., 2004). The rate of nonverbal communicative attempts at 2 years of age has been found to predict the level of expressive language at age 3 years and later at age 7 years (Charman et al., 2005). Sigman and McGovern (2005) found functional play skills, response to joint attention, and frequency of requests to be early childhood predictors of language skills in adolescence.

In contrast to cognitive level and language skills, ASD symptom severity appears to have limited predictive power in determining outcome (Fein et al., 1999; Stevens et al., 2000; Szatmari, Bryson, Boyle, Streiner, & Duku, 2003). Szatmari and associates (2003) found initial ASD symptoms to be weak predictors, whereas nonverbal intelligence and language ability were found to be more reliable predictors of outcome. Sutera et al. (2007) found no difference in ASD symptom severity at approximately 2 years of age (i.e., defined by total score on the CARS and the number of *DSM-IV-TR* symptoms endorsed) between children who had lost their ASD diagnoses over time and those who had retained their diagnoses. In sum, research suggests that individual child characteristics are important in predicting positive outcomes (i.e., decreases in ASD symptomatology) in children who retain their ASD diagnoses over time.

The Importance of Behavioral Intervention

Although individual child characteristics (e.g., early communication abilities, cognitive levels, social responsiveness) certainly play important roles in predicting outcome in children with ASDs, evidence supports the role of intensive behavioral intervention in facilitating positive outcomes in affected children. To date, behavior analytic (i.e., Applied Behavioral Analysis [ABA]) intervention is the only approach that has been established as being effective in producing significant, long-term improvements for children with ASDs (Smith, 1996). Specifically, not only has early intensive behavioral intervention been found to reduce stereotyped and disruptive behavior and to increase a variety of complex and functional skills in young children with ASDs (Matson, Benavidez, Compton, Paclawskyj, & Baglio, 1996), it has also resulted in improvements in intellectual functioning in affected children (Sallows & Graupner, 2005). A recent comparison of intensive behavior analytic intervention with other nonintensive and eclectic treatments for young children with ASDs indicated that children who received the intensive behavior analytic intervention had significantly higher mean scores across a variety of skill domains (e.g., cognitive, language, and adaptive skills) and significantly greater rates of learning at follow-up than children in both comparison groups (Howard, Sparkman, Cohen, Green, & Stanislaw, 2005). Sallows and Graupner (2005) reported similarly positive results.

Lovaas (1987) provided what appeared to be impressive evidence for "recovery" from ASDs, citing that 47% of his sample of 38 children with ASDs achieved typical intellectual and educational functioning after receiving intensive behavioral intervention (i.e., ABA). Intensive intervention was provided 40 hours per week for more than 2 years. Only 2% of the control group showed similar gains. Sigman and Ruskin (1999) followed a sample of 51 children originally diagnosed with ASDs at the mean age of 45 months from various research programs dating back to 1979. Seventeen percent of the children were found to have lost their ASD diagnoses over time at a mean age of 12.8 years. Although Sigman and Ruskin's (1999) finding was not as robust as that reported by

Lovaas (1987), which may be due in part to the fact that not all children in the former sample received intensive behavioral intervention, it nevertheless suggests that a sizable minority of children initially diagnosed with ASDs eventually lost their diagnoses, thereby achieving an "optimal outcome."

In an attempt to replicate Lovaas's (1987) findings, Smith, Groen, and Wynn (2000) compared children with ASDs who received an average of 24.5 hours per week of ABA therapy to a group who received only parent training. Results indicated that children who received ABA intervention evidenced greater improvement in cognitive and academic skills compared to their counterparts who received only parent training intervention. Consistent with other studies, these authors also found that children diagnosed with PDD-NOS made more gains than children diagnosed with Autistic Disorder, although neither treatment group was found to have made gains in adaptive skills.

IS "RECOVERY" POSSIBLE?

Although ample evidence exists supporting the notion that early intensive behavioral intervention is associated with positive gains in children with ASDs, it remains unclear whether early intervention is both necessary and sufficient with respect to "recovery" from ASDs. There are several cases in the literature describing children who had been diagnosed with ASDs and who over time had lost their diagnoses as they no longer met diagnostic criteria. However, "recovery" from ASDs remains a highly controversial phenomenon and is worthy of continued investigation for both theoretical and clinical reasons.

The Early Detection Study at the University of Connecticut, using the Modified Checklist for Autism in Toddlers (M-CHAT; Robins et al., 2001) to screen for ASDs in very young children, has contributed some findings relevant to this question. In this study, children are screened between the ages of 16 months and 30 months at 1) a pediatrician's office during a well-child visit, 2) initial intakes with an early intervention provider, or 3) because they have at least one older sibling already diagnosed with an ASD. The latter two groups comprise the higher risk sample, while the former is an unselected group. Children are excluded if their parents fill out the screener for the first time when they are younger than 16 months or older than 30 months, or if they have already received a diagnosis of autism or other developmental disorder (e.g., language disorder) by a certified professional.

The M-CHAT screener consists of 23 yes or no items that ask parents about aspects of their child's development. The items consist of questions about socialization, communication, and motor ability. Four of the items are reverse scored. Six of the items were determined to be "critical" for determining ASDs in toddlers based on discriminant functional analysis in the original paper. A child is considered to "screen positive" if he or she has concerning answers on at least three total screener items or at least two of the six critical items. Pediatricians can also flag children for whom an ASD is suspected. These children are seen for an evaluation regardless of whether they screen positive on the questionnaire.

When a child screens positive, his or her parents participate in a follow-up phone interview to review failed items and to confirm that their answers have not changed during the intervening weeks or months. The parents are invited to bring their child in for a developmental and diagnostic evaluation if the responses continue to indicate a positive screener. The evaluation consists of measures of adaptive functioning, cognitive ability, and autism diagnostic tests. These include the Vineland Adaptive Behavior Scales (VABS; Sparrow, Balla, & Cicchetti, 1984), the Autism Diagnostic Interview–Revised (ADI-R; Rutter, LeCouteur, & Lord, 2003), the Mullen Scales of Early Learning (Mullen, 1995), the

Autism Diagnostic Observation Schedule– Generic (ADOS-G; Lord, Rutter, DiLavore, & Risi, 1999), and the CARS (Schopler, Reichler, & Renner, 1988), as well a *DSM-IV-TR*–based clinical judgment of diagnosis (Volkmar, Chawarska, & Klin, 2005). All participants receive a follow-up screener between the ages of 42 months and 54 months. All children who had previously received an evaluation, as well as those who screen positive on the rescreener or who have been referred for possible ASDs in the interim, receive an evaluation.

The study has currently screened more than 6,000 participants, and approximately 1,500 follow-up screeners have been returned. To date, 424 children around the age of 2 years have received evaluations, and 58% of those children were given ASD diagnoses. In order to qualify for a developmental evaluation, children screened positive on the M-CHAT and failed a follow-up telephone interview. The children who screened positive on the M-CHAT and qualified for a developmental evaluation but did not receive ASD diagnoses were primarily diagnosed with various other developmental disorders (e.g., language delay, global developmental delay, regulatory disorder); very few ($n < 15$) have been diagnosed as typically developing. The current estimate of sensitivity is 85%–95%, while the current estimate of specificity is 87%.

Sutera et al. (2007) described a sample of 13 children in the Early Detection Study who were diagnosed with ASDs at approximately 2 years of age but who no longer met diagnostic criteria for ASD at 4 years of age. These children were said to have achieved an "optimal outcome," and by 4 years of age, they scored within the typical range on standardized measures of cognitive and adaptive functioning. Sutera et al. (2007) defined "optimal outcome" as follows: "(1) initially meeting *DSM-IV-TR* criteria for PDD-NOS or Autistic Disorder, *and* at follow-up (2) no longer meeting criteria for any ASD, and (3) functioning in the average range on standardized measures of cognition, language and adaptive skills." These authors examined whether various adaptive skills (e.g., communication, daily living, social, motor skills), cognitive ability, and symptom severity in these children when they were 2 years of age were useful predictors of "optimal outcome" (i.e., the loss of an ASD diagnosis) at the age of 4 years. They were compared to a sample of children who retained their ASD diagnoses ($n = 60$) and to a sample of children who had never been diagnosed with ASDs ($n = 17$) but who had screened positive on the M-CHAT and showed other delays such as global developmental delay or language delay. No significant differences among groups were found for age at initial evaluation/diagnosis or age at reevaluation. No differences were found between the group of children who achieved an "optimal outcome" and those who retained ASD diagnoses on measures of symptom severity, socialization, and communication obtained at the time of initial diagnosis at age 2. However, children with PDD-NOS were more likely to move off the autism spectrum than their counterparts diagnosed with Autistic Disorder. Specifically, 39% of the children initially diagnosed with PDD-NOS lost their diagnoses, whereas only 11% of the children diagnosed with Autistic Disorder moved off the spectrum. Better motor skills—noted by both parent report and direct testing—were found to be the most reliable factor differentiating the sample who achieved "optimal outcome" from those children who retained ASD diagnoses. A trend toward more developed daily living skills as defined by VABS Daily Living Skills Domain standard score in the group who achieved "optimal outcome" was also found. Thus, in this investigation, children who moved off the spectrum evidenced early impairments in socialization skills, communication skills and language ability, and individual symptoms and overall symptom severity comparable to the group of children who retained their ASD diagnoses

over time. While results of this investigation lend further support to the notion that some young children with ASDs may lose their diagnoses over time, these authors caution that predicting optimal outcome at a young age is extremely difficult, thus emphasizing the importance of high quality intensive intervention for all young children diagnosed with ASDs.

Although increasing evidence suggests that some children with ASDs may eventually lose their diagnoses, it is reasonable to expect that residual difficulties in the areas of attention, language, and socialization may persist in children who have achieved "optimal outcome."

Assessing Improved Outcomes

The area of improved outcomes was examined in a recent study by Kelley, Paul, Fein, and Naigles (2006b), who examined the language abilities of a group of children with optimal outcome. Kelley et al. (2006b) examined 14 children who were initially diagnosed with either Autistic Disorder or PDD-NOS between the ages of 13 months and 5 years by the third author (an experienced clinical neuropsychologist) using extensive parent interview, direct testing, and observation of the child. All of the children received intensive intervention for an average of 2–3 years. At the time of the study, the participants were between 5 and 9 years old and functioning independently in a typical, age-appropriate classroom with no educational support; in fact, many of the participants' teachers were reported to be unaware of the children's diagnostic histories. Two of the children continued to receive minimal home-based intervention services to prevent regression of learned skills and knowledge. A control group of typically developing children was individually matched on age and sex (with two females in each group). The groups were also matched on performance on the Test for Auditory Comprehension of

Language–Third Edition (TACL-3; Carrow-Woolfolk, 1999) vocabulary subtest.

Both groups were tested on various complex areas of language, including morphological, syntactical, lexical semantic, and pragmatic functioning. They were also given two basic theory of mind tasks, and their parents were interviewed about the children's adaptive behavior. The authors found that the primary areas of continued deficit were within the children's pragmatic language skills, although their vocabulary, adaptive communication skills, sentence memory, and grammatical and semantic skills were indistinguishable from the control group.

The optimal outcome group displayed increased difficulty distinguishing mental state verbs (i.e., guess versus think versus know). They also performed more poorly on a second order theory of mind task and on making verbal reasoning judgments, especially about animate objects. Although many of these tasks were not standardized, the authors reported that on the activities on which the optimal outcome group continued to have difficulties, these children were performing at levels reported for 3- or 4-year-olds.

On a narrative task, the experimental group was similar to the controls on general lexical variables or grammar. Their pragmatic performance was more varied. The experimental group was indistinguishable from the controls on repeating for emphasis, hedges, or using negatives for dramatic effect. Also, as both groups used few mental state or emotion words, there were no differences between the groups on those measures. Children in the optimal outcome group were less likely to give causal explanations for story events, were less likely to explain the characters' goals and motivations, and were more likely to misinterpret the pictures in the story and therefore provided incorrect narrative information. In addition, they often needlessly repeated themselves.

When the optimal outcome group's scores were correlated with symptom severity at initial diagnosis and current adaptive functioning, the authors found few significant results. The only measure that was correlated with initial severity was the false belief theory of mind task. This suggested that the potential for language outcome was independent of early symptom severity.

The authors did a follow-up study several years later when the children were between the ages of 9 and 12 years (Kelly et al., 2000a). This follow-up included comparison of the same children in the optimal outcome group with a high-functioning autism (HFA) group and a typically developing group, all matched for age and sex. The authors reported that the experimental groups were now even more similar in language ability to the typically developing control group than they were at ages 5–9 years. The only deficit that the authors found at this age (i.e., at least 4 years after being in an inclusive classroom and no longer meeting criteria for an ASD) was on a test of mental state verbs similar to the test done during the previous study (i.e., guess versus think versus know). On all other variables, the optimal outcome children were not significantly different from the typically developing control group, but they were higher functioning on many variables than the HFA group.

ATTENTIONAL DIFFICULTIES OF CHILDREN ON THE AUTISM SPECTRUM

In a case study analysis, Fein, Dixon, Paul, and Levin (2005) presented cases demonstrating the presence of residual attentional difficulties in 11 children (i.e., 9 boys, 2 girls), 3 of whom were initially clear cases of autism, and 8 of whom were clear cases of PDD-NOS that had evolved into clear cases of ADHD (i.e., 6 cases of ADHD, Inattentive Type and 5 cases of ADHD, Combined Type) in early to middle childhood. ASD diagnoses were made by the first author using *DSM-IV-TR* criteria on the basis of behavioral observation, neuropsychological testing, extensive parent interview, and teacher interview. Diagnoses of ADHD were also made by the first author using the ADHD Rating Scale–IV (DuPaul, Power, Anastopoulos, & Reid, 1998), as well as neuropsychological testing, behavioral observation, and parent and teacher interview. Consistent with the *DSM-IV-TR* criteria for ADHD, interviews were done to confirm that the behaviors consistent with ADHD were demonstrated in more than one setting and that these behaviors significantly interfered with adaptive skills and social adjustment.

Nine of the 11 cases, based on retrospective parental report, were documented to have the regressive type of autism, whereas 10 of the 11 children experienced recurrent ear infections. A majority of the children (i.e., 8 of 11) received intensive ABA treatment along with preschool services. As previously suggested, ABA treatments, which are designed to focus on ASD symptoms and teach skills systematically, may result in positive outcomes for children on the autism spectrum. Although the exact age at which the children's diagnostic transition took place was difficult to pinpoint, on average, children were 7–8 years old when the symptoms of PDD-NOS were no longer present and the presentation of ADHD was clear. Three of the 11 children's diagnoses evolved into ADHD between the ages of 6 and 7, with an additional three children having their diagnoses evolve by the age of 4–5. Many of the children demonstrated residual, mild features of ASDs, including some mild perseverative interests and mild motor stereotypies. Socially, these children demonstrated some awkwardness, which was more characteristic of aggressive, immature, and impulsive children with ADHD, rather than of children on the autism spectrum.

Based on the clinical development of the 11 children studied, the authors theorized four possibilities for the progression from a diagnosis of ASD to ADHD. The first possibility was that ASD and ADHD were comorbid disorders in this sample of children, such that when the more prominent ASD features were resolved with the help of ABA, the features of ADHD became increasingly prominent. The authors also discussed the possibility that these children represented a subtype of severe ADHD, which presents as ASD early in a child's development. A third possibility was that ASDs usually involve attentional impairments, along with the core symptoms of social and language impairment. As the core symptoms resolve, the attentional impairments that are part of the syndrome become more prominent and closely resemble the attentional features of primary ADHD. The fourth possibility was originally put forth by Kinsbourne (1991), who suggested that rather than being considered as a secondary symptom, the attentional features in children with ASDs should be considered a core deficit for children with ASD diagnoses. Therefore, given the centrality of these attentional impairments in children with ASDs, attentional features tend to persist even when other features such as social and language deficits have resolved. Kinsbourne (1991) postulated a clinical syndrome that includes elements of both PDD-NOS and ADHD—"the overfocused child." This clinical group is marked by a narrow focus of attention and social withdrawal in which these sets of behaviors serve to defend the child against an unstable arousal system. When considered in this way, ADHD and ASDs may lie on a continuum of arousal and stimulus-seeking resulting in a range from ADHD to typical to overfocused to PDD-NOS.

UNEXPLORED QUESTIONS

These recent studies and the previously mentioned outcome studies, in which a small percentage of children appeared to move off the autism spectrum, suggested that losing the behavioral features of ASDs is possible for some children. This research is obviously in its infancy. Many crucial questions remain completely unexplored. What percentage of young children with ASDs have the capacity to "recover" from the syndrome? What interventions are effective in promoting this change? Is there an age by which intervention must begin and how intense must it be? Do some children "recover" through maturation alone or is intervention necessary in all cases? What are the common residual conditions or impairments in "recovered" children (e.g., anxiety, depression, ADHD, OCD, eating problems, tics, social awkwardness, perseverative interests, language disability)? What factors in early childhood predict the possibility of "recovery" (e.g., genetic makeup, family history, cognitive functioning, symptom picture, motor functioning)? Are the children who have the potential for "recovery" those with the most structurally typical brains or those with a particular disease process or absence thereof?

There have been few speculations about the fundamental mechanism by which intervention can move children off the ASD spectrum. Dawson and Zanolli (2003) suggested that early intensive behavioral intervention works, at least in part, by pairing therapists with primary reinforcers, causing them to acquire secondary reinforcement value through conditioned reinforcement. This pairing reduces the social avoidance that may be primary in ASDs, which then results in a myriad of downstream effects.

The authors also discussed a deficit in face processing measured by evoked response potentials (ERPs) present in children with ASDs as an example of a social avoidance that for some children may be moderated through early intensive behavioral intervention, thereby producing better outcomes. Face processing represents a social phenomenon that "comes on line" for children with typical development around the age of 6 months because children at this age demonstrate the ability to success-

fully discriminate familiar from unfamiliar faces. Dawson and Zanolli (2003), along with other researchers, have hypothesized that experience-dependent cortical systems replace subcortical systems that enable early face processing. These neural changes rely on experience expectant developments, which occur during a sensitive period early in development in which the brain is ready to receive experiences with faces. Because of the early development and suggested sensitive period of development, an impairment in facial recognition (i.e., an aspect of social attention because a child must attune to the faces of others) may suggest early atypical brain functioning in children with ASDs.

The authors theorized that early intervention alters the face processing systems of the brain in two major ways. The first is by teaching the child to attend to social information and the second is conditioned reinforcement. As a result of the previously discussed pairing of reinforcement, early intensive behavioral intervention reinforces a child's attention to faces by making these interactions more rewarding and more frequent, thereby altering the child's motivational preferences. This pattern of increased face processing represents only one aspect of social attention that may be mediated by early intensive behavioral intervention. The authors discussed the possibility that early intensive behavioral intervention not only alters a child's behavioral performance, but may also facilitate a more typical trajectory of brain development (i.e., optimal outcome) in children on the autism spectrum. This theoretical approach is very promising and an excellent start. Two aspects of this model require further explication: how extended is the sensitive or plastic period for face processing? Given how early the face processing system develops, how can intervention that does not start until the age 3–4 years be effective? Second, although classical conditioning can explain how the social stimulus (i.e., the adult) can acquire secondary reinforcing value through pairing with primary reinforcers, the model must consider why extinction of this reinforcing value does not ensue when the reinforcers are unpaired (i.e., when the primary reinforcer is withdrawn).

Similarly, Mundy and Crowson (1997) suggested that a neurologically based deficit in social orienting is prevented from disrupting further neurological development by the social effects of early intervention. This disturbance in social orienting neurological processing may lead to an attenuation of the amount of social information that is provided as input to the developing nervous system of the child, which may then deprive the developing child with an ASD of the amount of social information or social stimulation needed for the normal shaping of neurological connections involved in the early process of social neurobehavioral development. Ongoing negative effects of the neurobiological processes lead to secondary neurological disturbances, which further deflect the trajectory of typical brain development. This increasingly deviant process is theorized to be mitigated by early intervention, which is dependent upon experiential building blocks, because early intervention may lessen the impact of attenuated social input on the developing nervous system of the child with an ASD by decreasing the effects associated with the secondary neurological disturbances. In addition, early intervention may provide the child with an experiential and neurological foundation that maximizes the likelihood that he or she will be able to make developmental gains as he or she catches up and moves toward a more typical neurodevelopmental path.

Plausible as these ideas are, they have not been subjected to any experimental verification. Other psychological mechanisms for the effects of early intervention could be posited, such as the prevention of interfering behaviors (e.g., repetitive movements, odd visual behaviors, perseverative sampling of the same aspects of the environ-

ment). The child may thus be forced to experience a more enriched and more typical environment, resulting in more typical cortical development and the possibility of more typical linguistic and social learning and behavior.

CONCLUSION

There is an enormous amount of difficult research ahead that is needed to answer some of these questions regarding the effectiveness of early intervention on children with ASDs. It should be emphasized that at the present time, the mechanisms behind successful intervention and the characteristics of children who might have the best outcome are completely unknown. This leaves clinicians in the position of advocating for the most intense and high quality intervention for all children, with the hope that those who can will move off the autism spectrum and the remaining majority will nevertheless have the best possible outcome they can achieve.

REFERENCES

American Academy of Pediatrics, Council on Children with Disabilities, Section on Developmental Behavioral Pediatrics, Bright Futures Steering Committee and Medical Home Initiatives for Children With Special Needs Project Advisory Committee. (2006). Identifying infants and young children with developmental disorders in the medical home: An algorithm for developmental surveillance and screening. *Pediatrics, 118*(1), 405–420.

American Psychiatric Association. (2000). *Diagnostic and statistical manual of mental disorders* (4th ed., text rev.). Washington, DC: Author.

Baird, G., Charman, T., Baron-Cohen, S., Cox, A., Swettenham, J., Wheelwright, S., et al. (2000). A screening instrument for autism at 18 months of age: A six-year follow-up study. *Journal of the American Academy of Child and Adolescent Psychiatry, 39*, 694–702.

Baron-Cohen, S., Cox, A., Baird, G., Swettenham, J., & Nightingale, N. (1996). Psychological markers in the detection of autism in infancy in a large population. *British Journal of Psychiatry, 168*(2), 158–163.

Bono, M.A., Daley, T., & Sigman, M. (2004). Relations among joint attention, amount of intervention, and language gain in autism. *Journal of Autism and Developmental Disorders, 34*, 494–505.

Carrow-Woolfolk, E. (1999). *Test of Auditory Comprehension of Language–Third Edition (TACL-3)*. Austin, TX: PRO-ED.

Charman, T., & Baird, G. (2002). Practitioner review: Diagnosis of autism spectrum disorder in 2- and 3-year-old children. *Journal of Child Psychology and Psychiatry, 43*, 289–305.

Charman, T., Taylor, E., Drew, A., Cockerill, H., Brown, J., & Baird, G. (2005). Outcome at 7 years of children diagnosed with autism at age 2: Predictive validity of assessments conducted at 2 and 3 years of age and pattern of symptom change over time. *Journal of Child Psychology and Psychiatry, 46*, 500–513.

Cox, A., Klein, K., Charman, T., Baird, G., Baron-Cohen, S., Swettenham, J., et al. (1999). Autism spectrum disorders at 20 and 42 months of age: Stability of clinical and ADI-R diagnosis. *Journal of Child Psychology and Psychiatry and Allied Disciplines, 40*(5), 719–732.

Dawson, G., & Zanolli, K. (2003). Early intervention and brain plasticity in autism. In G. Bock & J. Goode (Eds.), *Autism: Neural basis and treatment possibilities. Novartis Foundation Symposia* (pp. 266–297). New York: Wiley Inter-Science.

DeMyer, M.K., Barton, S., DeMyer, W.E., Norton, J.A., Allen, J., & Steele, R. (1973). Prognosis in autism: A follow-up study. *Journal of Autism and Childhood Schizophrenia, 3*(3), 199–246.

DuPaul, G., Power, T., Anastopoulos, A., & Reid, R. (1998). *ADHD Rating Scale–IV: Checklists, norms, and clinical interpretation*. New York: Guilford Press.

Eaves, L., & Ho, H. (2004). Brief report: Stability and change in cognitive and behavioral characteristics of autism through childhood. *Journal of Autism and Developmental Disorders, 26*, 557–569.

Fein, D., Dixon, P., Paul, J., & Levin, H. (2005). Brief report: Pervasive developmental disorder can evolve into ADHD: Case illustrations. *Journal of Autism and Developmental Disorders, 35*(4), 525–534.

Fein, D., Stevens, M., Dunn, M., Waterhouse, L., Allen, D., Rapin, I., et al. (1999). Subtypes of

Pervasive Developmental Disorder: Clinical characteristics. *Child Neuropsychology, 5*(1), 1–23.

Filipek, P., Accardo, P., Baranek, G., Cook, Jr., E., Dawson, G., Gordon, B., et al. (1999). The screening and diagnosis of autism spectrum disorders. *Journal of Autism and Developmental Disorders, 29*(6), 439–475.

Gabriels, R.L., Hill, D.E., Pierce, R.A., Rogers, S.J., & Wehner, B. (2001). Predictors of treatment outcome in young children with autism: A retrospective study. *Autism, 5*, 407–429.

Gillberg, C. (1990). Autism and pervasive developmental disorders. *Journal of Child Psychology and Psychiatry, 31*, 99–119.

Gillberg, C., Ehlers, S., Schaumann, H., Joacobsen, G., Dahlgren, S., Lindblom, R., et al. (1990). Autism under age 3 years: A clinical study of 28 cases referred for autistic symptoms in infancy. *Journal of Child Psychology and Psychiatry, 6*, 921–934.

Gillberg, C., & Steffenburg, S. (1987). Outcome and prognostic factors in infantile autism and similar conditions: A population-based study of 46 cases followed through puberty. *Journal of Autism and Developmental Disorders, 17*(2), 273–287.

Howard, J., Sparkman, C., Cohen, H., Green, G., & Stanislaw, H. (2005). A comparison of intensive behavioral analytic and eclectic treatments for young children with autism. *Research in Developmental Disabilities, 26*, 359–383.

Kelley, E., Paul, J., Fein, D., & Naigles, L. (2006a). *Language profiles of high-functioning children with autism and children with a history of autism: What factors contribute to an optimal outcome?* Unpublished Doctoral Dissertation, University of Connecticut, Storrs.

Kelley, E., Paul, J., Fein, D., & Naigles, L. (2006b). Residual language deficits in optimal outcome children with a history of autism. *Journal of Autism and Developmental Disorders, 36*, 807–828.

Kinsbourne, M. (1991). Overfocusing: An apparent subtype of attention-deficit/hyperactivity disorder. In N. Amir, I. Rapin, & D. Braski (Eds.), *Pediatric neurology: Behavior and cognition of the child with brain dysfunction* (Vol. 1, pp. 18–35). *Pediatric Adolescent Medicine*. Basel: Karger.

Koegel, R.L., Koegel, L.K., & McNerney, E.K. (2001). Pivotal areas in intervention for autism. *Journal of Clinical Child Psychology, 30,* 19–32.

Koegel, L.K., Koegel, R.L., Shoshan, Y., & McNerney, E.K. (1999). Pivotal response intervention II: Preliminary long-term outcomes data. *Journal of the Association for Persons with Severe Handicaps, 24,* 186–198.

Lockyer, L., & Rutter, M. (1969). A five- to fifteen-year follow-up study of infantile psychosis: III. Psychological aspects. *British Journal of Psychiatry, 115,* 865–882.

Lockyer, L., & Rutter, M. (1970). A five- to fifteen-year follow-up study of infantile psychosis: IV. Patterns of cognitive ability. *British Journal of Social and Clinical Psychology, 9,* 152–163.

Lord, C. (1995). Follow-up of two-year-olds referred for possible autism. *Journal of Child and Adolescent Psychiatry, 36,* 1365–1382.

Lord, C., Rutter, M., DiLavore, P., & Risi, S. (1999). *Autism Diagnostic Observation Schedule–WPS edition.* Los Angeles: Western Psychological Services.

Lord, C., Storoschuk, S., Rutter, M., & Pickles, A. (1993). Using the ADI-R to diagnose autism in preschool children. *Infant Mental Health Journal, 14*(3), 234–252.

Lotter, V. (1974a). Social adjustment and placement of autistic children in Middlesex: A follow-up study. *Journal of Autism and Childhood Schizophrenia, 4*(1), 11–32.

Lotter, V. (1974b). Factors related to outcome in autistic children. *Journal of Autism and Childhood Schizophrenia, 4*(3), 263–277.

Lovaas, I. (1987). Behavioral treatment and normal educational and intellectual functioning in young autistic children. *Journal of Counseling and Clinical Psychology, 55,* 3–9.

Matson, J.L., Benavidez, D.A., Compton, L.S., Paclawskyj, T., & Baglio, C. (1996). Behavioral treatment of autistic persons: A review of research from 1980 to the present. *Research in Developmental Disabilities, 17,* 433–465.

Moore, V., & Goodson, S. (2003). How well does early diagnosis of autism stand the test of time? Follow-up study of children assessed for autism at age 2 and development of an early diagnostic service. *Autism, 7,* 47–63.

Mullen, E. (1995). *Mullen Scales of Early Learning.* Circle Pines, MN: American Guidance Service.

Mundy, P., & Crowson, M. (1997). Joint attention and early social communication: Implications for research on intervention with autism. *Journal of Autism and Developmental Disorders, 27,* 653–676.

Osterling, J., & Dawson, G. (1994). Early recognition of children with autism: A study of first birthday home videotapes. *Journal of Autism and Developmental Disorders, 24,* 247–257.

Robins, D., Fein, D., Barton, M., & Green, J. (2001). The modified checklist for autism in toddlers: An initial study investigating the early detection of autism and pervasive developmental disorders. *Journal of Autism and Developmental Disorders, 31*(2), 131–144.

Rogers, S. (2001). Diagnosis of autism before the age of 3. *International Review of Research in Mental Retardation, 23,* 1–31.

Rutter, M., Greenfeld, D., & Lockyer, L. (1967). A five to fifteen year follow-up study of infantile psychosis: II. Social and behavioral outcome. *British Journal of Psychiatry, 113,* 1183–1199.

Rutter, M., LeCouteur, A. & Lord, C. (2003). *Autism Diagnostic Interview–Revised.* Los Angeles: Western Psychological Services.

Sallows, G.O., & Graupner, T.D. (2005). Intensive behavioral treatment for children with autism: Four-year outcome and predictors. *American Journal on Mental Retardation, 110*(6), 417–438.

Schopler, E., Reichler, R.J., DeVellis, R.F., & Daly, K. (1980). Toward objective classification of childhood autism: Childhood Autism Rating Scale (CARS). *Journal of Autism and Developmental Disorders, 10*(1), 91–103.

Schopler, E., Reichler, R., & Renner, B. (1988). *The Childhood Autism Rating Scale.* Los Angeles: Western Psychological Services.

Sigman, M., & McGovern, C.W. (2005). Improvement in cognitive and language skills from preschool to adolescence in autism. *Journal of Autism and Developmental Disorders, 35,* 15–23.

Sigman, M., & Ruskin, E. (1999). *Continuity and change in the social competence of children with autism, Down syndrome, and developmental delays.* Boston: Blackwell Publishing.

Smith, T. (1996). Are other treatments effective? In C. Maurice, G. Green, & S.C. Luce (Eds.), *Behavioral intervention for young children with autism: A manual for parents and professionals.* Austin, TX: PRO-ED.

Smith, T., Groen, A.D., & Wynn, J.W. (2000). Randomized trial of intensive early intervention for children with pervasive developmental disorder. *American Journal on Mental Retardation, 105,* 269–285.

Sparrow, S.S., Balla, D.A., & Cicchetti, D.V. (1984). *Vineland Adaptive Behavior Scales.* Circle Pines, MN: American Guidance Service.

Stevens, M.C., Fein, D.A., Dunn, M., Allen, D., Waterhouse, L.H., Feinstein, C., et al. (2000). Subgroups of children with autism by cluster analysis: A longitudinal examination. *Journal of the American Academy of Child and Adolescent Psychiatry, 39,* 346–352.

Stone, W.L., Lee, E.B., Ashford, L., Brissie, J., Hepburn, S.L., Coonrod, E.E., et al. (1999). Can autism be diagnosed accurately in children under 3 years? *Journal of Child Psychology and Psychiatry and Allied Disciplines, 40*(2), 219–226.

Sutera, S., Pandey, J., Esser, E., Rosenthal, M., Wilson, L., Barton, M., et al. (2007). Predictors of optimal outcome in toddlers diagnosed with autism spectrum disorders. *Journal of Autism and Developmental Disabilities, 37*(1), 98–107.

Szatmari, P., Bryson, S.E., Boyle, M.H., Streiner, D.L., & Duku, E. (2003). Predictors of outcome among high functioning children with autism and Asperger syndrome. *Journal of Child Psychology and Psychiatry, 44*(4), 520–528.

Volkmar, F., Chawarska, K., & Klin, A. (2005). Autism in infancy and early childhood. *Annual Review of Psychology, 56,* 315–36.

Volkmar, F., Klin, A., Siegel, B., Szatmari, P., Lord, C., Campbell, M., et al. (1994). Field trial for autistic disorder in DSM-IV. *American Journal of Psychiatry, 151,* 1361–1367.

Volkmar, F., Lord, C., Bailey, A., Schultz, R., & Klin, A. (2004). Autism and pervasive developmental disorders. *Journal of Child Psychology and Psychiatry, 45*(1), 135–170.

World Health Organization. (1994). *International Classification of Diseases, tenth revision (ICD-10).* Geneva: Author.

13

Autism Spectrum Disorders

A Conceptualization

Pasquale J. Accardo

Several theories attempt to clarify the core deficit in autism spectrum disorders (ASDs) and then derive the widely diverse developmental and behavioral symptomatology from that core deficit. Although each theory succeeds in explaining many behaviors, none has convincingly addressed the entire gamut. Similarly, a number of subdivisions of the autism spectrum have been proposed, but none of these nosologies successfully relates to etiology, treatment responsiveness and long-term outcome. The present conceptualization will not attempt to resolve these areas of controversy, but will instead present a rough working model of ways to think about ASDs that can be used to address the most serious issue for the primary health care provider—screening and early diagnosis.

HISTORICAL PERSPECTIVE

When Kanner first described autism in 1943 (Table 13.1), there was no other disorder with which it could be even approximately compared. Some of the observed behaviors recalled similar symptoms in schizophrenia, depression, and severe neglect (Wing, 1997). Later research would place ASDs solidly in the category of neurodevelopmental disorders, but in 1943, the only two such disabilities were cerebral palsy (CP) and mental retardation (now referred to as intellectual disability [ID]). The excellent motor skills present in most younger children with ASDs ruled out any degree of

CP, whereas the advanced performance of Kanner's subjects on the Seguin form board, a measure of nonverbal intelligence, seemed to exclude ID.

Neurodevelopmental disorders that presented with uneven cognitive profiles were relatively unknown at mid-century. The late nineteenth century had identified the extremely rare syndrome of *dyslexia* (i.e., a severe reading deficit in the presence of average to above average general intelligence), but this had not yet been expanded into the broader entity of learning disabilities. At the time, dyslexia was still receiving psychoanalytic explanations. Language disorders such as acquired aphasias had long been recognized in adults, but developmental language disorders presenting in children had gone unrecognized.

Strauss's pioneering studies of brain-damaged children described an increasing number of behaviors associated with ASDs at the extreme end of the spectrum of brain damage (Strauss & Lehtinen, 1947), but it would be three decades before the spectrum of neurodevelopmental disorders would develop sufficiently for clinicians and researchers to recognize where ASDs fit into the broader classification of childhood disability.

CLINICAL PRESENTATION

The clinical diagnosis of an ASD requires a child to present with significant impairments in communication, socializa-

Table 13.1.   Kanner's (1943) description of autism

Inability to relate to people
Failure to use language to communicate
Obsessive desire to maintain sameness
Fascination with inanimate objects
Good rote memory
Parents who were variously described as perfectionistic, rigid, intelligent, obsessive, detached, and cold ("refrigerator" parents)

ization, as well as with some occasional repetitive/restrictive behaviors. ASDs are considered when children's difficulties in the relevant areas represent more significant delays than can be explained by their general cognitive level. The uneven developmental pattern in ASDs can occur at levels of intelligence all the way from gifted to severely impaired.

tion, and repetitive/restrictive behaviors (Table 13.2, Columns 1–3). A problem in the early identification of ASDs is that children with severe general cognitive impairment will present with significant problems in communication and social-

Kanner's (1943) original separation of ASDs from ID turned out to be premature. By the mid-1980s, approximately 85% of people diagnosed with ASDs were also considered to have an ID. Because of the evolving criteria and increased sensitivity to diagnoses of ASDs, many children with

Table 13.2.   Behavioral features of autism

Qualitative impairment in social interaction	Qualitative impairment in communication	Atypical (restrictive, repetitive) behaviors	Sensory integration symptoms	Attention-deficit/ hyperactivity disorder (ADHD) behaviors
No eye contact	Mutism	Absence of pretend play	Selective about menu and the texture, color, and temperature of food, as well as its position on a plate	Hyperactivity
Poor eye contact	Language delay	Preoccupation with parts of objects		Constant, often purposeless movement
"In own little world"	Echolalia: immediate, delayed; movie scripts, books	Lines up/sorts toys		Impulsivity
No peer interaction		Water play		Daredevil behavior
Peer interaction limited to gross motor activities	Refers to self in third person	Perseveration	Tactile (overly touchy, likes to feel specific things/textures— e.g., hair)	Emotional outbursts
	Pronominal reversal	Flapping		Inattention; sometimes gets overfocused on objects or unusual aspects of objects
No reciprocity or sharing	Language regression	Stereotypies		
Does not read faces	Equinus gait	Rocking	Tactile aversive (dislikes certain textures/things— e.g., sand, tags in clothes)	
Limited or no facial or emotional expressivity	Acts as if deaf	Head banging		
	No protodeclarative pointing ("joint attention")	Self-injurious behavior		
Treats people like objects (climbs over people as if they were furniture/ things)	Good rote memory	Spinning/twirling		
	Poor pragmatic language/conversational skills	Likes fans		
Laughs inappropriately		Stiff/noncuddly baby with arching		
	Lack of communicative intent/lack of frustration over failure to communicate	Inflexible routines/rituals		
		Preservation of sameness		
	Masters very few signs	Insensitivity to pain		

Columns 1–3 describe behaviors under the three impairment categories necessary for a diagnosis of an autism spectrum disorder. It should be noted that many communication and socialization items could appear in either column. The primary language deficit is in the social use of language, whereas the primary socialization deficit relates to communicating with others. The behaviors in Column 4 suggest the possibility of an additional impairment category of sensory integration disorder; by extension it is possible to classify some of these behaviors under Column 3, but that would not help in identifying an appropriate treatment resource. As discussed in the chapter text, all children with a pervasive developmental disorder exhibit sufficient behavioral features to qualify for a diagnosis of ADHD (Column 5).

milder impairments are being identified such that the percentage of comorbid ID is approximating, although still above, 50%. It is this improved identification that has contributed to the perception of an "autism epidemic" (Shattuck, 2006).

This scenario is similar to what occurred when learning disabilities were first separated from ID. The mid-twentieth century saw the identification of the "eight-hour-retarded child" (i.e., the child who was intellectually impaired during his or her 8 hours in a classroom, but who for the remainder of the nonschool day and for his or her entire life outside of and after school was actually both competent and intelligent). Such children had language disorders or language-based learning disabilities that were misdiagnosed as ID by the older versions of the Stanford-Binet Intelligence Test, which were heavily weighted in favor of verbal abilities. It is still common to find young school-age children placed in slow classes for "developmental delay" when their only assumed delay is an immature attention span; they can actually learn at age-appropriate levels, but they have difficulty cooperating with the classroom routine and structure, which impairs their ability to consistently demonstrate what they have learned. Once again, the misclassification of an uneven cognitive/developmental pattern is made because of the assumption of smooth, level delay patterns. ASDs would seem to be best characterized as the last identified and most extreme pattern of *uneven* cognitive developmental patterns.

ASDs still share components with the spectrum of neurodevelopmental disabilities.

- *Cerebral palsy:* Toe walking occurs as a transient normal variant, but it is more common in children with most developmental disabilities, especially in those with language disorders, and it is most prolonged and striking in children with ASDs (Accardo, 1997; Accardo, Morrow, Heaney, Whitman, & Tomazic, 1992;

Accardo & Whitman, 1989). Unlike the toe walking associated with CP, there are no neuromotor findings (e.g., spasticity in the lower extremities, increased deep tendon reflexes, upgoing Babinski reflexes). Over time, one occasionally encounters the eventual shortening of the Achilles tendons from the persistent toe walking present in children with ASDs.

- *Intellectual disability:* Many children with ASDs are comorbid for ID. The degree of ID may represent one of the best prognostic indicators with regard to responsiveness to therapeutic intervention (Coplan & Jawad, 2005). Professionals frequently discount intelligence testing in preschool children with ASDs, where it can be difficult, although not impossible, to obtain valid test results. When a child with an ASD succeeds in cooperating with the examiner, positive or high results can be considered valid. Failures must be evaluated on a case-by-case basis with regard to the degree of cooperation and comprehension obtained. Alternately, too much weight should not be given to splinter skills or isolated savant skills unless there is evidence to support generalization to nonverbal intelligence.

- *Attention-deficit/hyperactivity disorder (ADHD):* The *Diagnostic and Statistical Manual of Mental Disorders, Fourth Edition, Text Revision* (*DSM-IV-TR*; American Psychiatric Association, 2000) system precludes the diagnosis of ADHD in children with a pervasive developmental disorder (PDD), but clinically most children with a PDD display all the clinical and behavioral findings of ADHD (Table 13.2, Column 5). Precluding a separate diagnosis for ADHD makes sense only if it is understood that almost all children with a PDD also have ADHD.

- *Learning disabilities:* Children with ASDs frequently test higher in nonverbal problem-solving abilities or performance intelligence quotient (IQ) scores. Thus, they perform much better in mathematics than in reading. Alternately, children with Asperger syndrome (AS) have a cognitive and behavioral profile similar to children with right-brain learning disabilities (Asperger, 1991).

- *Language disorders:* All children with ASDs have significant communication disorders. Communication disorders can be divided along three closely interrelated language streams—expressive language (i.e., what the child can say), receptive language (i.e., what speech the child understands), and pragmatic language (i.e., all the nonverbal components of human communication, including facial expression, gesture, body posture, pausing, and intonation). The main reason that the core deficit in ASDs has been classified as a deficit in socialization is the lack of impaired communication at age 3 years in children identified with AS. However, all people with AS eventually demonstrate significant deficits in pragmatic language. Whether or not they have language disorders, all people have better receptive language than expressive language skills. The reverse only appears to occur in ASDs when children's rote expression seems to be more advanced than their receptive skills. Such echoing or parroting, however, is not true communication. Many of the characteristic features of ASDs can be alternately considered to be problems with the social use of language (i.e., socialization impairments) or pragmatic language deficits (i.e., communication impairments), which are either communication or socialization deficits.

SCREENING

In recent years, increasing emphasis has been placed on the early identification of ASDs since intensive treatment has been demonstrated to be most effective when begun during the preschool years. Whereas ASDs are not often diagnosed until just before the age of 36 months, most ASD cases will be identifiable by 24 months. There is increasing pressure from parent groups for primary care physicians to routinely screen for ASDs to facilitate early identification and treatment. At present, there is no ideal screening instrument or protocol for ASDs (Committee on Children with Disabilities, 2001a). The absence of such an instrument is significant because the pediatric health care provider remains the only professional who routinely has consistent and repeated contact with all children from birth to age 3 years.

There are a number of screening tests (Table 13.3), but these are not sufficiently sensitive and specific to warrant universal usage. Many await validation. There seems to be a chronic tendency for instruments to overidentify children with developmental disorders other than ASDs and to miss children with the milder ASD variants. In addition, problems often exist with the application of these tests in the pediatric clinic setting. Administration times of greater than 5–10 minutes are unacceptable. Instruments that rely entirely on parent questionnaires

---

Table 13.3. Autism screening instruments

Autism Behavior Checklist (ABC; Krug, Arick, & Almond, 1980)

Autism Screening Questionnaire (ASQ; Berument, Rutter, Lord, Pickles, & Bayley, 1999)

Checklist for Autism in Toddlers (CHAT; Baron-Cohen, Wheelwright, Cox, Baird, Charman, Swettenham, et al., 2000)

Communication and Symbolic Behavior Scales Developmental Profile™ (CSBS DP™), First Normed Edition, Infant-Toddler Checklist (Wetherby & Prizant, 2002)

Modified Checklist for Autism in Toddlers (M-CHAT; Robins, Fein, Barton, & Green (2001)

Pervasive Developmental Disorder Screening Test (PDDST) Stage One (Siegel, 2004)

Screening Tool for Autism in Two-Year Olds (STAT; Stone, Coonrod, & Ousley, 2000)

Social Communicative Questionnaire (SCQ; Rutter, Bailey, & Lord, 2003)

require a certain reading level, and even more importantly, a mindset that can respond accurately to behavioral questions that may require fairly subtle distinctions. Judging social interactions in 2-year-old toddlers who have had no formal exposure to structured peer group settings can be quite difficult. Limited social interaction presents on the autism spectrum along a gradient, with the most severe cases treating all human beings like blocks of wood. Children with milder cases actually interact reasonably well with their parents and siblings, whereas children with the mildest cases can interact socially with everyone except their age peers.

Closer examination of the components of several existing screening instruments may provide a useful perspective (Tables 13.4 and 13.5). Pretend play and joint attention stand out as major markers for the early identification of ASDs. Nevertheless, items such as these may not represent the most practical or useful approach for the pediatric office setting. A fair amount of interpretation is required by both the parents and the physician. The evolution of joint attention may not exhibit as rigid a timetable as suggested by the information presented in Table 13.6, and this would contribute to a weakening of both its sensitivity and specificity for the identification of ASDs. If later research succeeds in demonstrating that joint attention can be formatted into such a timetable, it would certainly represent the single most effective early marker for the identification of ASDs. In lieu of formally validated screening tests,

Table 13.4. Checklist for Autism in Toddlers (CHAT) items—by history (A) and by observation (B)—that are most sensitive to a diagnosis of autism

A5: pretend play

A7: protodeclarative pointing/point to something interesting—to share interest

B2: looks at something pointed to

B3: pretend play

B4: point to something named

Source: Baron-Cohen, Allen, and Gillberg (1992).

Table 13.5. Modified Checklist for Autism in Toddlers (M-CHAT) items most sensitive to autism

2. Does your child take an interest in other children?

7. Does your child ever use his/her index finger to point, to indicate interest in something?

9. Does your child ever bring objects over to you (parent) to show you something?

13. Does your child imitate you?

14. Does your child respond to his/her name when you call?

15. If you point at a toy across the room, does your child look at it?

Source: Robins, Fein, Barton, and Green (2001).

researchers have recommended checklists of findings to help clinicians make early identifications (Table 13.7). Instead of recommending a specific screening test, the Committee on Children with Disabilities (2001b) suggested that the practitioner explore aspects of the children's communicative and social interactive behavior by using a series of 16 exploratory questions, many of which are open ended, so the interview process can easily take 15–30 minutes and thus not qualify as a screening test by both the time requirement and the lack of a dichotomous outcome (Table 13.8).

One of the first decisions that must be made regarding the identification of a developmental disorder is the age at which it can be identified with a reasonable degree of certitude. Behaviors typical in children younger than 1 year of age who later qualify

Table 13.6. Joint attention

Responding Joint Attention (RJA) [passive skills]	
8 months	Gaze monitoring: child looks to where mother is looking
10–12 months	Follow a point: child looks to where mother is pointing
Initiating Joint Attention (IJA) [active skills]	
12–14 months	Proto-imperative pointing: child points to desired object
14–16 months	Proto-declarative pointing: child "comments" on object pointed to
14–16 months	Showing: child demonstrates something interesting

Sources: Johnson (2004) and Mundy and Burnette (2005).

Table 13.7. Early markers for autism

Red flags	Five early signs of autism
No babbling by 12 months	Does the baby respond to his or her name when called by caregiver?
No pointing or other gestures by 12 months	Does the young child engage in joint attention?
No single words by 16 months	Does the child imitate others?
No two-word spontaneous utterances by 24 months	Does the child respond emotionally to others?
Loss of any language or social skills at any age	Does the baby engage in pretend play?

Sources: Choueiri and Bridgemohan (2005) and Kasari and Wong (2002).

for a diagnosis of autism (Table 13.9) have been identified, but it is doubtful whether these behaviors can be considered diagnostic. Failure to turn to one's name at 1 year of age is again suspicious and too restrictive a base for a diagnosis. Although ASDs must be diagnosable by 3 years of age, most children will exhibit sufficient characteristic symptoms between 18 and 24 months of age. Clinicians should recall the three major groups of behaviors characteristic of ASDs (i.e., impairments in communication, socialization deficits, and fixations). If evaluating social interactions is problematic, then it seems logical to resort to language as an initial marker. This is especially appropriate because it allows for an association of an ASD with an existing screening procedure.

Communication disorders are the single most common developmental problem in children. Approximately 80% of all children receiving early intervention services qualify for speech therapy (Accardo et al., 1999). Pediatricians routinely assess children's language development at well-child checkups during the second year of life. The two most critical (i.e., "sudden death") milestones are the absence of words at 18 months of age and the absence of two-word phrases and a vocabulary of less than 50 words at 24 months of age.

Children with ASDs present with one of three language patterns (Accardo, 2000, 2002, 2004):

1. No words at 24 months (more significant if words that had been present at 18 months were later "lost")

2. A vocabulary of fewer than 50 words and no two-word phrases at 24 months (more significant if words that had been present at 18 months were "lost" prior to 24 months)

3. A vocabulary of more than 50 words and the use of two-word phrases, but with the additional presence of a significant percentage of echoing

These language milestones are part of a routine developmental surveillance

Table 13.8. The pediatrician should ask the parent whether the child . . .

Speaks as well as his or her peers
Makes good eye contact
Responds selectively to his or her name
Acts as if in own world
Tunes others out
Has a social smile that can be elicited reciprocally
Communicates wants
Follows simple commands
Shows things
Points to interesting objects or events
Has long, severe tantrums
Has repetitive, odd, stereotypic behaviors
Has an unusual attachment to inanimate objects
Plays alone
Plays with toys in an unusual manner
Engages in pretend play

Source: Committee on Children with Disabilities (2001b).

Table 13.9. Behavioral features in children younger than 12 months of age who later qualify for a diagnosis of autism

Does not anticipate being picked up
Does not demonstrate affection toward familiar people
Shows no interest in nonsibling children/peers
Does not reach for familiar person
Does not play simple interaction games

Source: Klin, Volkmar, and Sparrow (1992).

(Accardo & Capute, 1979, 2005; Capute & Accardo, 1996a, 1996b), except for the fact that one must specifically inquire as to the percentage of a child's utterances that are echoed or repeated. Starting from the presentation of several specific language markers at the age of 24 months, one can add on several other characteristics of ASDs to yield a screening *protocol*—as opposed to a screening test—that should be manageable in the busy office setting.

SCREENING PROTOCOL FOR AUTISM SPECTRUM DISORDERS

Figure 13.1 presents a protocol that can be used in screening for ASDs (see the appendix at the end of this chapter for a photo-

---

Screening Protocol for Autism Spectrum Disorders

Child's name _____ Date _____

Age _____ Sex _____ Race _____

Diagnosis
_____ None (typical)
_____ Communication disorder
_____ Developmental delay
_____ Autism spectrum disorder possible
_____ Other

Part A

1.	50-word vocabulary/two-word sentences	Yes/NA	(0)	No	(1)
2.	Echolalia	No/NA	(0)	Yes	(1)
3.	Mutism	No	(0)	Yes	(2)
4.	Regression	No	(0)	Yes	(1)

Part B

1.	Family history of autism, PDD-NOS, AS, depression, bipolar disorder	No	(0)	Yes	(1)
2.	Autism, PDD, AS in a sibling	No	(0)	Yes	(1)
3.	Toe walking (by history)	No	(0)	Yes	(1)
4.	Eye contact	Good	(0)	Poor	(1)
5.	Reads faces	Yes	(0)	No	(1)
6.	Flapping	No	(0)	Yes	(1)
7.	Picky eater	No	(0)	Yes	(1)

Part C

1.	OFC > 1.5 *SD* above mean	No	(0)	Yes	(1)
2.	Posteriorly rotated ears	No	(0)	Yes	(1)
3.	Toe walking (by observation)	No	(0)	Yes	(1)

Total score: _____

From Rogers, B.T., & Accardo, P.J. (2005). The clinical use of the Capute Scales. In P.J. Accardo & A.J. Capute, *The Capute Scales: Cognitive Adaptive Test/Clinical Linguistic & Auditory Milestone Scale (CAT/CLAMS)* (p. 32). Baltimore: Paul H. Brookes Publishing Co.; Copyright © 2008 Kennedy Fellows Association; adapted by permission. In *Autism Frontiers: Clinical Issues and Innovations,* edited by Bruce K. Shapiro & Pasquale J. Accardo (2008, Paul H. Brookes Publishing Co., Inc.).

Figure 13.1. A screening protocol for autism spectrum disorders. (From Rogers, B.T., & Accardo, P.J. [2005]. The clinical use of the Capute Scales. In P.J. Accardo & A.J. Capute, *The Capute Scales: Cognitive Adaptive Test/Clinical Linguistic & Auditory Milestone Scale [CAT/CLAMS]* [p. 32]. Baltimore: Paul H. Brookes Publishing Co.; Copyright © 2008 Kennedy Fellows Association; adapted by permission.) (*Key:* PDD-NOS = pervasive developmental disorder-not otherwise specified; AS = Asperger syndrome; OFC = occipitofrontal circumference; *SD* = standard deviation.)

copiable version). Each protocol item has a strong correlation—usually a greater than 50% overlap is reported—with the presence of an ASD. The process is divided into three sections:

1. Part A: Communication Screen
2. Part B: History
3. Part C: Physical Examination

Part A: Communication Screen

Part A involves a preliminary language history of four questions. Because receiving a diagnosis of autism requires language delay or deviance, a score of 0 on this section ends the screening.

1. Typically developing 2-year-old children have a vocabulary of more than 50 words and are also beginning to put two words together in short sentences or phrases. Failure to attain both of these milestones is considered reason for automatic referral for formal language assessment. Clinicians are helped by the fact that the two milestones are linked or associated such that they both occur together (i.e., one does not occur without the other). Score 1 point if either milestone is absent.

2. If more than 20% of a child's utterances are repeated, echoed, or parroted, then language deviance is present. Score 1 point if the child presents with more than 20% echoing.

3. Mutism, the absence of any spoken language, is scored 2 points because it masks both items A1 and A2. (If the child receives a score of 2 for mutism, then items A1 and A2 should be coded as 0 or "not applicable".)

4. Score 1 point if regression is present (i.e., the child's vocabulary has decreased by at least half in the period between 12 and 24 months).

Part B: History

Part B asks for further historical data concerning variables known to be associated with ASDs.

1. Is there a family history of ASDs, pervasive developmental disorder-not otherwise specified (PDD-NOS), AS, major depression, bipolar disorder, or schizophrenia? The presence of one close (i.e., first or second degree) relative with one of these conditions is scored 1 point.

2. Is there an observed or diagnosed presence of autism, PDD-NOS, or AS in any of the child's siblings? Such a presence is scored 1 point (in addition to B1).

3. When the child first started walking, did he or she tend to walk on his or her toes (i.e., an equinus gait, or "toe walking") for at least 3 months? Score 1 point if the answer is yes.

4. When the child does attempt to communicate, does he or she look at the recipient? Score 1 point if eye contact is indirect (e.g., the child looks at the recipient's mouth or just past the recipient's head), fleeting, or absent.

5. Can the child read, understand, and/or appropriately respond to the emotional expressions on the faces of others (i.e., does the child smile back when a parent smiles at him or her, pause when the parent frowns or looks stern, smile or laugh when the parent makes a silly face)? Score 1 point if the answer is no.

6. When the child gets excited or distressed, does he or she tend to flap his or her hands while held in a "surrender" posture? Score 1 point if the answer is yes.

7. If one were to list all the solid foods that their child eats, is the total number of items less than 20? Score 1 point if the child eats less than 20 different solid foods.

Part C: Physical Examination

Part C contains several observational items to be completed as part of the physical examination.

1. Does the child's head circumference (occipitofrontal circumference [OFC]) measure greater than 1.5 standard deviation (*SD*) above the mean for age? Score 1 point for OFC > + 1.5 *SD*. Although many developmental disabilities are associated with microcephaly, one of the earliest signs of autism may be a rapidly enlarging head late in the first year or early in the second year of life (Accardo, 2001; Fidler, Bailey, & Smalley, 2000; Gilberg & de Souza, 2002).

2. Are the child's ears rotated posteriorly more than 10 degrees from the vertical? Score 1 point if the answer is yes. Gillberg and Coleman (2000) reported that more than half of children with autism have such a marker.

3. Has the child been observed to toe walk? Score 1 point if the answer is yes (in addition to B3).

Scores on this screening protocol can range from 0 to 13. Generally, children with ASDs do not score below 3, and they typically score above 5. These cutoffs are based on clinical experience. Research is needed to demonstrate the best cutoff score for ASDs.

Items A1, A3, B1, B2, C1, and C2 would typically be included in the 2-year-old well-child checkup. The questions for Part A and the questions and examinations for Parts B and C should take no longer than 2 minutes.

▨ CONCLUSION

The employment of an early screening device assumes continuity in the pattern of the evolution of a neurodevelopmental disorder. In fact, CP and mild ID can rarely be identified in the first year of life unless they are very severe. The nature of developmental processes makes the identification of milder variants fairly difficult. Sowell (1997, 2001) collected reports of many cases of children who seemed to be delayed in language early on but who later did not exhibit any diagnosable disability. As many as half of the children who present with expressive language delay at the age of 2 years can completely catch up with no therapeutic intervention by the age of 3 years.

Screening tests assume to target the basic underlying deficit in ASDs. This, in turn, presumes that the wide variety of ASDs are unitary. A comparison with other major categories of neurodevelopmental disorders makes such an assumption highly unlikely. For every child who qualifies for a diagnosis of an ASD, Gaussian distribution of multiply determined traits would suggest at least five other children with some features of ASDs who would not qualify for formal ASD diagnoses. The items selected for a screening test may also commonly occur in these borderline ASD cases and thus yield a very poor specificity.

Most research on screening for ASDs relies on the use of populations of at-risk children (i.e., those who have siblings with ASDs). This assumes—but does not document—continuity with the population of children-at-large to be screened. Such research will be most helpful in identifying items that may be of use in less selected populations but that must be tested separately before general usage can be recommended. It is imperative that the rush toward earlier identification not confuse the presence of risk markers with diagnosis.

▨ REFERENCES

Accardo, P.J. (1997). On one's toes about developmental language disorders. *Journal of Pediatrics, 130*, 509–510.

Accardo, P.J. (2000). Diagnostic issues in autism. In P.J. Accardo, C. Magnusen, & A.J. Capute

(Eds.), *Autism: Clinical and research frontiers* (pp. 103–131). Timonium, MD: York Press.

Accardo, P.J. (2000). Early diagnosis of autism and Asperger syndrome. *AAP Grand Rounds, 3*, 41–42.

Accardo, P.J. (2001). Macrocephaly and autism. *AAP Grand Rounds, 5*, 29.

Accardo, P.J. (2002). The child who does not talk: A pediatric overview. In P.J. Accardo, B.T. Rogers, & A.J. Capute (Eds.), *Disorders of language* (pp. 113–124). Timonium, MD; York Press.

Accardo, P.J. (2004). Screening and diagnosis for autistic spectrum disorders. In B. Gupta (Ed.), *Autistic spectrum disorders in children* (pp. 125–148). New York: Marcel Dekker.

Accardo, P.J., & Capute, A.J. (1979). *The pediatrician and the developmentally delayed child: A clinical textbook on mental retardation. Monographs in developmental pediatrics* (Vol. 2). Baltimore: University Park Press.

Accardo, P.J., & Capute, A.J. (2005). *The Capute Scales: Cognitive Adaptive Test/Clinical Linguistic & Auditory Milestone Scale*. Baltimore: Paul H. Brookes Publishing Co.

Accardo, P.J., Morrow, J., Heaney, M.S., Whitman, B.Y., & Tomazic, T. (1992). Toe walking and language development. *Clinical Pediatrics, 31*, 158–160.

Accardo, P.J., et al. (1999). *Clinical practice guideline: Report of the recommendations: Communication disorders, assessment, and intervention for young children (Age 0–3 years)*. Albany: New York State Department of Health.

Accardo, P.J., & Whitman, B.Y. (1989). Toe walking: A marker for language disorders in the developmentally disabled. *Clinical Pediatrics, 28*, 347–350.

American Psychiatric Association. (2000). *Diagnostic and statistical manual of mental disorders* (4th ed., text rev.). Washington, DC: Author.

Asperger, H. (1991). 'Autistic psychopathy' in childhood (U. Frith, Trans.). In U. Frith (Ed.), *Autism and Asperger syndrome* (pp. 37–92). Cambridge, United Kingdom: Cambridge University Press. (Orignal work published 1944)

Baron-Cohen, S., Allen, J., & Gillberg, C. (1992). Can autism be detected at 18 months? The needle, the haystack, and the CHAT. *British Journal of Psychiatry, 161*, 839–843.

Baron-Cohen, S., Wheelwright, S., Cox, A., Baird, G., Charman, T., Swettenham, J., et al. (2000).

Early identification of autism by the Checklist for Autism in Toddlers (CHAT). *Journal of the Royal Society of Medicine, 93*(10), 521–525.

Berument, S.K., Rutter, M., Lord, C., Pickles, A., & Bayley, A. (1999). Autism Screening Questionnaire: Diagnostic validity. *British Journal of Psychiatry, 175*, 444–451.

Capute, A.J., & Accardo, P.J. (1996a). The infant neurodevelopmental assessment: A clinical interpretive manual for CAT-CLAMS in the first two years of life: Part 1. *Current Problems in Pediatrics, 26*, 238–257.

Capute, A.J., & Accardo, P.J. (1996b). The infant neurodevelopmental assessment: A clinical interpretive manual for CAT-CLAMS in the first two years of life: Part 2. *Current Problems in Pediatrics, 26*, 279–306.

Choueiri, R., & Bridgemohan, C. (2005). To make the biggest difference, screen early for autism spectrum disorders. *Contemporary Pediatrics, 22*, 54–64.

Committee on Children with Disabilities. (2001a). The pediatrician's role in the diagnosis and management of autistic spectrum disorder in children. *Pediatrics, 107*, 1221–1226.

Committee on Children with Disabilities. (2001b). Technical report: The pediatrician's role in the diagnosis and management of autistic spectrum disorder in children. *Pediatrics, 107*. Retrieved from http://www.pediatrics.org/cgi/content/full/107/5/e85

Coplan, J., & Jawad, A.F. (2005). Modeling clinical outcome of children with autistic spectrum disorders. *Pediatrics, 116*, 117–122.

Fidler, D.J., Bailey, J.N., & Smalley, S.L. (2000). Macrocephaly in autism and other pervasive developmental disorders. *Developmental Medicine and Child Neurology, 42*, 737–740.

Filipek, P.A., Accardo, P.J., Ashwal, S., Baranek, G.T., Cook, E.H., Jr., Dawson, G., et al. (2000). Practice parameter: Screening and diagnosis of autism: Report of the Quality Standards Subcommittee of the American Academy of Neurology and the Child Neurology Society. *Neurology, 55*, 468–479.

Filipek, P.A., Accardo, P.J., Baranek, G.T., Cook, E.H., Jr., Dawson, G., Gordon, B., et al. (1999). The screening and diagnosis of autistic spectrum disorders. *Journal of Autism and Developmental Disorders, 29*, 437–482.

Gillberg, C., & Coleman, M. (2000). *The biology of the autistic syndromes*. London: Mac Keith Press.

Gilberg, C., & de Souza, L. (2002). Head circumference in autism, Asperger syndrome, and ADHD: A comparative study. *Developmental Medicine and Child Neurology, 44,* 296–300.

Johnson, C.P. (2004). Early clinical characteristics of children with autism. In V.B. Gupta (Ed.), *Autistic spectrum disorders in children* (pp. 85–123). New York: Marcel Dekker.

Kanner, L. (1943). Autistic disturbances of affective contact. *Nervous Child, 2,* 217–250.

Kasari, C., & Wong, C. (2002). Five early signs of autism. *EP Magazine.* November, 60–62.

Klin, A., Volkmar, F.R., & Sparrow, S.S. (1992). Autistic social dysfunction: Some limitations of the theory of mind hypothesis. *Journal of Child Psychology, Psychiatry, and Allied Disciplines, 33,* 861–876.

Krug, D.A., Arick, J.R., & Almond, P.J. (1980). Behavior checklist for identifying severely handicapped individuals with high levels of autistic behavior. *Journal of Child Psychology and Psychiatry and Allied Disciplines, 21*(3), 221–229.

Mundy, P., & Burnette, C. (2005). Joint attention and neurodevelopmental models of autism. In F.R. Volkmar, R. Paul, A. Klin, & D. Cohen (Eds.), *Handbook of autism and pervasive developmental disorders* (pp. 650–681). New York: John Wiley & Sons.

Robins, D.L., Fein, D., Barton, M.L., & Green, J.A. (2001). The Modified Checklist for Autism in Toddlers: An initial study investigating the early detection of autism and pervasive developmental disorders. *Journal of Autism and Developmental Disorders, 31,* 131–144.

Rogers, B.T., & Accardo, P.T. (2005). The clinical use of the Capute Scales. In P.J. Accardo & A.J. Capute, *The Capute Scales: Cognitive Adaptive Test/Clinical Linguistic & Auditory Milestone Scale (CAT/CLAMS)* (pp. 29–40). Baltimore: Paul H. Brookes Publishing Co.

Rutter, M., Bailey, A., & Lord, C. (2003). *Social Communication Questionnaire (SCQ).* Los Angeles: Western Psychological Services.

Shattuck, P.T. (2006). The contribution of diagnostic substitution to the growing administrative prevalence of autism in US special education. *Pediatrics, 117,* 1028–1037.

Siegel, B. (2004). *Pervasive Developmental Disorder Screening Test, Second Edition (PDDST–II), Stage One.* San Antonio, TX: Harcourt Assessment.

Sowell, T. (1997). *Late-talking children.* New York: Basic Books.

Sowell, T. (2001). *The Einstein syndrome: Bright children who talk late.* New York: Basic Books.

Stone, W.L., Coonrod, E.E., & Ousley, O.Y. (2000). Brief report: Screening Tool for Autism in Two-Year-Olds (STAT): Development and preliminary data. *Journal of Autism and Developmental Disorders, 30*(6), 607–612.

Strauss, A.A., & Lehtinen, L.E. (1947). *Psychopathology and education of the brain-injured child.* New York: Grune & Stratton.

Wetherby, A.M., & Prizant, B.M. (2002). *Communication and Symbolic Behavior Scales Developmental Profile™ (CSBS DP™), first normed edition.* Baltimore: Paul H. Brookes Publishing Co.

Wing, L. (1997). The history of ideas on autism: Legends, myths and reality. *Autism, 1,* 13–23.

Screening Protocol for
Autism Spectrum Disorders

Screening Protocol for Autism Spectrum Disorders

Child's name _____ Date _____

Age _____ Sex _____ Race _____

Diagnosis   _____ None (typical)

_____ Communication disorder

_____ Developmental delay

_____ Autism spectrum disorder possible

_____ Other

Part A

1.	50-word vocabulary/two-word sentences	Yes/NA	(0)	No	(1)
2.	Echolalia	No/NA	(0)	Yes	(1)
3.	Mutism	No	(0)	Yes	(2)
4.	Regression	No	(0)	Yes	(1)

Part B

1.	Family history of autism, PDD-NOS, AS, depression, bipolar disorder	No	(0)	Yes	(1)
2.	Autism, PDD, AS in a sibling	No	(0)	Yes	(1)
3.	Toe walking (by history)	No	(0)	Yes	(1)
4.	Eye contact	Good	(0)	Poor	(1)
5.	Reads faces	Yes	(0)	No	(1)
6.	Flapping	No	(0)	Yes	(1)
7.	Picky eater	No	(0)	Yes	(1)

Part C

1.	OFC > 1.5 *SD* above mean	No	(0)	Yes	(1)
2.	Posteriorly rotated ears	No	(0)	Yes	(1)
3.	Toe walking (by observation)	No	(0)	Yes	(1)

Total score: _____

From Rogers, B.T., & Accardo, P.J. (2005). The clinical use of the Capute Scales. In P.J. Accardo & A.J. Capute, *The Capute Scales: Cognitive Adaptive Test/Clinical Linguistic & Auditory Milestone Scale (CAT/CLAMS)* (p. 32). Baltimore: Paul H. Brookes Publishing Co.; Copyright © 2008 Kennedy Fellows Association; adapted by permission. In *Autism Frontiers: Clinical Issues and Innovations,* edited by Bruce K. Shapiro & Pasquale J. Accardo (2008, Paul H. Brookes Publishing Co., Inc.).

Index

Page numbers followed by *t* and *f* indicate tables and figures, respectively.